EVERYDAY FASHIONS OF THE THIRTIES

As Pictured in Sears Catalogs

Edited by Stella Blum

DOVER PUBLICATIONS, INC., NEW YORK

Dedication

After editing the final selection of material to be included in this book, Stella Blum died. For more than ten years, first as Curator of the Costume Institute of the Metropolitan Museum, New York, later as Director of the Kent State University Museum, Ohio, Mrs. Blum, working closely with Dover Publications, developed a distinctive series of books on fashion that benefited from her scholarship and insight. As a colleague and friend, she will be greatly missed. Her books will always reflect her unique contribution to costume history. The publisher dedicates this volume to her memory.

Published in Canada by General Publishing Company, Ltd., 30 Lesmill Road, Don Mills, Toronto, Ontario.
Published in the United Kingdom by Constable and Company, Ltd.

Everyday Fashions of the Thirties as Pictured in Sears Catalogs is a new work, first published by Dover Publications, Inc., in 1986.

Manufactured in the United States of America
Dover Publications, Inc., 31 East 2nd Street, Mineola, N.Y. 11501

Library of Congress Cataloging-in-Publication Data
Main entry under title:

Everyday fashions of the thirties as pictured in Sears catalogs.

1. Costume—United States—History—20th century. 2. Sears, Roebuck and Company—Catalogs. I. Blum, Stella. II. Sears, Roebuck and Company.
GT615.E92 1986 391′.00973 86-1072
ISBN 0-486-25108-X (pbk.)

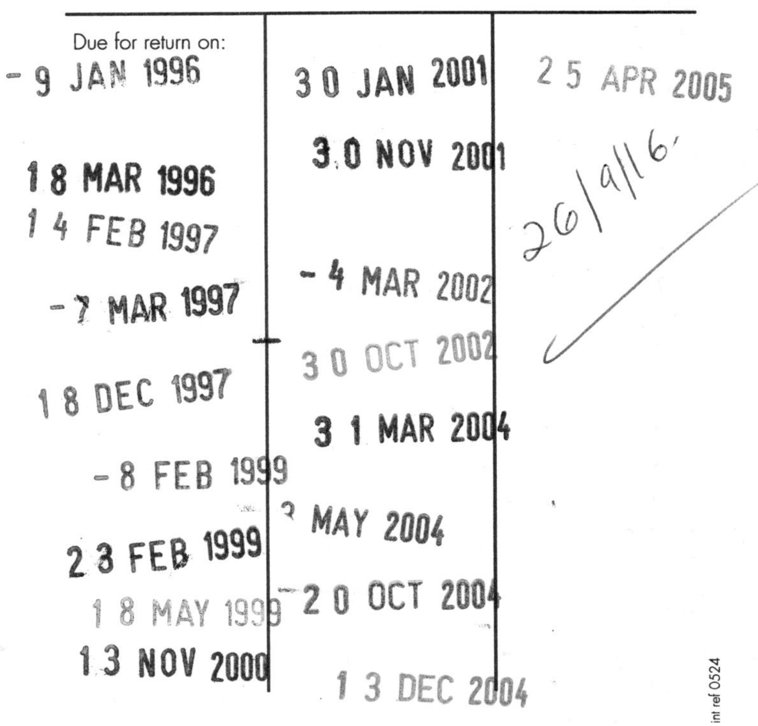
UNIVERSITY OF WESTMINSTER
Failure to return or renew overdue books may result in suspension of borrowing rights at all University of Westminster libraries.
Due for return on:
- 9 JAN 1996
18 MAR 1996
14 FEB 1997
- 7 MAR 1997
18 DEC 1997
- 8 FEB 1999
23 FEB 1999
18 MAY 1999
13 NOV 2000
30 JAN 2001
30 NOV 2001
- 4 MAR 2002
30 OCT 2002
31 MAR 2004
MAY 2004
- 20 OCT 2004
13 DEC 2004
25 APR 2005
26/9/16.
int ref 0524
Information Resource Services Harrow IRS Centre
Watford Road Northwick Park Harrow HA1 3TP
Telephone 0171 911 5885

27 0009577 X

Publisher's Note

Slicing off history in easily digestible units of decades is a useful device, but one that has its pitfalls, for it can easily obscure the broader sweep of time, with its long-developing trends. The thirties, however, are neatly framed by two events: the crash of 1929, with the attendant Great Depression, and the outbreak of world hostilities in 1939.

One might be tempted to think that the financial deprivations suffered by most people during the Depression would have brought fashion to a halt, but it continued, although the catalogs of Sears, Roebuck and Co., from which this anthology has been assembled, reflected the economic tumble.

In fall 1929, advertising copy had been light and breezy: "The newest styles, the most recent designs, and the very latest in colorings and finishes. . . ." (A change in buying patterns in the mid-twenties had, however, necessitated an approach, emphasizing low price and good value, that had not been prominent at the beginning of the decade.) In the spring 1930 catalog, the import of what had happened had not yet been fully realized: A full page of electrical gadgets designed "to drive drudgery from your home" seems to assume continued prosperity.

In the fall 1930 catalog, reality had made its mark: "Thrift is the spirit of today. Reckless spending is a thing of the past." Finally, in the fall 1932 catalog: "These are not ordinary times. . . . Of greatest importance today are the costs of the necessities of life. . . . We realize that economy dictates that women must sew more this year. . . . Repairing, rather than replacing, will be the order in many families. . . . We recognize the struggle that is taking place everywhere to make ends meet." (In point of fact, even though Sears knew that women would be mending, patching and making from scratch rather than ordering ready-made clothes, they offered a narrower range of materials than they had before the Depression.)

That fashions *did* change, and that people, whatever their circumstances, did try their best to follow them, is a potent argument for the view of fashion as a psychological and sociological necessity. How else can one justify a change in style that called for dresses made of *more* cloth than prior to the Depression?

The twenties had been a decade of liberation; a revolution in manners had occurred after World War I. Women enjoyed a new freedom that was mirrored in their dress. The restriction of the boned corset had been eliminated, the hemline had risen to give women unhampered ease in walking, the feminine ideal had evolved into a boyish form. Men's clothing also tended toward increased informality.

By the late twenties, hemlines began to fall and the waistline, which had dropped to the hips, was returning to its natural position. There was a move away from the boyish flapper to a softer, more feminine form. In the early thirties the hemline dropped very low, then was lifted slightly and remained at that position until the end of the decade, when skirts shortened. For a while the bottom of the dress was allowed to flair in flounces. Puffs were worn on upper sleeves and squarish shoulders were emphasized to contrast with the silhouette's sensuously molded torso. Long dresses for evening wear replaced the flamboyant short beaded gowns that had characterized the twenties.

In men's fashions the waist was suppressed; the wide trousers that had been so popular in the twenties continued to be worn in sporty or collegiate styles, reaching a 22-inch width, but by the late thirties, although trousers were still of a generous cut, the width was modified.

Women's cloche hats, another trademark of the twenties, disappeared, their place being taken by berets, pillboxes and brimmed hats, frequently worn at a jaunty angle. Turbans later gained popularity.

The movies provided one of the major escapes from the harsh realities of the Depression, so it was natural that the sales gimmick of marketing accessories (and some dresses) endorsed by such stars as Loretta Young, Claudette Colbert and Fay Wray should be expanded from pre-Depression days. Even children's clothing found its own star—Shirley Temple—for promotion.

Women's sportswear developed further. Although most apparel had become more feminine, in sportswear masculine forms continued to be adapted: middy slacks, sportsuits, leather jackets. The tailored suit was also favored, especially in business, where masculine dress was equated with seriousness of intent.

In the spring 1930 catalog women's overalls were first introduced—a harbinger of Rosie the Riveter, the image that was to dominate the first half of the next decade.

EVERYDAY FASHIONS OF
THE THIRTIES

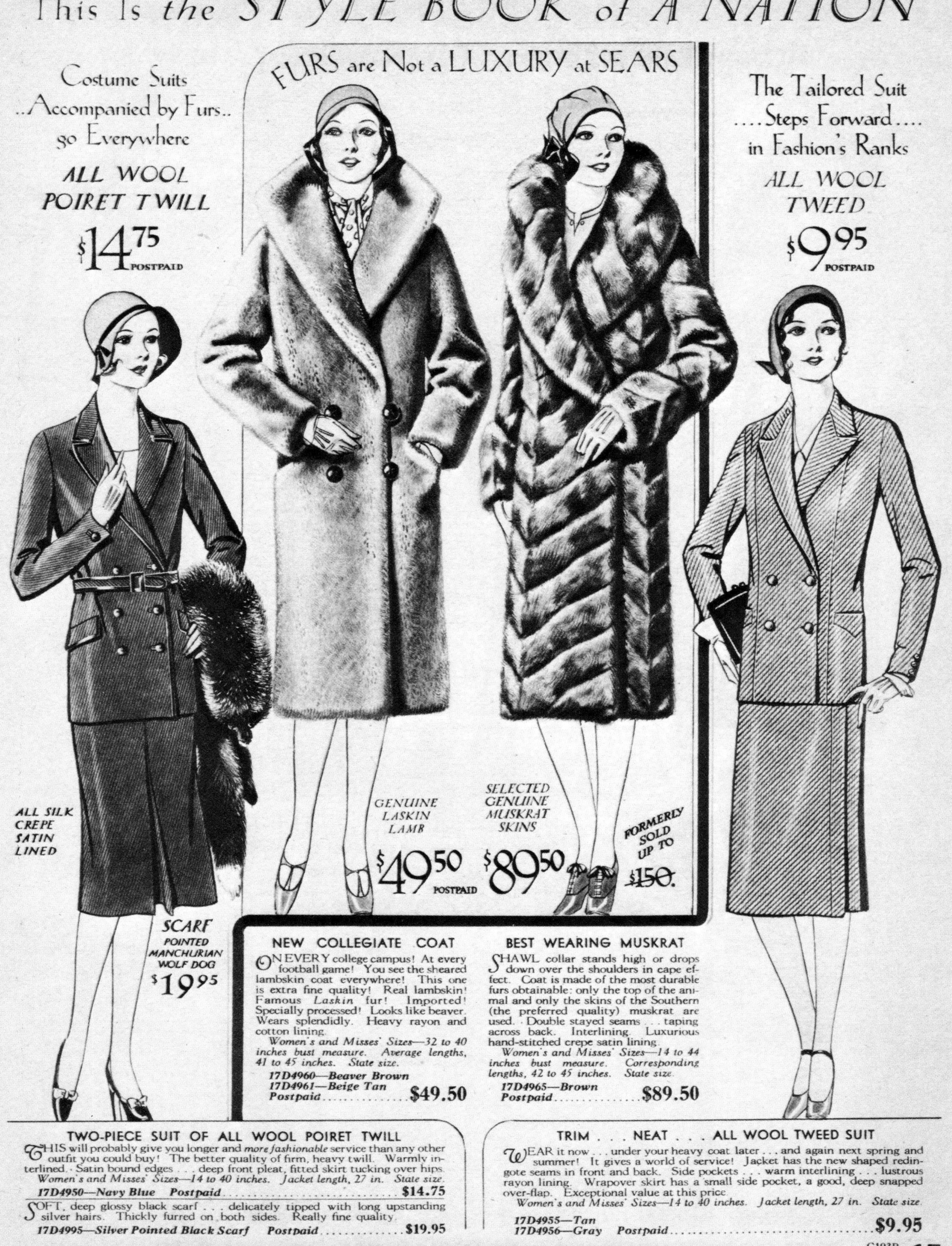

This Is the STYLE BOOK of A NATION

Costume Suits ..Accompanied by Furs.. go Everywhere

ALL WOOL POIRET TWILL

$14.75 POSTPAID

FURS are Not a LUXURY at SEARS

The Tailored Suit ....Steps Forward.... in Fashion's Ranks

ALL WOOL TWEED

$9.95 POSTPAID

ALL SILK CREPE SATIN LINED

GENUINE LASKIN LAMB

$49.50 POSTPAID

SELECTED GENUINE MUSKRAT SKINS

$89.50

FORMERLY SOLD UP TO ~~$150.~~

SCARF POINTED MANCHURIAN WOLF DOG

$19.95

NEW COLLEGIATE COAT

ON EVERY college campus! At every football game! You see the sheared lambskin coat everywhere! This one is extra fine quality! Real lambskin! Famous *Laskin* fur! Imported! Specially processed! Looks like beaver. Wears splendidly. Heavy rayon and cotton lining.

Women's and Misses' Sizes—32 to 40 inches bust measure. Average lengths, 41 to 45 inches. State size.

17D4960—Beaver Brown
17D4961—Beige Tan
Postpaid **$49.50**

BEST WEARING MUSKRAT

SHAWL collar stands high or drops down over the shoulders in cape effect. Coat is made of the most durable furs obtainable: only the top of the animal and only the skins of the Southern (the preferred quality) muskrat are used. Double stayed seams . . . taping across back. Interlining. Luxurious hand-stitched crepe satin lining.

Women's and Misses' Sizes—14 to 44 inches bust measure. Corresponding lengths, 42 to 45 inches. State size.

17D4965—Brown
Postpaid **$89.50**

TWO-PIECE SUIT OF ALL WOOL POIRET TWILL

THIS will probably give you longer and *more fashionable* service than any other outfit you could buy! The better quality of firm, heavy twill. Warmly interlined. Satin bound edges . . . deep front pleat, fitted skirt tucking over hips.

Women's and Misses' Sizes—14 to 40 inches. Jacket length, 27 in. State size.

17D4950—Navy Blue Postpaid **$14.75**

SOFT, deep glossy black scarf . . . delicately tipped with long upstanding silver hairs. Thickly furred on both sides. Really fine quality.

17D4995—Silver Pointed Black Scarf Postpaid **$19.95**

TRIM . . . NEAT . . . ALL WOOL TWEED SUIT

WEAR it now . . . under your heavy coat later . . . and again next spring and summer! It gives a world of service! Jacket has the new shaped redingote seams in front and back. Side pockets . . . warm interlining . . . lustrous rayon lining. Wrapover skirt has a small side pocket, a good, deep snapped over-flap. Exceptional value at this price.

Women's and Misses' Sizes—14 to 40 inches. Jacket length, 27 in. State size.

17D4955—Tan
17D4956—Gray Postpaid **$9.95**

.... ORDER BLANKS ARE IN BACK OF THIS CATALOG ....

C103P B-K-MN **17**

FROCKS FOR MISSES DISPLAY NEW LINES OF SMARTNESS
A
"TWIN-PRINT" ENSEMBLE
$6.98 POSTPAID
B
IMPORTED ALL SILK JAPANESE PONGEE
$4.98 POSTPAID
D
ALL SILK FLAT CREPE
$7.98 POSTPAID
E
"GEM-O-SHEER" RAYON CHIFFON
$7.98 POSTPAID
F
RAYON AND COTTON FLAT CREPE
$4.98 POSTPAID
WE PAY THE POSTAGE
C
ALL SILK FLAT CREPE
$10.95 POSTPAID
G
ALL SILK GEORGETTE CREPE
$10.95 POSTPAID

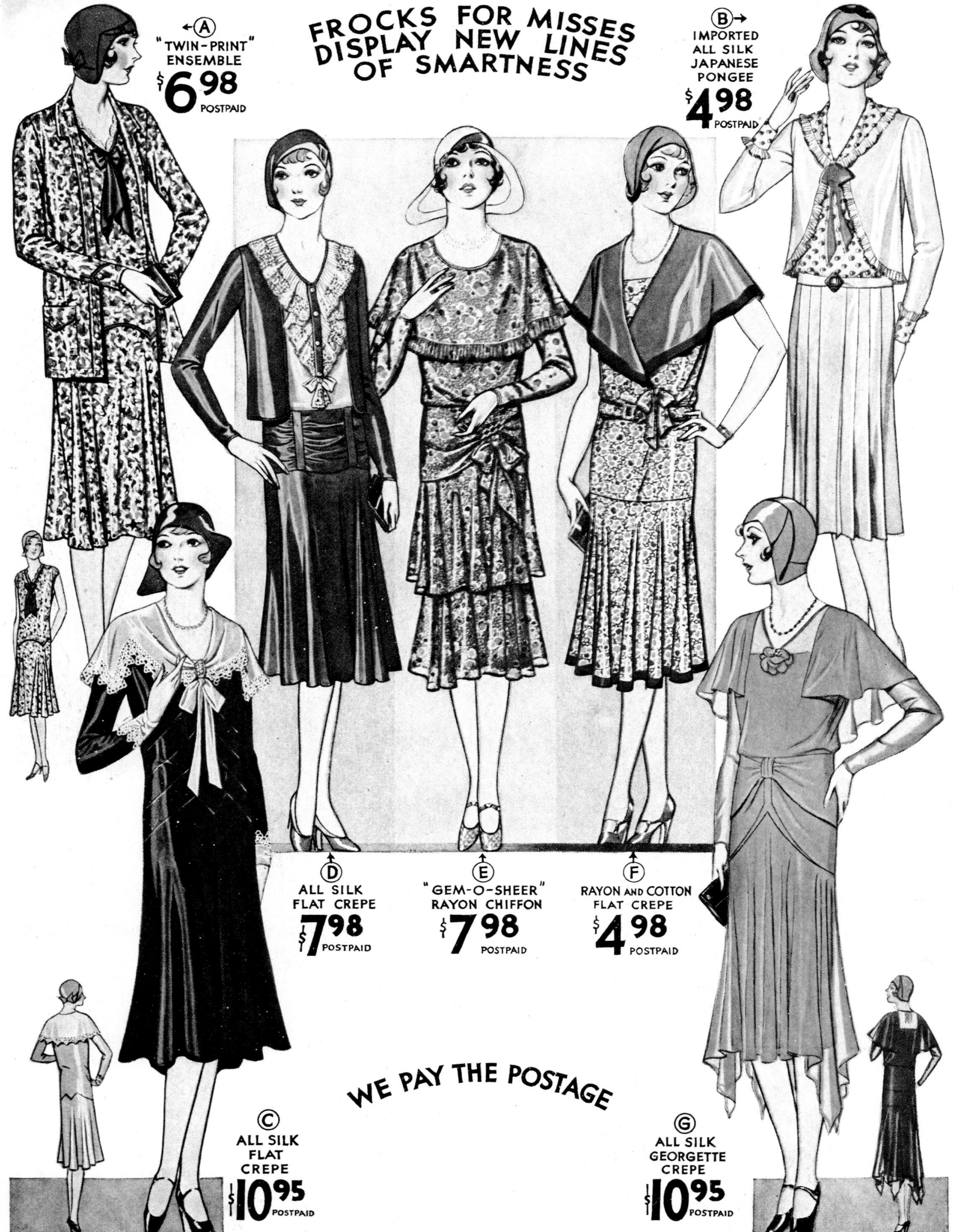

WE GUARANTEE TO SATISFY YOU AND SAVE YOU MONEY

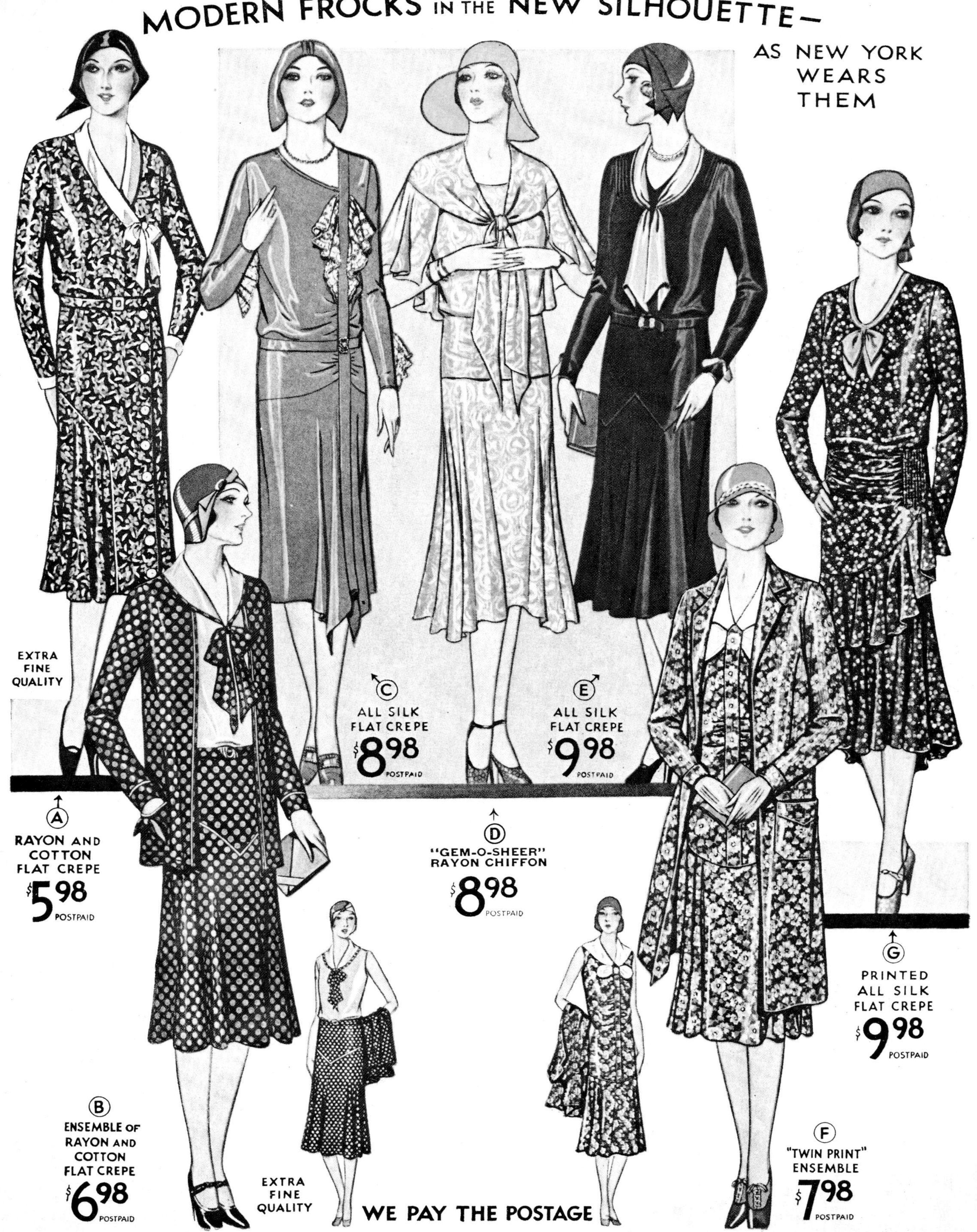
MODERN FROCKS IN THE NEW SILHOUETTE—
AS NEW YORK WEARS THEM
EXTRA FINE QUALITY
A
RAYON AND COTTON FLAT CREPE
$5.98 POSTPAID
C
ALL SILK FLAT CREPE
$8.98 POSTPAID
E
ALL SILK FLAT CREPE
$9.98 POSTPAID
D
"GEM-O-SHEER" RAYON CHIFFON
$8.98 POSTPAID
G
PRINTED ALL SILK FLAT CREPE
$9.98 POSTPAID
B
ENSEMBLE OF RAYON AND COTTON FLAT CREPE
$6.98 POSTPAID
EXTRA FINE QUALITY
WE PAY THE POSTAGE
F
"TWIN PRINT" ENSEMBLE
$7.98 POSTPAID

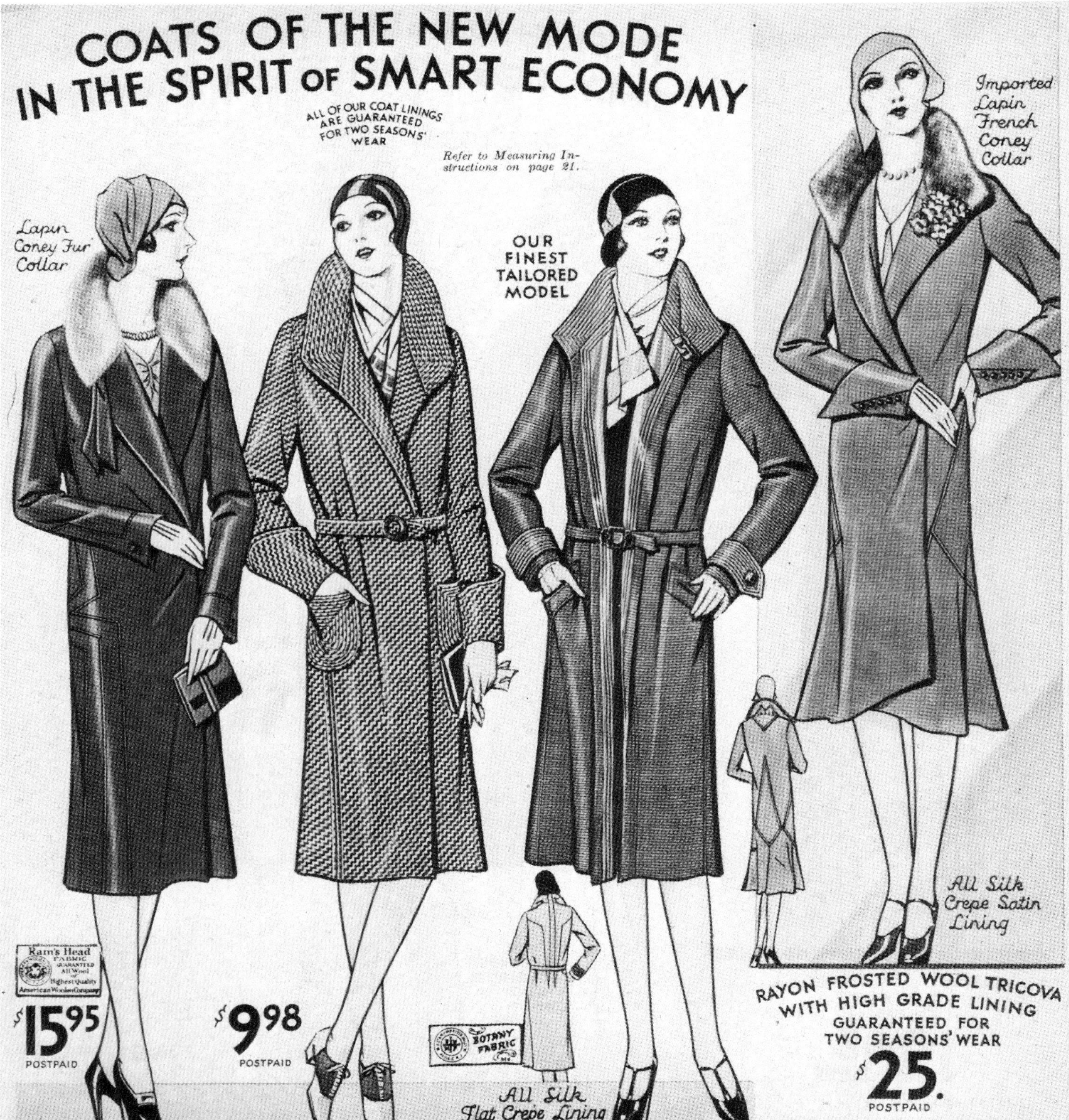

RAM'S HEAD FINE ALL WOOL BROADCLOTH

17V8510—*Tan*
17V8511—*Black*
17V8512—*Navy Blue*

THIS coat can be vain of its looks and proud of its excellence. It shows smartly patterned tailored seamings at sides and on sleeves. Collared with the new honey beige Lapin French Coney fur with streamer tabs adding a chic finishing note. Has Satin de Chine (silk and cotton) lining.

Women's and Misses' Sizes—34 to 46 inches bust measure. Corresponding lengths, 42 to 45 inches. State bust measure.

WOOL AND SILK FANCY TWEED

17V8515—*Tan*

SNUGLY belted—patch pocketed—and smartly tailor stitched in the manner of those dashing English sports coats. The fabric is a new small weave fancy tweed (nine-tenths wool, one-tenth silk). Seamings at the sides and back and a bow finish under the collar are other style notes of interest. Has strong Sateen lining.

Women's and Misses' Sizes —34 to 44 inches bust measure. Corresponding lengths, 41 to 44 inches. State bust measure.

ALL WOOL REPBLOOM A BOTANY FABRIC

$19.98 POSTPAID

17V8520—*Navy Blue*
17V8521—*Tan*

EVEN a custom tailored coat can offer you no more in smartness, fabric and expert workmanship. A model for discriminating women! A "quality" coat in every sense! This is our very finest tailored style. Every detail proves its excellence to you! The fabric is glossy, firmly corded, high quality repp from the famous Botany Mills. The style is not only trim and correct for all occasions—it is *distinctive!* It is strapped, seamed and artfully tailor stitched. The lining and tuxedo facings are of matching heavy All Silk Flat Crepe.

Women's and Misses' Sizes—34 to 44 inches bust measure. Corresponding lengths, 42 to 45 inches. State bust measure.

17V8525—*Deer Tan* 17V8526—*Black*

A LOVELY coat! It is so flattering in line—so chic and typical of the new 1930 mode—that you will surely be enchanted with it. Note the smart cut of the model—its geometric seamings—its graceful low placed flare. Even the button trimmed cuffs have a dashing air of newness, and the fur collar of Lapin French Coney fur—so fashionable this season—adds a luxurious note of elegance. A colorful flower cluster appears on one lapel. It is beautifully tailored of a fine weave cloth (nine-tenths wool and one-tenth Rayon frosted). Lined with richly lustrous All Silk Crepe Back Satin.

Women's and Misses' Sizes—34 to 44 inches bust measure. Corresponding lengths, 42 to 45 inches. State bust measure.

FOR INDEX AND GENERAL INFORMATION, SEE PINK PAGES IN CENTER OF BOOK P158B C-K-MN 49

AS FASHIONABLE AS THOUGH THEY COST TWICE AS MUCH

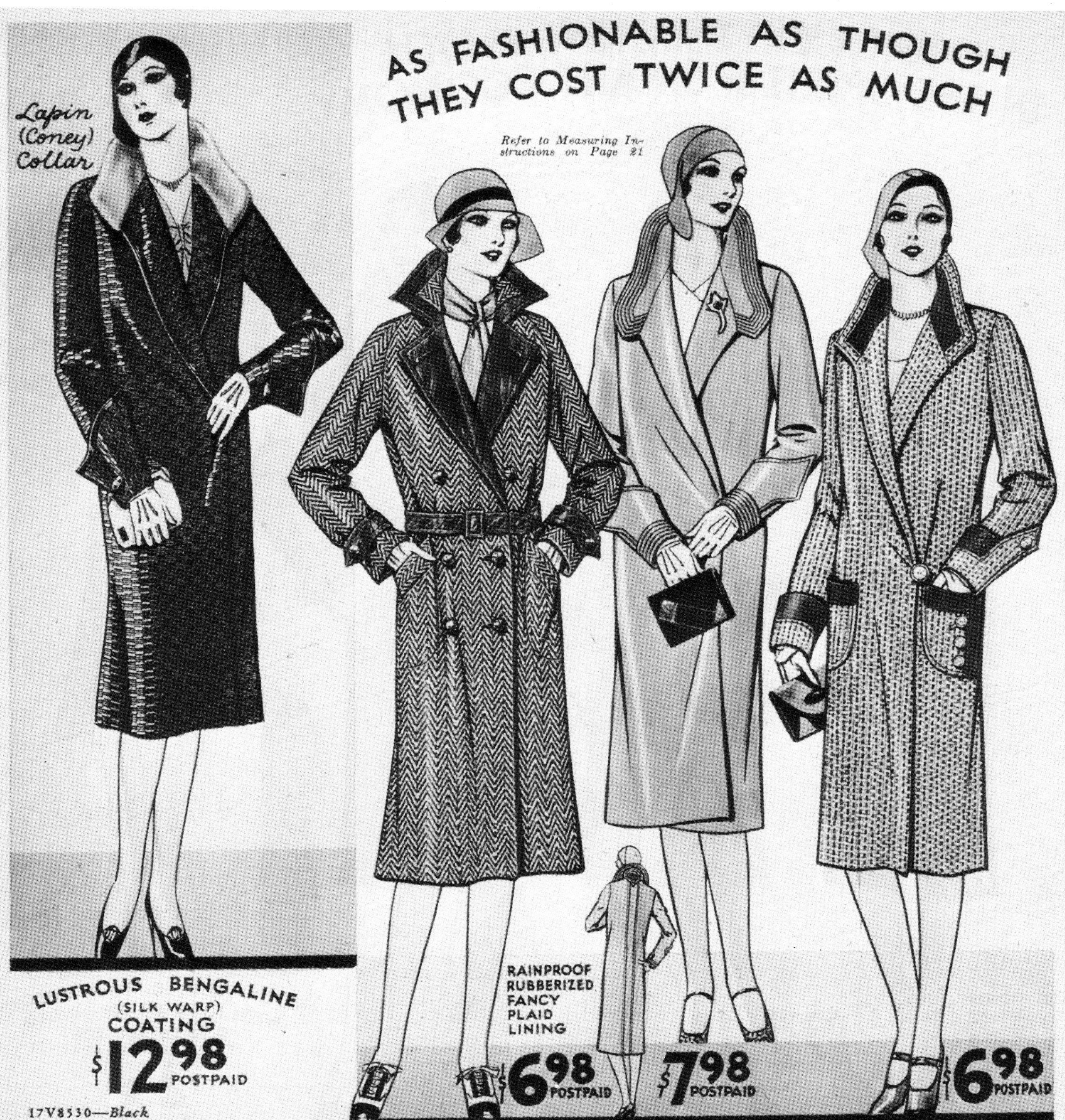

LUSTROUS BENGALINE (SILK WARP) COATING

$12.98 POSTPAID

17V8530—*Black*

FOR dress wear—choose this black coat of shimmering beauty collared in effective contrast with honey beige Lapin French Coney—one of the most fashionable furs this season. It is a lovely model of flattering lines—so rich in appearance that one could easily imagine it costing twice as much as $12.98. The coat is made of heavy, durable grade, fancy weave lustrous Bengaline (silk warp—cotton filling)—and gains added chic with tailor stitched Satin bandings on its attractive cavalier style cuffs and front facings. The back is Satin piped and the collar trimmed with perky self bow. Has a guaranteed Rayon and cotton lining.

Women's and Misses' Sizes—34 to 44 inches bust measure. Corresponding lengths, 42 to 45 inches. State bust measure.

ALL OF OUR COAT LININGS ARE GUARANTEED FOR TWO SEASONS' WEAR

COTTON TWEED ALL-WEATHER SPORT COAT

17V8535—*Tan*
17V8536—*Gray*

A NEW idea in sports fashion! Smartly attired in this swagger double breasted coat—one can easily have a nonchalant disregard for wind, dampness or rain—and look equally dashing when the sun is shining.

Has contrasting color leatherette trimmings, light brown on tan and black on gray. Fancy plaid lined and rubber interlined. A rare bargain at $6.98.

Women's and Misses' Sizes—34 to 44 inches bust measure. Corresponding lengths, 42 to 45 inches. State bust measure.

HALF WOOL BROADCLOTH COATING

17V8540—*Tan*

DON'T judge the true worth of this good looking coat by its very low price. It is one of our special money saving offers! Made of smooth textured Broadcloth coating (half wool and balance cotton).

The coat is cut on smart modern lines, carefully tailored and neatly trimmed with stitchings and seaming. Lined with durable Sateen.

Women's and Misses' Sizes—34 to 46 inches bust measure. Corresponding lengths, 42 to 45 inches. State bust measure.

FANCY TRAVEL TWEED THREE-FOURTHS WOOL

17V8545—*Tan*

A SWAGGER styled coat—and a good coat! In fact, it is exceptional for so low a price. Made of a new small patterned fancy Tweed (nearly three-fourths wool balance Rayon and cotton) which is guaranteed to give sturdy wear—it is neatly tailored—and lined with strong Sateen. Attractively trimmed with wool mixed Broadcloth and novelty buttons.

Women's and Misses' Sizes—34 to 44 inches bust measure. Corresponding lengths, 41 to 44 inches. State bust measure.

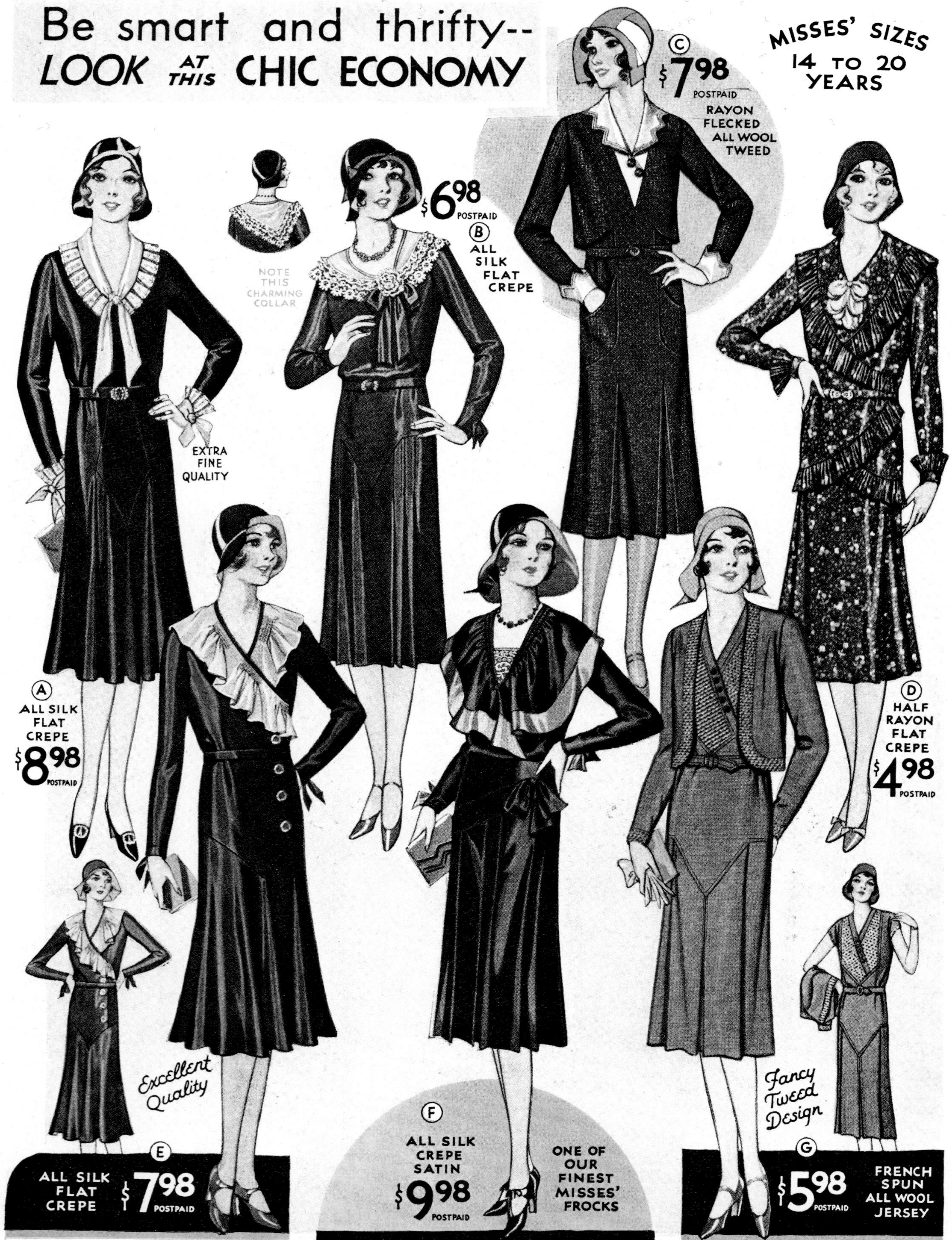

Be smart and thrifty--
LOOK AT THIS CHIC ECONOMY
MISSES' SIZES 14 TO 20 YEARS
$7.98 POSTPAID
RAYON FLECKED ALL WOOL TWEED
$6.98 POSTPAID
B ALL SILK FLAT CREPE
NOTE THIS CHARMING COLLAR
EXTRA FINE QUALITY
A ALL SILK FLAT CREPE $8.98 POSTPAID
D HALF RAYON FLAT CREPE $4.98 POSTPAID
Excellent Quality
Fancy Tweed Design
E ALL SILK FLAT CREPE $7.98 POSTPAID
F ALL SILK CREPE SATIN $9.98 POSTPAID
ONE OF OUR FINEST MISSES' FROCKS
G $5.98 POSTPAID FRENCH SPUN ALL WOOL JERSEY
44 C106 P-B-K-MN ITEMS ON THESE PAGES SHIPPED..POSTAGE PAID BY SEARS, ROEBUCK and CO.

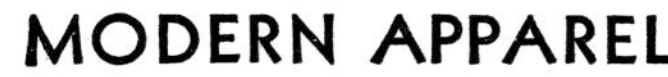

SEMI-MADE

TAILORED BY EXPERTS
FOR YOUR CONVENIENCE

Only the following simple seams requiring your personal adjustment are left for you to complete:

1. *Sleeve seam.*
2. *Side seams.*
3. *Seam where sleeve is set in.*
4. *Cuff and sleeve hem.*
5. *Skirt hem.*

STATE SIZE

And send us these measurements:

Bust.
Hip.
Sleeve length from under arm to wrist.
Dress length from back of neck to bottom of skirt.

We allow for seams and hems so **be sure to state exact measurements.**

AN ASTOUNDING NEW STYLE IDEA!

A huge success in the FASHION CONSCIOUS STYLE CENTERS, and predicted to be the most successful style idea ever advanced. Most helpful and economical to the woman who wishes to be well dressed.

Here is what you receive:

A The smartest, most correct garment styles we could buy from one of America's finest designers.

B Expertly cut out, and all the difficult tailoring, stitching, pleating and tucking skillfully completed by a manufacturer who tailors only very fine retail garments that sell for $25.00 to $50.00.

C Most careful attention to details of design, workmanship, color combinations and other style touches, which are so difficult to obtain on home made garments.

D Very fine materials which are never put into cheap garments.

E And with all this, the opportunity to fit these wonderful styles to yourself as you complete the few easy seams left for you to do. Only those seams which allow you to make personal adjustments are left for you.

F We require four simple measurements (see instructions to the left). We require about seven days to furnish you this service.

G We believe your saving is at least a third over similar quality, style and workmanship in finished garments elsewhere.

H Full instructions sent with each garment. Even the inexperienced can complete the few simple seams left to do.

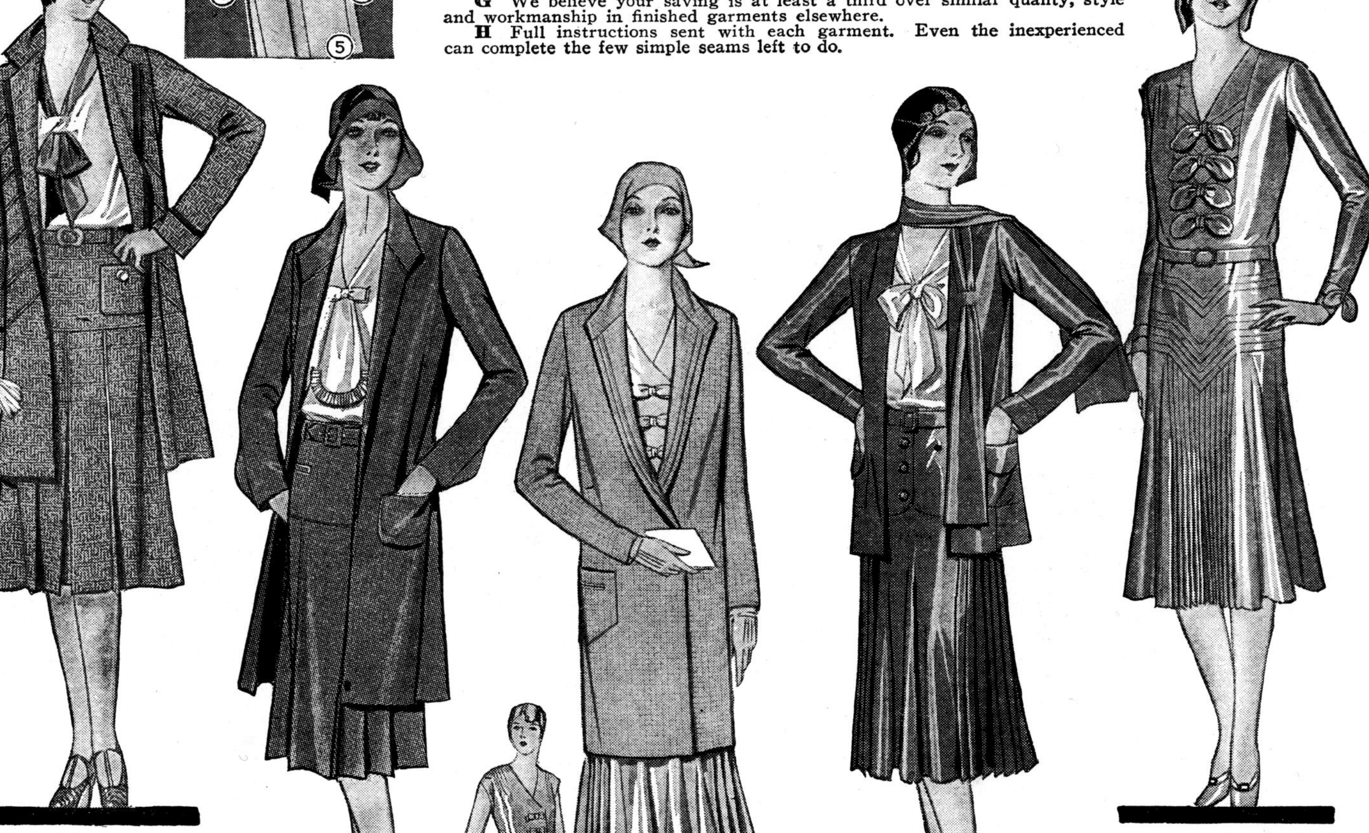

Semi-Made All Wool Tweed Ensemble

$14.75 Post paid

Consists of a silk blouse, tweed skirt and three-quarter length coat. To complete the coat and blouse it is necessary only to set in the sleeves, join the sleeve seams and turn up the hems. The skirt is complete except to join the pleated part to the yoke, join the side seams and put in the hem. The tweed is our Finest All Wool Quality 14V3094. The silk is our finest all Silk Flat Crepe 14V6763. The narrow bandings of the coat are of fine Wool Crepe. Buckles, buttons and snap fasteners are included.

14V3001—Colors: Tan Tweed with Eggshell blouse; Blue Tweed with Pearl white blouse; Green Tweed with Eggshell blouse.

Semi-Made garment cut in sizes 34, 36, 38 and 40-inch bust. Misses' sizes, 14, 16 and 18 years. State color and measurements.

Semi-Made Covert Cloth Ensemble

$14.75 Post paid

Blouse of All-Silk Flat Crepe, 14V6763. Coat and Skirt of our Finest All Wool Covert Cloth, 14V3107.

14V3002—Comes in colors: **Black, Navy, Garland (dark) green or Tan, all with Eggshell blouse.**

Semi-Made garment cut in sizes, 34, 36, 38 and 40 inches bust. Misses' sizes, 14, 16 and 18 years. State color and measurements.

Semi-Made Tennis Ensemble

Postpaid $14.75

A graceful waistline frock and a charming coat. Coat is made of our Finest All Wool Basket Weave 14V3492. Frock is of our Finest All Silk Flat Crepe 14V6763. Just join side seams, set in the sleeves, attach cuffs and turn up hem.

14V3003—Colors: **White, Garland green, Pink, China (medium) blue or Canary (bright) yellow.**

Semi-Made garment cut in sizes 34, 36, 38 and 40-inch bust. Misses' sizes, 14, 16 and 18 years. State color and measurements.

Semi-Made All Silk Jacket Suit

$19.75 Post paid

Fashioned of our Finest All Silk Flat Crepe 14V6763. It features new style details with its finger tip jacket, graceful scarf, tuck-in blouse and flared and pleated yoke skirt.

14V3004—Comes in colors: **Brown, Navy or Rose beige, all with Eggshell blouse.**

Semi-Made garment in sizes 34, 36, 38 and 40-inch bust. Misses' sizes, 14, 16 and 18 years. State color and measurements.

Semi-Made All Silk Flat Crepe Frock

$10.95 Post paid

A symmetrical column of bows—a normal waistline—a longer skirt of rippling flares and tiny pleats set on an intricately cut and tucked yoke—in its entirety, an obviously 1930 frock!

It is developed of Our Finest All Silk Flat Crepe 14V6763, and it is complete except to set in the sleeves, to turn up the cuffs (and hems) and to join the side seams. The gay little bows, the neckline, the tucks and the skirt are skillfully completed for you. Buttons and snap fasteners are included.

14V3005—Colors: **Black, Bleu royale, Garland green, China (medium) blue or Rose beige.**

Semi-Made garment cut in sizes 34, 36, 38 and 40-inch bust. Misses' sizes, 14, 16 and 18 years. State color and measurements.

Order Blanks Are in Back of This Catalog

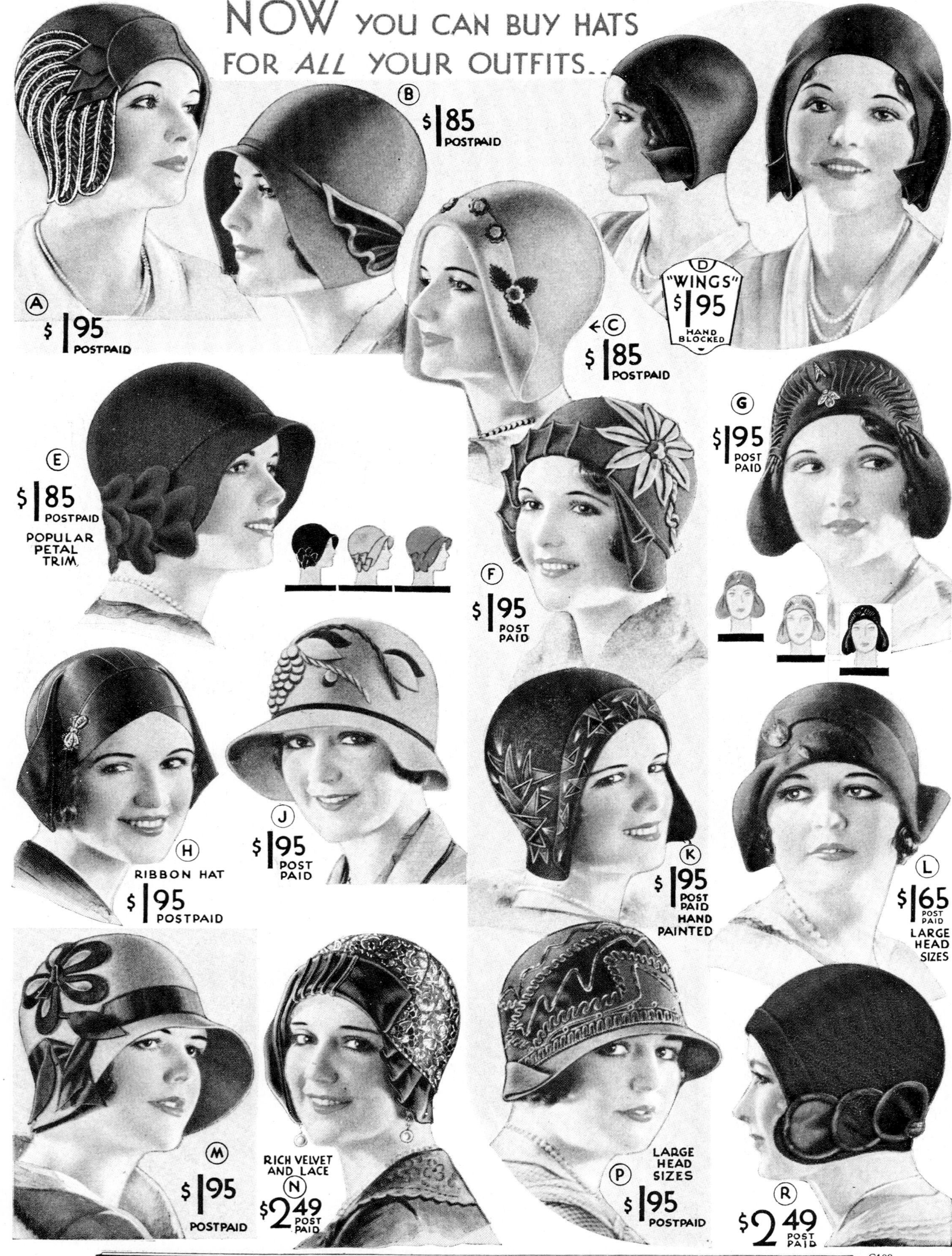

Order Blanks Are in Back of This Catalog

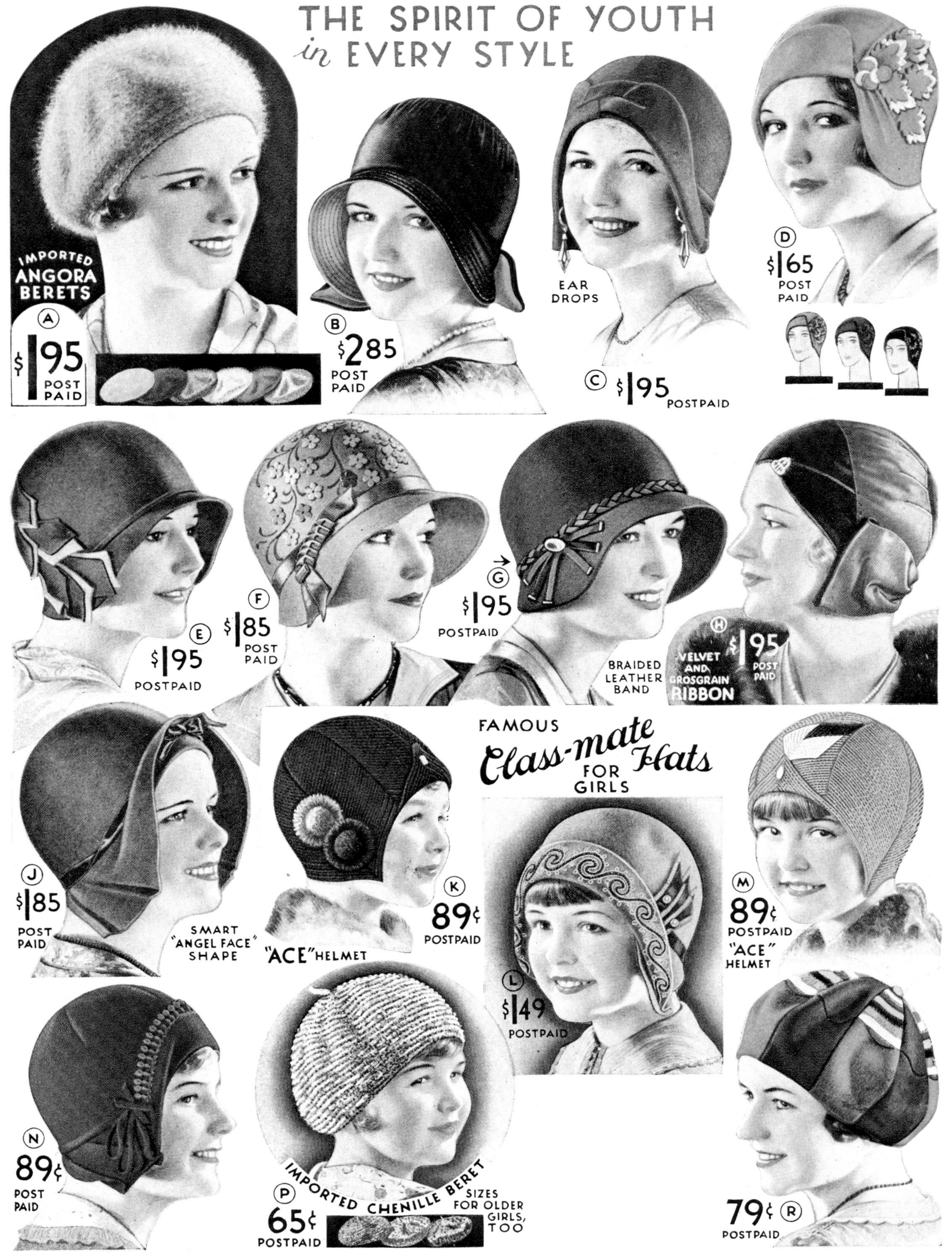

Items on These Pages Shipped POSTAGE PAID by Sears, Roebuck and CO.

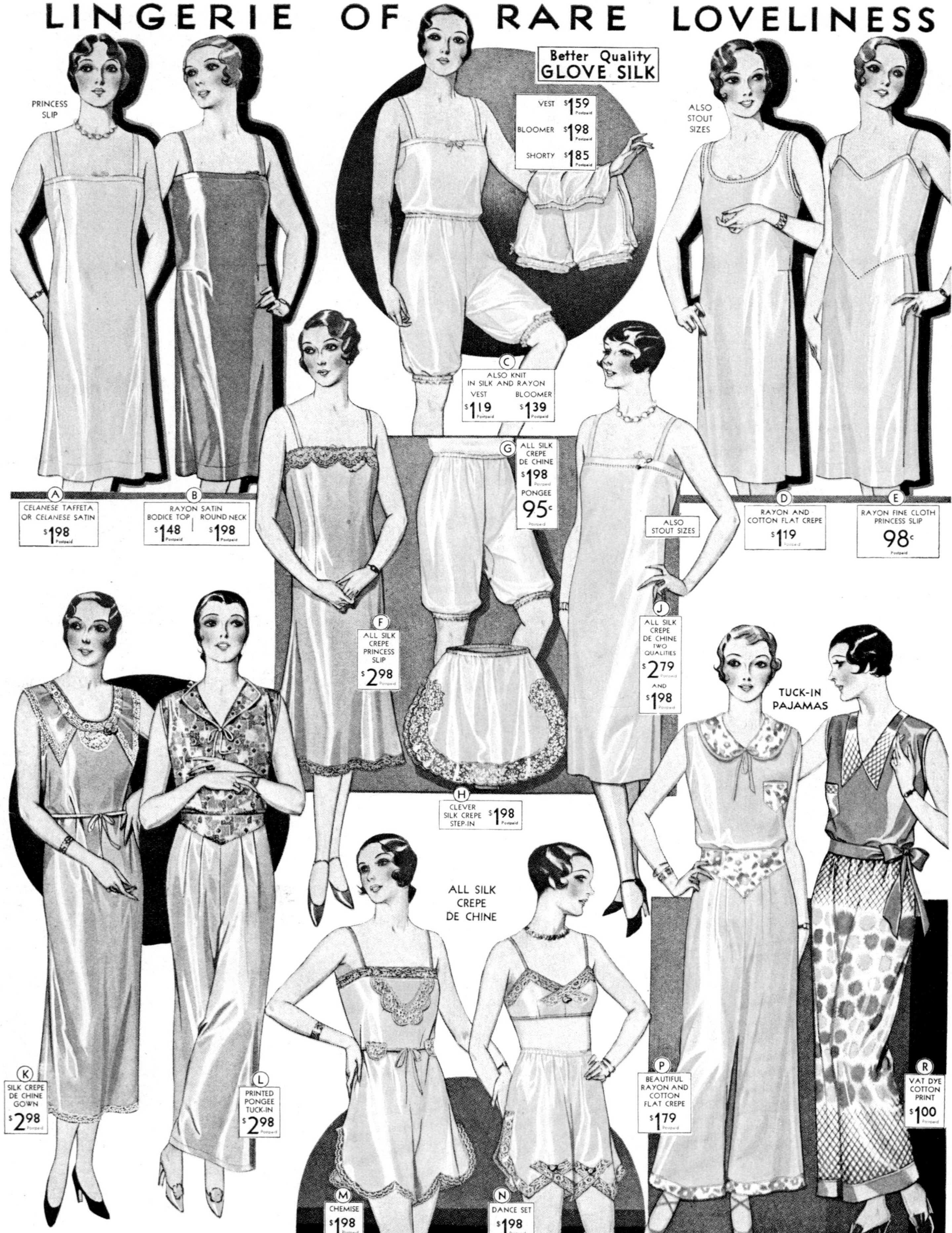

LINGERIE OF RARE LOVELINESS
PRINCESS SLIP
Better Quality GLOVE SILK
VEST $1.59 Postpaid
BLOOMER $1.98 Postpaid
SHORTY $1.85 Postpaid
ALSO STOUT SIZES
C
ALSO KNIT IN SILK AND RAYON
VEST $1.19 Postpaid
BLOOMER $1.39 Postpaid
G
ALL SILK CREPE DE CHINE $1.98 Postpaid
PONGEE 95c Postpaid
A
CELANESE TAFFETA OR CELANESE SATIN $1.98 Postpaid
B
RAYON SATIN
BODICE TOP $1.48 Postpaid
ROUND NECK $1.98 Postpaid
D
RAYON AND COTTON FLAT CREPE $1.19 Postpaid
E
RAYON FINE CLOTH PRINCESS SLIP 98c Postpaid
ALSO STOUT SIZES
F
ALL SILK CREPE PRINCESS SLIP $2.98 Postpaid
J
ALL SILK CREPE DE CHINE TWO QUALITIES $2.79 Postpaid AND $1.98 Postpaid
TUCK-IN PAJAMAS
H
CLEVER SILK CREPE STEP-IN $1.98 Postpaid
ALL SILK CREPE DE CHINE
K
SILK CREPE DE CHINE GOWN $2.98 Postpaid
L
PRINTED PONGEE TUCK-IN $2.98 Postpaid
P
BEAUTIFUL RAYON AND COTTON FLAT CREPE $1.79 Postpaid
R
VAT DYE COTTON PRINT $1.00 Postpaid
M
CHEMISE $1.98 Postpaid
N
DANCE SET $1.98 Postpaid

Items on These Pages Shipped POSTAGE PAID by Sears, Roebuck and CO.

NIGHTWEAR of CHARM and GRACE

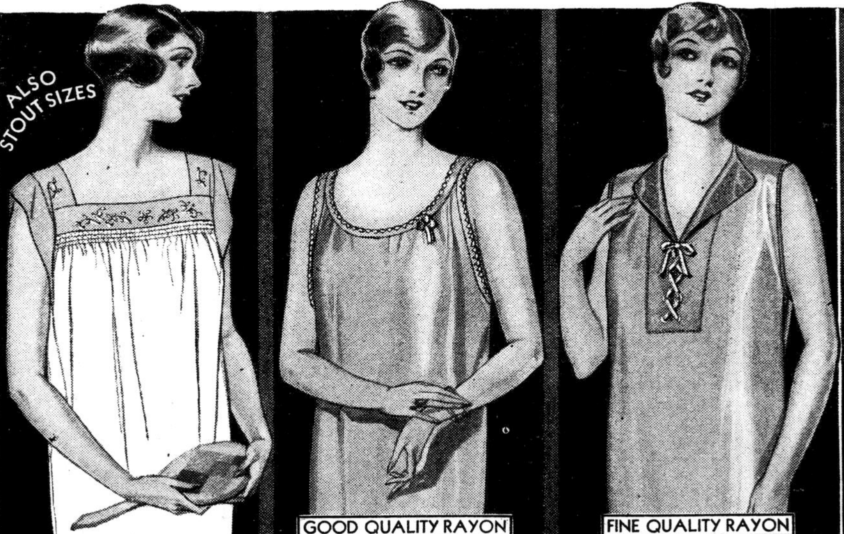

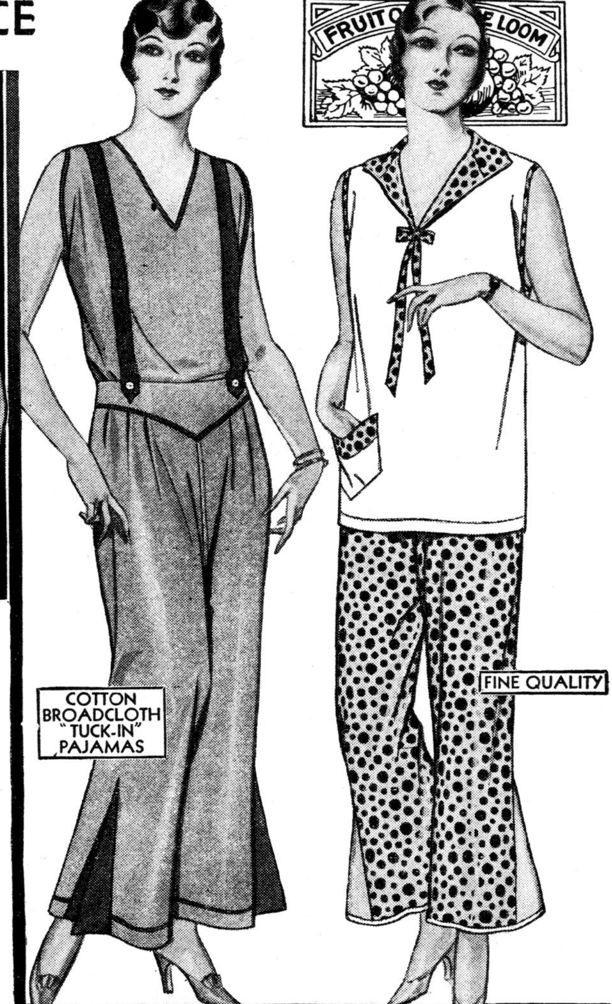

38V1168—White and flesh. **38V1169**—Flesh and white. **69¢** Postpaid
Sizes, 34 to 44 inches bust measure. State size.

Stout Sizes

38V1170—White and flesh. **79¢** Postpaid
Sizes, 46 to 54 inches bust measure. State size.

A truly remarkable value for attractive style and worth while saving. This neat Gown made of **standard quality nainsook** has the comfortable Jenny neck decorated with dainty Lorraine embroidery work in pastel shades. Bands at top and arm openings are of contrasting color. Shirring across front. Full cut. Bargain!

38V1182—Flesh. **38V1183**—Peach. **38V1184**—Blue. **$1.00** Postpaid
Sizes, 32 to 40 inches bust measure. State size.

Quality has not been sacrificed in this Rayon Gown. It is much superior to the usual **knit Rayon** gown offered at this price. Our sizes are standard, and workmanship is of the best. Its most becoming simplicity is varied by a tiny flower. The round neck and roomy armholes are finished with neatly tailored touches. A quality value far surpassing this low price. **Have you seen the other styles of beautiful Rayon underwear offered to you on our pages? They are excellent values, and the prices are so low!**

38V1158—Peach. **38V1159**—Flesh. **$1.39** Postpaid
Sizes, 34 to 44 inches bust measure. State size.

Another charmer in lovely **knit Rayon,** featuring both style and value. Note the contrasting Rayon crepe collar set off by the clever lacing effect. You'll want this pretty Slipover Gown all the more when you consider how low we've priced it for a gown of such really fine quality and workmanship. Just right for those seeking something "just a little better," who still like to save money.

38V1180—Blue. **38V1181**—Peach. **$1.00** Postpaid
Sizes, 34 to 44 in. bust measure. State size.

Even Pajamas have their flare and suggest themselves as new ways to lounge fashionably and sleep comfortably. This "tuck-in style," of good **quality cotton broadcloth,** is made quite tricky, with its "suspender" banding of contrasting color, buttoning onto trousers. The bell bottoms provided with inserts are in keeping with the prevailing Pajama styles. Smart "V" neck, and smartly sleeveless.

38V1175—Blue and white. **38V1176**—Green and white. **$1.79** Postpaid
Sizes, 34 to 44 inches bust measure. State size.

These modish Slipover Pajamas follow the vogue for bright color bubble dots to achieve unusual jauntiness! They're practical, too, made of **"Fruit of the Loom" cotton broadcloth,** an extra fine fabric, in two tub fast colors that stand many washings and wear unusually well. **Plain white sleeveless** jacket shows contrasting material in collar, string tie, armhole bindings and the **wide** bell trousers of dotted broadcloth attain their flare through triangular inserts of white. Unusually good value! Such a delightful gift!

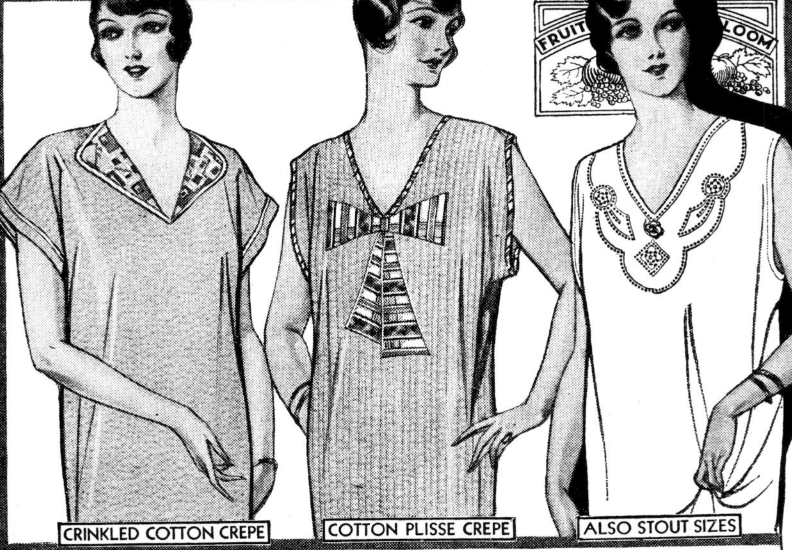

ALSO STOUT SIZES

38V1151—Flesh. **38V1152**—Orchid. **38V1153**—Peach. **79¢** Postpaid
Sizes, 34 to 44 inches bust measure. State size.

Exceptional lingerie value is embodied in this Slipover Gown of ultra-practical **crinkled cotton crepe.** An unusually attractive style in dainty colors that are reliably tub fast. **Needs no ironing!** Flat sewed-down reveres of fancy printed crepe are a pleasing bit of color contrast adding to the style effectiveness of this becoming model. Comfortably cut, with kimono sleeves finished in a tiny turnback cuff.

38V1160—Peach. **38V1161**—Orchid. **98¢** Postpaid
Sizes, 34 to 44 inches bust measure. State size.

Conspicuously smart, yet very practical. **Plisse crinkled cotton crepe,** that requires no ironing, fashions this dainty Gown that proves its flair for fashion with an appliqued bow of colorful modernistic design! "V" neck bound in the same smart material. Ideal for everyday use. Washed in a jiffy. So inexpensive the thrifty woman will buy now!

38V1162—White. **$1.00** Postpaid
Sizes, 34 to 44 in. bust measure. State size.

Stout Sizes. **38V1163**—White. **$1.27**
Sizes, 46 to 54 inches bust measure. State size.

Made of the famous **"Fruit of the Loom" nainsook** in an exquisitely soft, fine quality. This inexpensive Slip-On Gown carries every assurance of distinctive value! In effective contrast to the striking simplicity of its style, is a tasteful trim of fancy hemstitching and rich handmade lace medallions. A dainty ribbon rosette.

Regular Sizes

38V1007—White. **79¢** Postpaid
Sizes, 34 to 44 in. bust. State size.

Stout Sizes

38V1008—White. **97¢** Postpaid
Sizes, 46 to 54 in. bust. State size.

Favored open front Gown **of standard quality nainsook**—worth more than its cost in comfort and service. Series of pin tucks vary the simplicity of the yoke. Double back yoke.

38V1188—White. **49¢** Postpaid
Sizes, 34 to 44 in. bust measure. State size.

You will be amazed that a garment of this quality can be sold at so low a price. **Standard quality nainsook** is used to fashion this Jenny neck style Gown, trimmed with a pretty lace medallion and shirring across back and front, and finished with hemstitching.

"How to Order" and Other Information – See Index for Page

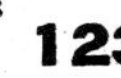

GIVE NEGLIGEE!

Cheery-Comfortable-Practical and SO MUCH LOWER PRICED at SEARS

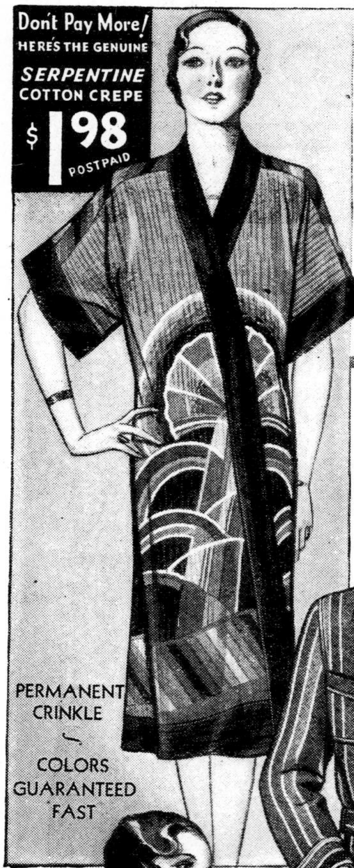

Don't Pay More! HERE'S THE GENUINE *SERPENTINE* COTTON CREPE $1.98 POSTPAID

COMPARE! See What You SAVE at SEARS

BRILLIANT, vivid, modernistic coats in cotton crepe! Guaranteed washable! Smarter and more serviceable than much higher priced kimonos. *Women's and Misses' Sizes—34 to 44 in. bust measure. State size.*

27D5815—Black Ground
27D5816—Red Ground
Postpaid....$1.98

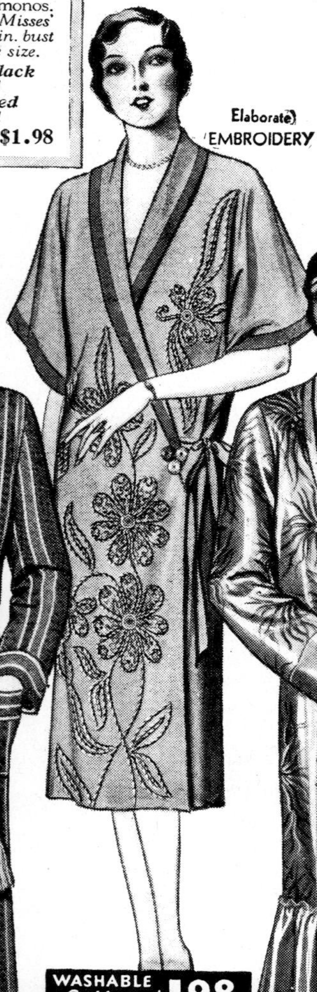

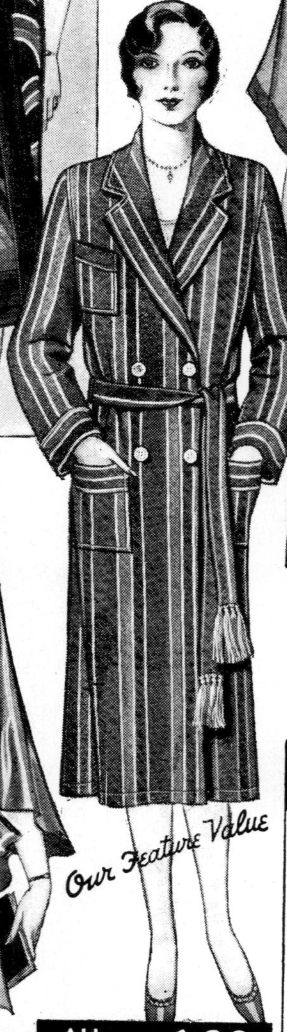

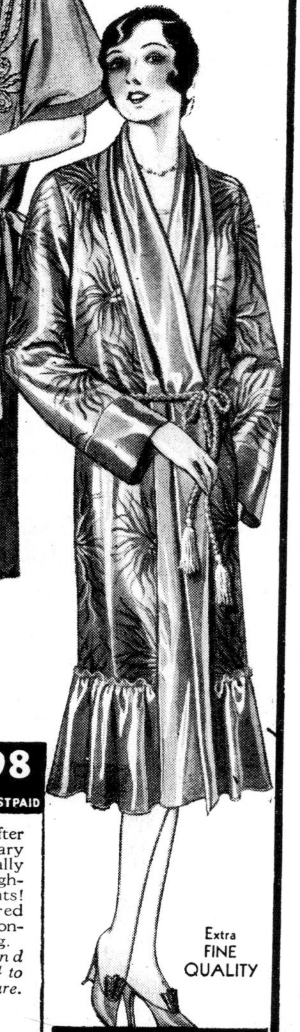

PERMANENT CRINKLE — COLORS GUARANTEED FAST

Elaborate EMBROIDERY

WASHABLE Cotton Box Loom CREPE $1.98 POSTPAID

FINER and softer than ordinary qualities! Generally found in much higher priced garments! Bonaz embroidered flower sprays. Contrasting trimming. *Women's and Misses' Sizes—34 to 44 in. bust measure. State size.*

27D5817—Rose
27D5818—Copenhagen Blue
Postpaid....$1.98

Our Feature Value

ALL WOOL FLANNEL $6.98 POSTPAID

A BETTER robe than ever! Really low priced! Good heavy all-wool striped flannel! Fast colors. Warm, smart, double-breasted front, three pockets, deep, notched collar give a trim, mannish effect. *Women's and Misses' Sizes—34 to 46 inches bust measure. State size.*

31D5819—Rose Fancy
31D5820—Blue Fancy
31D5821—Lavender Fancy **$6.98**

Extra FINE QUALITY

RAYON TWILL SATIN $5.98 POSTPAID

LOOKS like hand-painted satin! Guaranteed washable! One of our most beautiful robes! Brilliant surface is over-spread with flower print! Far more beautiful and rich-looking than the price implies. *Women's and Misses' Sizes—34 to 44 inches bust measure. State size.*

31D5825—Peach
31D5826—Rose
31D5827—Blue **Postpaid $5.98**

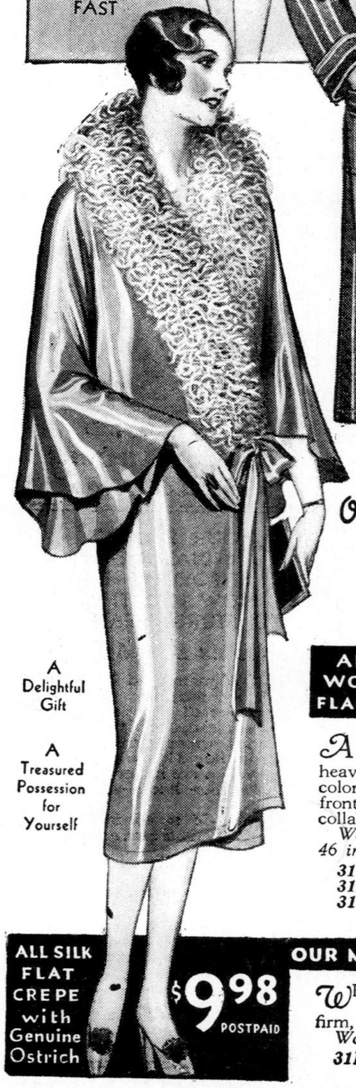

A Delightful Gift

A Treasured Possession for Yourself

ALL SILK FLAT CREPE with Genuine Ostrich $9.98 POSTPAID

OUR MODEST PRICE TAKES IT OUT OF THE "LUXURY" CLASS

WE'VE never had such a beautiful negligee at this low price! Fluffy, feathery curls of genuine ostrich! A lovely, soft frame for the face! Fine, firm, all silk Flat Crepe. New, graceful cape-cut sleeves! *Women's and Misses' Sizes—34 to 44 inches bust measure. State size.*

31D5828—Light Blue **31D5829—Rose** **Postpaid....$9.98**

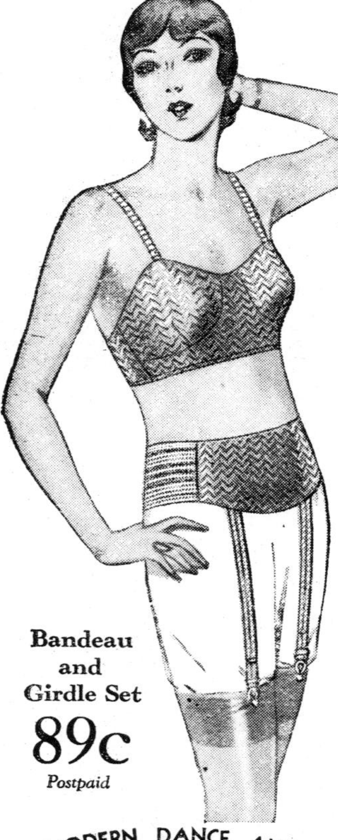

Bandeau and Girdle Set 89c Postpaid

MODERN DANCE AND ATHLETIC SET

For Slender Figures

UPLIFT BANDEAU, of Rayon figured pink cotton material, elastic and hooks at back. Silk ribbon straps. Side closing girdle to match with elastic sides.

18V427—Bandeau } Set,
18V428—Girdle.. } *Postpaid* 89c
State bust and waist size.
18V428—Girdle only. *Postpaid* 49c
State waist size.
Bandeau not sold separately.

Bandeau in even bust sizes, 30 to 38 inches. Girdle in all waist sizes, 24 to 30; also 32 and 34 inches.

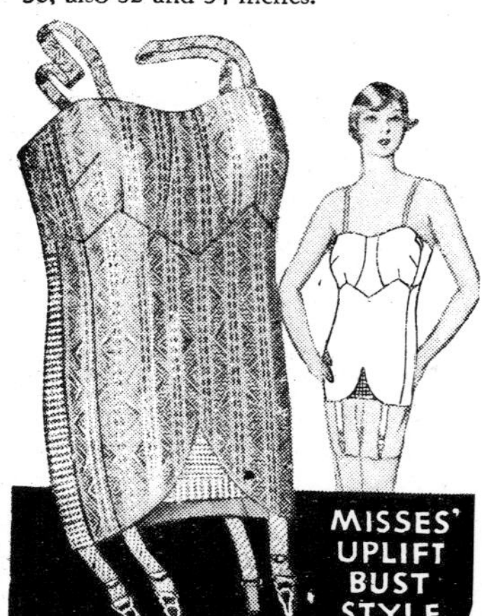

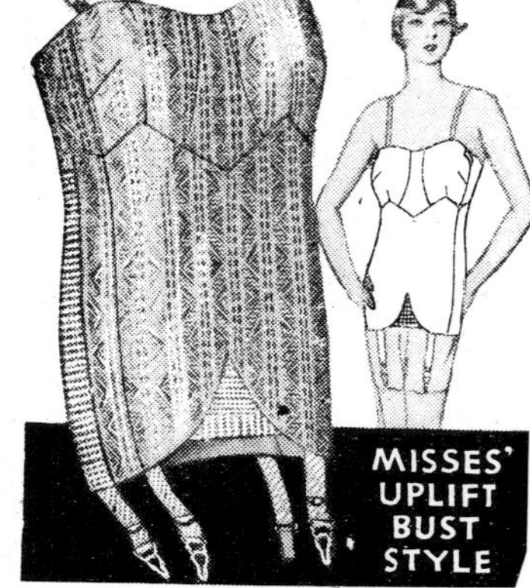

A GLOVE for Every Ensemble

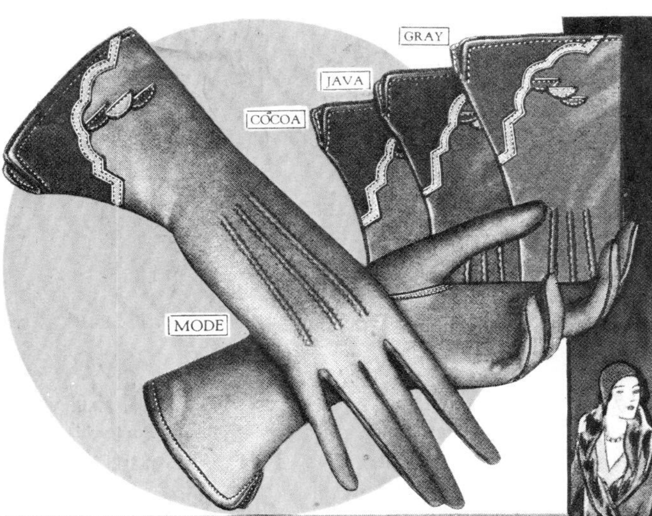

BRADLEY GLOVES

59c A PAIR
Postpaid

33D3260—Cocoa.
33D3261—Gray.
33D3262—Mode.
33D3263—Java.

Sizes, 6 to 8½. Half sizes. State size. Style—quality, charm, serviceability, all combined at a price hardly ever equaled. The material is very good quality, washable, cotton **chamoisuede fabric.** Tailored in the newest 3½-button length. Modish flared cuffs with contrasting binding and the same clever two-tone applique trim that's shown on gloves of much higher price. New hairline stitching in contrasting color adds interest to the backs! A trim, smooth imported glove—priced appealingly low

98c A PAIR
POSTPAID

33D3295—Mode.
33D3296—Sunset.
33D3297—Java.

Sizes, 6 to 8½. Half sizes. State size. Rare distinction and fine value! The Vogue boasts no smarter style than these semi-gauntlet **Imported Slip-on Gloves** of **washable shrunk** cotton **Chamoisuede fabric.** Authentically styled after the latest European fashion creations. The flare cuffs have contrasting color binding and insert gores jauntily laced at the sides Kip knot seams, and smooth neat Kip-bolton thumbs.

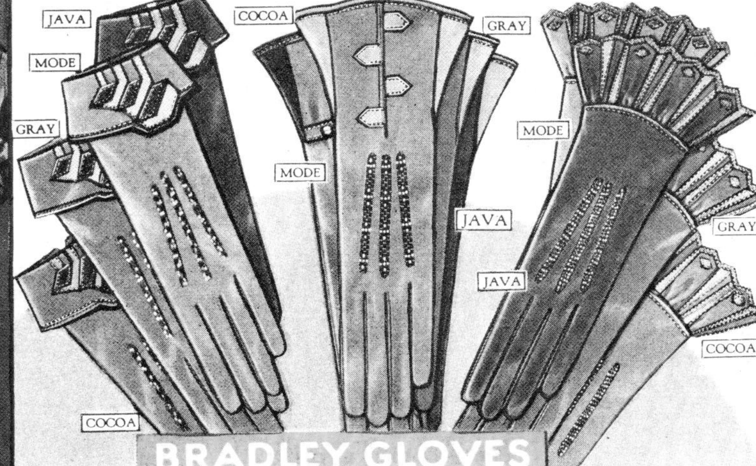

BRADLEY GLOVES

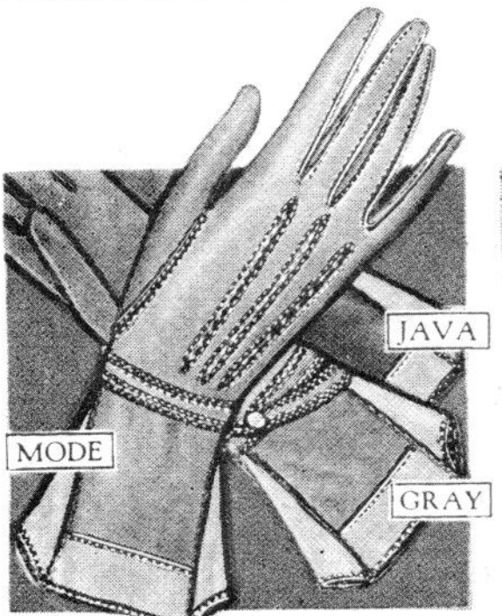

A New Mode

98c A PAIR
Postpaid

33D3315 Mode.
33D3316 Gray.
33D3317 Java

Sizes, 6 to 8½. Half sizes. Be sure to state size. To prove their unusual style effectiveness, these **Imported** Gloves of very fine quality washable pre-shrunk cotton **Chamoisuede Fabric,** introduce a smart flare into their cuffs by side inserts of contrasting color with matching band at top. There's a smart little wrist strap with contrasting color piping and hairline stitching and one clasp fastener. The latest fancy two-tone stitched backs; Kip-knot seams and Bolton thumbs.

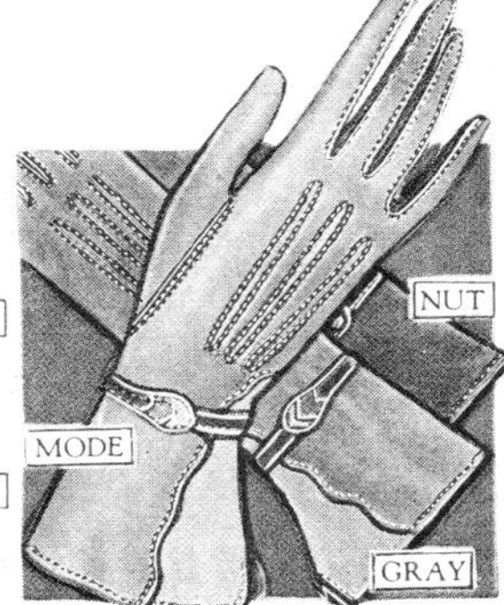

Very Chic!

$1.39 A PAIR
Postpaid

33D3340 Mode.
33D3341 Gray.
33D3342 Nut.

Sizes, 6 to 8½. Half sizes. Be sure to state size. Postpaid. Made of **very fine quality, washable, cotton chamoisuede fabric, double woven**—a style creation by one of the foremost European designers. This imported skilfully tailored slip-on has a novel insert gore of contrasting color. Cuff and gore is edged with contrasting color to match the all-around piping trimmed wrist strap with its touches of smart applique and pearl button clasp. Neatly stitched backs. Kip-knot seams and bolton thumbs.

Two-Tone Applique

49c A PAIR
Postpaid

33D3245 Cocoa.
33D3246 Gray.
33D3247 Mode.
33D3248—Java.

Sizes, 6 to 8½. Half sizes. Be sure to state size.

Ever so smartly styled of good quality, **washable,** cotton **chamoisuede fabric** with the latest design in turnback scalloped cuffs with a fancy two-tone applique trim. The scallops are outlined in clever two-tone stitching, and the backs are beautifully embroidered in the new two-tone contrast effect. One clasp fastener. Remarkably attractive and decidedly serviceable. Imported Gloves. Remember, they're easily washable, too.

Yes! Modern!

79c A PAIR
Postpaid

33D3270 Cocoa.
33D3271 Gray.
33D3272 Mode.
33D3273 Java.

Sizes, 6 to 8½. Half sizes. State size.

Real glove charm—from the contrasting color gores on both sides to the matching fancy applique and piping on the backs! New! Note the clasp fastened semi-strap, with its touches of contrasting piping! Neatly tailored of very good quality Chamoisuede cotton fabric that washes beautifully. The smartest imported glove. Embroidered backs.

Smart Flare Cuffs

69c A PAIR
Postpaid

33D3290 Cocoa.
33D3291 Gray.
33D3292 Mode.
33D3293 Java.

Sizes, 6 to 8½. Half sizes. Be sure to state size.

With such very smart gloves obtainable at a price so appealingly low, no woman will want to be without at least one pair of these **Imported Gloves** of very good quality, **washable, Chamoisuede** cotton **fabric.** The fancy scalloped flare cuffs show touches of modish contrasting color applique. Backs are embroidered in dainty two-tone effect. One clasp fastener. Chic and yet so practical.

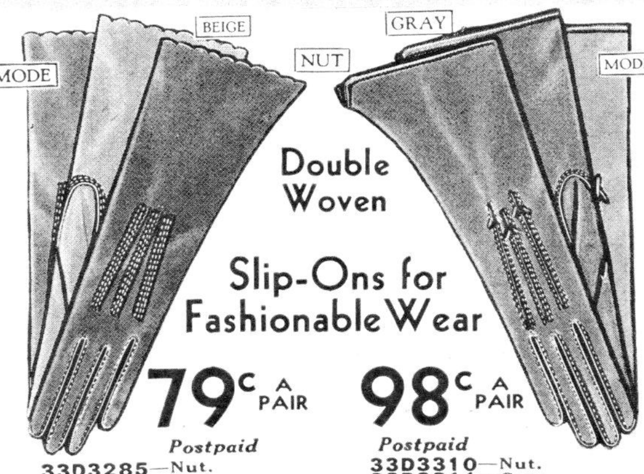

Double Woven

Slip-Ons for Fashionable Wear

79c A PAIR
Postpaid

33D3285—Nut.
33D3286—Mode.
33D3287—Beige.

Sizes, 6 to 8½. Half sizes. Be sure to state size. Postpaid. A fashionably plain **Imported slip-on** made of very fine quality, **washable, double woven,** cotton **chamoisuede fabric.** A trimly styled glove suitable for wear with any costume. Daintily pinked tops and stitched backs vary its distinctive simplicity. Kip knot seams.

98c A PAIR
Postpaid

33D3310—Nut.
33D3311—Gray.
33D3312—Mode.

Sizes, 6 to 8½. Half sizes. Be sure to state size. Postpaid. The **washable, double-woven Chamoisuede cotton fabric** in these new **Imported Slip-on** Gloves is of exceptionally fine quality. Cuffs are smartly trimmed with a tiny edging of contrasting color. Kip-knot sewed seams; Kip-bolton thumbs. Hand drawn spear backs.

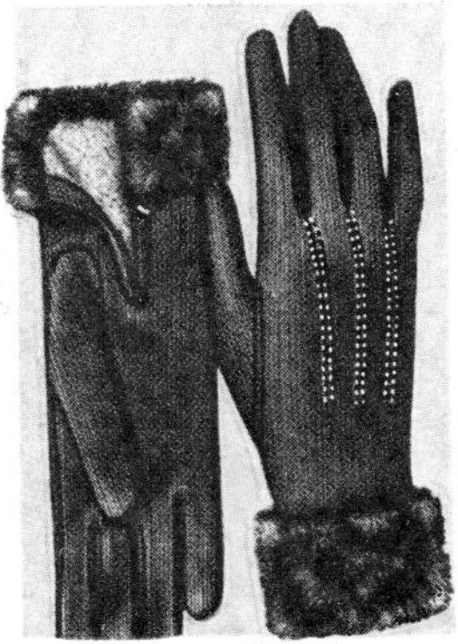

Jersey Cloth

49c A Pair
Postpaid

33D3620 Brown.

Sizes, 6 to 8½. Half sizes. State size.

A splendid glove of fine quality closely woven jersey cloth. Snug and comfortingly warm with heavy fleeced lining and cuffs of thick warm fur. This model is surprisingly low priced.

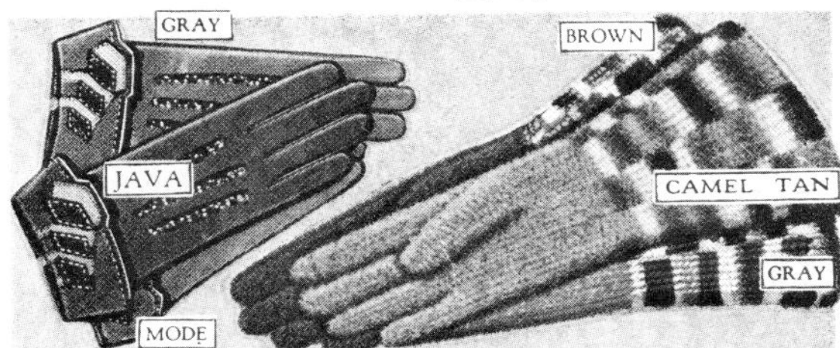

Smart Styles for the Miss

49c A PAIR
Postpaid

33D3730 Mode.
33D3731 Gray.
33D3732 Java.

Ages, 5 to 12 years. State age. Misses' imported gloves of **good quality, washable,** cotton **chamoisuede fabric.** Striking scalloped turndown cuffs with two-tone applique.

49c A PAIR
Postpaid

33D3780 Camel tan.
33D3781 Brown.
33D3782 Gray.

Ages, 5 to 14 years. State age. Misses' Imported Gauntlet Gloves of good quality warm brushed yarns of about two-thirds wool, balance cotton. Seamless knit. Gay colored cuffs.

How to Measure Your Hand for Size

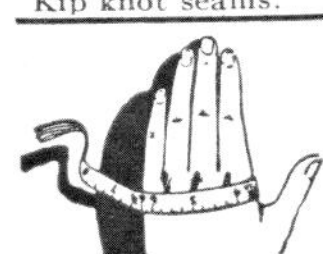

GIVE GLOVE SIZE. HOLD HAND OUT FLAT WITH FINGERS TOUCHING, THUMB RAISED; draw ordinary tape measure close but not tight all around hand as shown in illustration (do not include thumb). The number of inches shown by this measurement is your correct glove size. Tape measure furnished free on request.
Women's sizes in Fabric and Lined Kid Gloves: 6, 6½, 7, 7½, 8 and 8½.
Women's sizes in Unlined Kid Gloves: 6, 6¼, 6½, 6¾, 7, 7¼, 7½, 7¾, and 8.
For Glove sizes for Children 5 to 14 years of age, GIVE AGE OF CHILD.

Order Blanks Are in Back of This Catalog

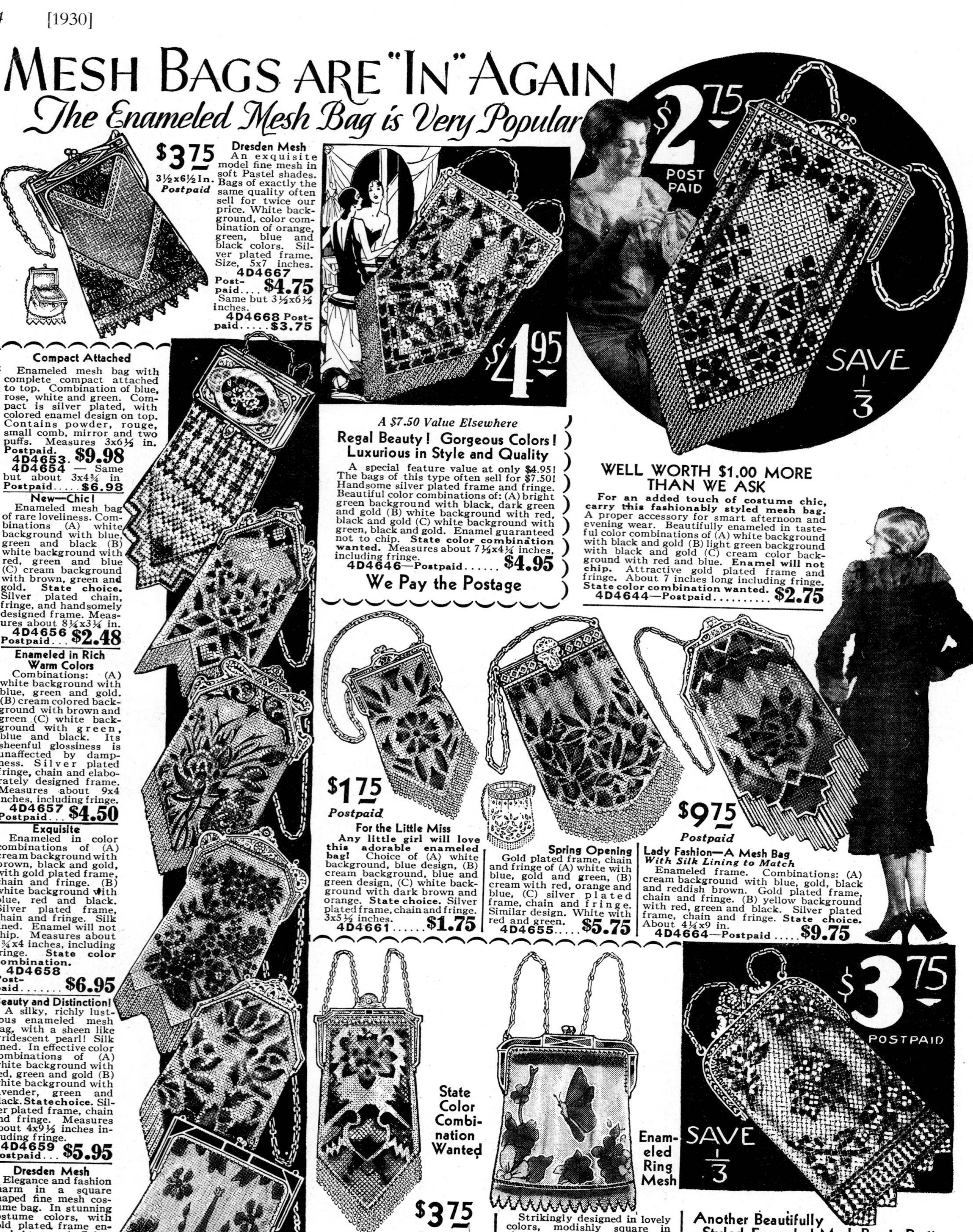

MESH BAGS ARE "IN" AGAIN

The Enameled Mesh Bag is Very Popular

$3.75 3½x6½ In. Postpaid

Dresden Mesh
An exquisite model fine mesh in soft Pastel shades. Bags of exactly the same quality often sell for twice our price. White background, color combination of orange, green, blue and black colors. Silver plated frame. Size, 5x7 inches.
4D4667 Postpaid.... $4.75
Same but 3½x6½ inches.
4D4668 Postpaid..... $3.75

$4.95

$2.75 POST PAID

SAVE 1/3

Compact Attached
Enameled mesh bag with complete compact attached to top. Combination of blue, rose, white and green. Compact is silver plated, with colored enamel design on top. Contains powder, rouge, small comb, mirror and two puffs. Measures 3x6½ in.
Postpaid.
4D4653. $9.98
4D4654 — Same but about 3x4¾ in
Postpaid..... $6.98

New—Chic!
Enameled mesh bag of rare loveliness. Combinations (A) white background with blue, green and black (B) white background with red, green and blue (C) cream background with brown, green and gold. **State choice.** Silver plated chain, fringe, and handsomely designed frame. Measures about 8¼x3¼ in.
4D4656 Postpaid... $2.48

Enameled in Rich Warm Colors
Combinations: (A) white background with blue, green and gold. (B) cream colored background with brown and green (C) white background with green, blue and black. Its sheenful glossiness is unaffected by dampness. Silver plated fringe, chain and elaborately designed frame. Measures about 9x4 inches, including fringe.
4D4657 Postpaid... $4.50

Exquisite
Enameled in color combinations of (A) cream background with brown, black and gold, with gold plated frame, chain and fringe. (B) white background with blue, red and black. Silver plated frame, chain and fringe. Silk lined. Enamel will not chip. Measures about 8¾x4 inches, including fringe. **State color combination.**
4D4658 Postpaid....... $6.95

Beauty and Distinction!
A silky, richly lustrous enameled mesh bag, with a sheen like irridescent pearl! Silk lined. In effective color combinations of (A) white background with red, green and gold (B) white background with lavender, green and black. **State choice.** Silver plated frame, chain and fringe. Measures about 4x9½ inches including fringe.
4D4659 Postpaid... $5.95

Dresden Mesh
Elegance and fashion charm in a square shaped fine mesh costume bag. In stunning costume colors, with gold plated frame enameled to match. Color choice (A) black and white (B) blue and white (C) green and white (D) brown and white. **State choice.** Impressive quality, and excellent good taste! Measures 5x6 inches.
4D4660 Postpaid... $5.75

A $7.50 Value Elsewhere

Regal Beauty! Gorgeous Colors! Luxurious in Style and Quality

A special feature value at only $4.95! The bags of this type often sell for $7.50! Handsome silver plated frame and fringe. Beautiful color combinations of: (A) bright green background with black, dark green and gold (B) white background with red, black and gold (C) white background with green, black and gold. Enamel guaranteed not to chip. **State color combination wanted.** Measures about 7½x4¼ inches, including fringe.
4D4646—Postpaid...... $4.95

We Pay the Postage

WELL WORTH $1.00 MORE THAN WE ASK

For an added touch of costume chic, carry this fashionably styled mesh bag. A proper accessory for smart afternoon and evening wear. Beautifully enameled in tasteful color combinations of (A) white background with black and gold (B) light green background with black and gold (C) cream color background with red and blue. **Enamel will not chip.** Attractive gold plated frame and fringe. About 7 inches long including fringe. **State color combination wanted.**
4D4644—Postpaid.......... $2.75

$1.75 Postpaid

For the Little Miss
Any little girl will love **this adorable enameled bag!** Choice of (A) white background, blue design, (B) cream background, blue and green design, (C) white background with dark brown and orange. **State choice.** Silver plated frame, chain and fringe. 3x5½ inches.
4D4661...... $1.75

Spring Opening
Gold plated frame, chain and fringe of (A) white with blue, gold and green, (B) cream with red, orange and blue, (C) silver plated frame, chain and fringe. Similar design. White with red and green.
4D4655..... $5.75

$9.75 Postpaid

Lady Fashion—A Mesh Bag
With Silk Lining to Match
Enameled frame. Combinations: (A) cream background with blue, gold, black and reddish brown. Gold plated frame, chain and fringe. (B) yellow background with red, green and black. Silver plated frame, chain and fringe. **State choice.** About 4½x9 in.
4D4664—Postpaid..... $9.75

$3.75 POSTPAID

SAVE 1/3

State Color Combination Wanted

$3.75 Postpaid

Brilliant Glossy Enamel Finish
Color choice of: (A) cream background with blue, purple, rose and black. (B) white background with light blue, purple, gold and black. (C) cream background with light green, red and gold. 3½x8¼ in. Gold plated frame, chain and fringe.
4D4665 Postpaid........... $3.75

Enameled Ring Mesh

Strikingly designed in lovely colors, modishly square in shape, with an appearance of rare style and quality! Color choice of (A) white background with blue, green, yellow and rose, blue frame (B) white background with brown, yellow, green and rose, brown frame (C) white background with green, yellow and rose, green frame. Enamel frames, modernistically designed. To carry on "dress up" occasions.
4D4666 Postpaid.......... $4.75

Another Beautifully Styled Enameled Mesh Bag in Pretty Colorings and Patterns

Has a light blue background with gold and darker blue color design. Gold plated frame. Enamel guaranteed not to chip. An exceptional value at this price.
4D4645—3½x5¾ inches.
Postpaid.................. $3.75
Pattern similar to above with same colorings.
4D4647—4¼x6 inches.
Postpaid.................. $4.75

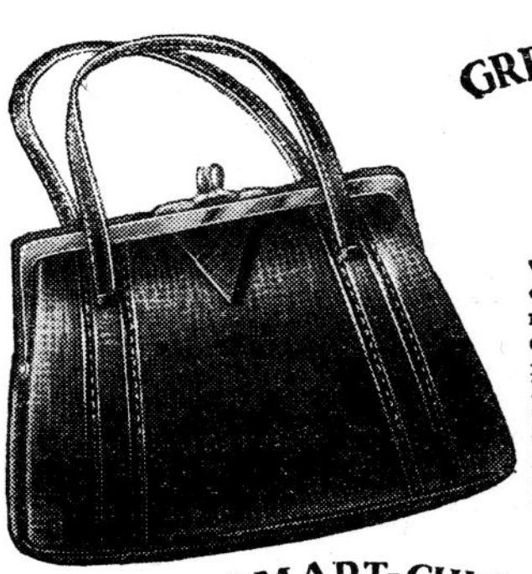

GREAT FAVORITE

POST PAID $2.45

18V1501—Brown with gold color frame, or Black with gun-metal frame. State color. Large and roomy, genuine cowhide. Soft, pliable swagger handles. Strong frame. Inner swinging change purse. Mirror. Good lining. Size, 9x6½ inches.

SMART-CHIC

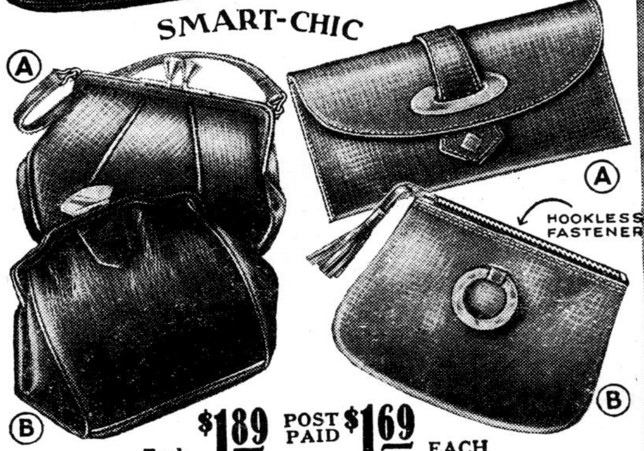

Each $1.89

A18V1502—Top Handle.
B18V1503—Back Strap.
Colors: Suntan, Brown sugar, or Black. State color. Genuine calf leather. Inner swinging change purse. Mirror. Neatly lined. 7½x5½ in.

POST PAID $1.69 EACH

A18V1504 — Underarm Back Strap. Size, 8½x4½ in.
B18V1505 — Hookless Fastener. Back Strap. Size, 7½x5 inches.
Colors: Suntan, Brown sugar, Garland (medium) green, Nautical blue, Danger (medium) red, or Black. State color. Made of soft, pliable, genuine calf leather.

SERVICEABLE

POST PAID $1.98

18V1506
Colors: Brown or Black. State color. Smooth cowhide top strap purse. Hand laced flap. Embossed design. Three compartments. Neatly lined. Mirror. Size, 9½x5¼ inches.

GREAT VALUE

POST PAID 85¢

18V1507
Colors: Brown or Black. State color. Durable artificial leather, back strap. Three compartments. Neatly lined. Mirror. Size, 8½x 5½ inches.

MODERNISTIC

18V1508
Modernistic shaded colors: Brown, Green, Blue, Red or Black. State color. Popular back strap. "Kafsted" artificial leather. Snap fastener. Two pockets. Mirror and coin purse. Piping to match. Size, 8x5 in.

48¢ POSTPAID

SPANISH CRAFT BAGS

IN COLORS

GENUINE IMPORTED STEERHIDE

ART LACED—POPULAR DESIGNS—HAND COLORED

Our New Feature. Embossed Initials
Coin purses of these seven styles will be embossed with two or three initials. Print initials.

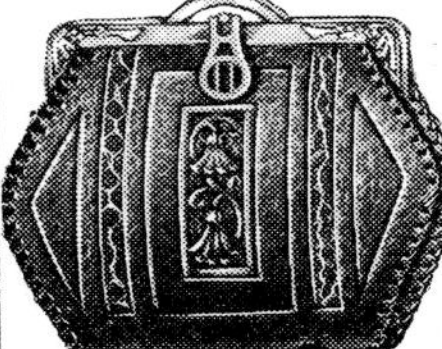

Compares With $10.00 Values Elsewhere $6.95 Postpaid

18V1406½ — Blended Brown, Gold Color frame.
18V1405½ — Blended Blue, Silver Color frame.
A great favorite. Design resembles hand tooling. "Art" hand lacing. Safety "Turn-Loc" frame, suede lined, beveled mirror. Size, 6¾x7 in. Print initials desired.

SMART "BACK-STRAP" STYLE

POSTPAID $6.95

18V1419½ Blended Brown with Gold Color frame.
18V1418½—Blended Blue with Silver Color frame.
Neat design resembles hand tooling. "Art" hand lacing. Size, 7½x5½ inches. Print initials to be embossed on purse.

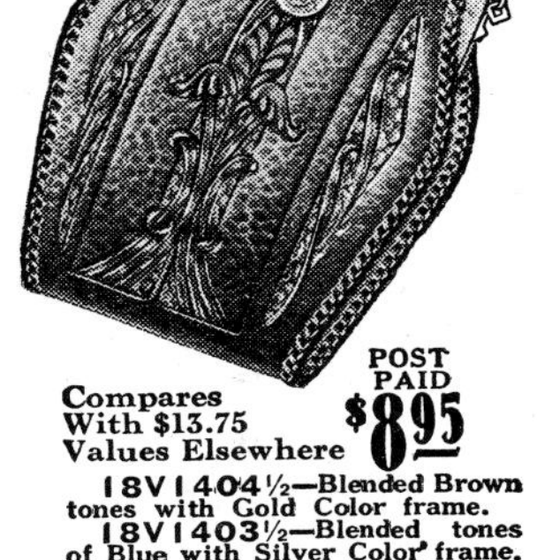

Compares With $13.75 Values Elsewhere POST PAID $8.95

18V1404½—Blended Brown tones with Gold Color frame.
18V1403½—Blended tones of Blue with Silver Color frame.
Our famous special. Popular design resembles hand tooling. "Art" hand lacing encircles entire bag and handle. Safety "Turn-Loc" frame, suede lined, beveled mirror, your initials embossed on coin purse. Print initials desired. Size, 7x8 inches.

OUR GREAT OFFER

$5.00 EACH POSTPAID

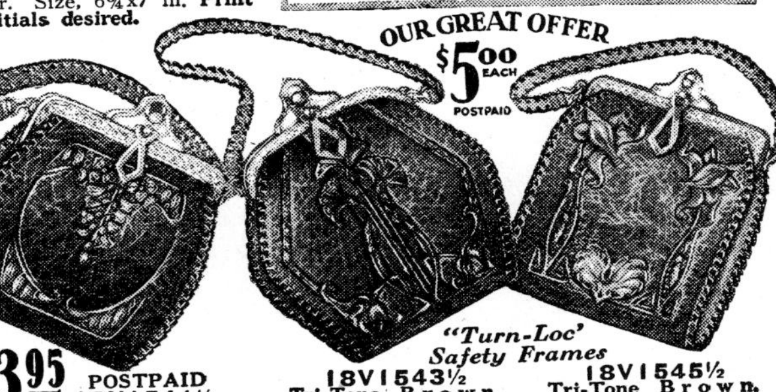

"Turn-Loc" Safety Frames

$3.95 POSTPAID

18V1541½ Tri-Tone Brown, Gold Color frame.
18V1542½ — Blended Blue tones, Silver Color frame.
Leather lined. Mirror. Size, 5¼x5¼ in. Print initials.

18V1543½ Tri-Tone Brown, Gold Color frame.
18V1544½ Blended Blue tones, Silver Color frame.
"Art" laced. Mirror and coin purse. Print initials. Size, 6¾x6 inches. $5.00

18V1545½ Tri-Tone Brown, Gold Color frame.
18V1546½ Blended Blue tones, Silver Color frame.
"Art" lacing, suede lined, mirror, coin purse. Print initials. 5½x5¾ in...$5.00

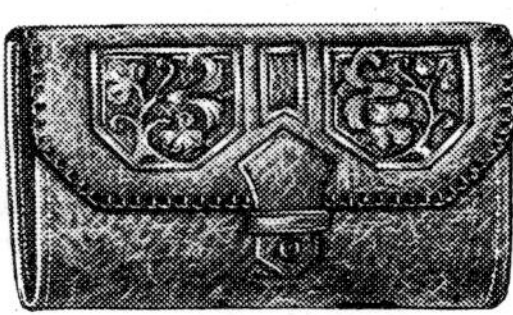

POST PAID $2.98

18V1428½ — Blended tones of Brown. Size, 7x5 inches.
18V1427½ — Blended tones of Blue. Size, 7x5 inches.
Popular back strap frameless purse. Embossed design. Flap is hand laced, snap fastener, separate coin compartment, mirror, suede lined. Print initials desired to be embossed on purse.

THREE-COMPARTMENT BAG

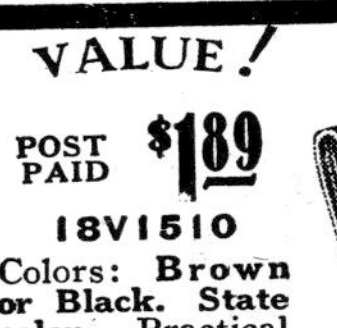

POST PAID $2.89

18V1509—Colors: Brown sugar or Black. State color.
Unusual offering in large and roomy size calf leather bag. Three spacious compartments. Semi-leather covered clasping frame. Durable top handle. Good quality lining. Mirror and coin purse in pocket. Size, 9¾x6¾ inches.

VALUE!

POST PAID $1.89

18V1510
Colors: Brown or Black. State color. Practical pin grain leather, back strap purse. Neatly lined. Three compartments. Mirror. Size, 8x5 inches.

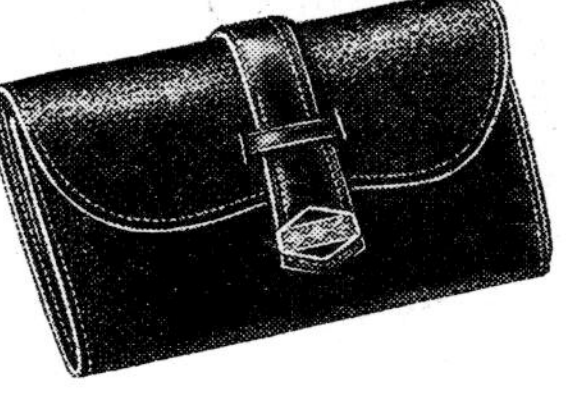

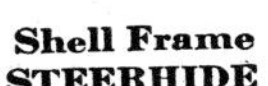

Shell Frame STEERHIDE

18V1511—Back strap steerhide purse with heavy shell (simulated) frame. Beige (tan) color. Embossed design. Change purse, mirror. Good lining. Size, 8x5½ inches.

STEERHIDE BAG

SHELL FRAME $2.89 POST PAID

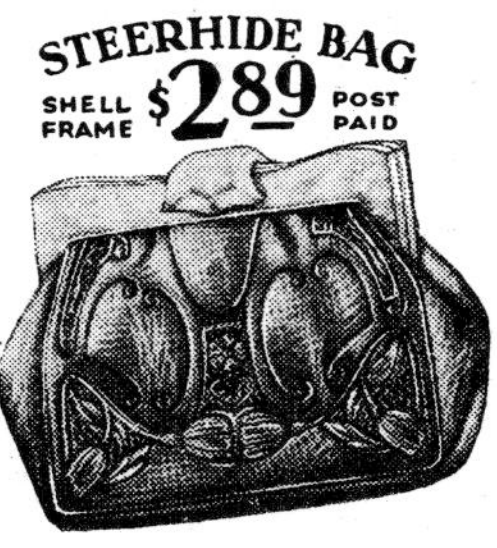

BAGS FOR THE YOUNGSTERS

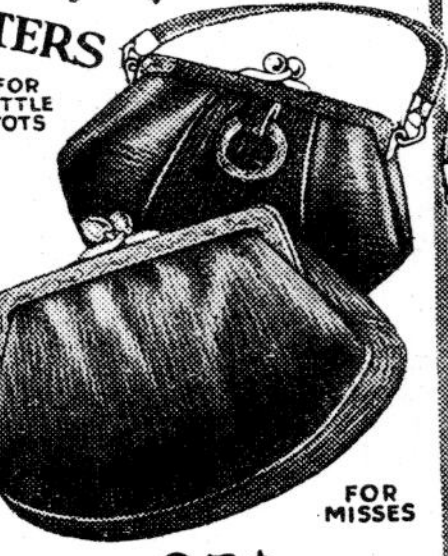

FOR LITTLE TOTS

FOR MISSES

Choice Each 99¢ POST PAID

For Girls 8 to 12 Years

18V1512A—Top Handle.
18V1513B—Back Strap.
Genuine leather. Smart and stylish. Durable gold color frames. Assorted colors. Neatly lined. Mirror. Size, 7x5 in.

48¢ POST PAID

For Girls 8 to 10 Years

18V1514
Popular style, top strap purse of artificial leather. Assorted colors. Three compartments. Mirror. Size, 6½x3¾.

Choice Each 25¢ POST PAID

18V1515 — Top Handle. Size, 5½x4.
18V1516—Back Strap. Size, 6½x4.
Big value, artificial leather purses in assorted colors.

WONDER VALUES

CHOICE 98¢ EACH POSTPAID

18V1517
Colors: Brown, or Black. State color. Large and roomy top handle, durable artificial leather. Covered frame. Attractive ornamented pull tab. Inner swinging change purse. Good durable lining. Size, 8¾x6 inches.

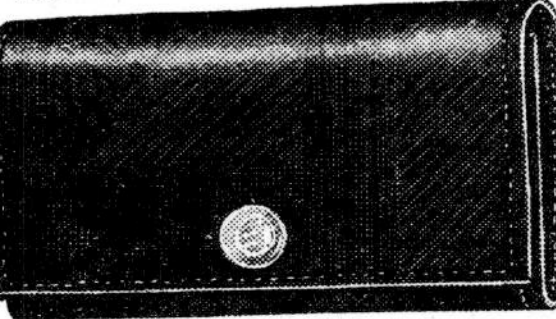

18V1518
Colors: Brown or Black. State color. Newest and practical style underarm back strap purse.

98¢ Large shell (simulated) button snap fastener. Three compartments. Durable lining. Mirror. Size, 9½x5 inches.

NEW GATE FRAME TAPESTRY

98¢ POST PAID

18V1519 — Popular style silver color gate-frame tapestry bag in assorted patterns. Chain link handle. Roomy size. Mirror and coin purse. Size, 6½x7½ inches.

• THE VERY LATEST • IN FINE COMPACTS

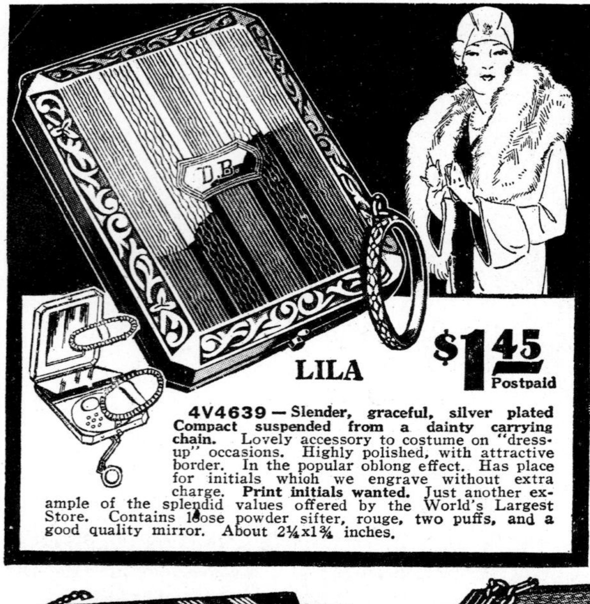

LILA

$1.45 Postpaid

4V4639—Slender, graceful, silver plated Compact suspended from a dainty carrying chain. Lovely accessory to costume on "dress-up" occasions. Highly polished, with attractive border. In the popular oblong effect. Has place for initials which we engrave without extra charge. Print initials wanted. Just another example of the splendid values offered by the World's Largest Store. Contains loose powder sifter, rouge, two puffs, and a good quality mirror. About 2¼x1¾ inches.

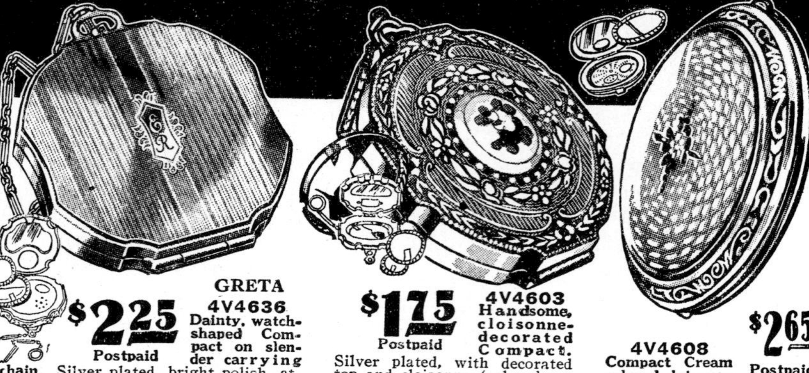

GRETA

$2.25 Postpaid

4V4636 Dainty, watch-shaped Compact on slender carrying chain. Silver plated, bright polish, attractive border. Contains loose powder sifter, rouge, two puffs and mirror. Size, about 2x2 in. Any initial engraved without extra charge. Print initial.

$1.75 Postpaid

4V4603 Handsome, cloisonne-decorated Compact. Silver plated, with decorated top and cloisonne (colored enamel) center. Has carrying hain. About 2 inches in diameter. Contains loose powder sifter, rouge, mirror and double puff.

$2.65 Postpaid

4V4608 Compact Cream colored cloisonne enamel on solid silver top. Loose powder sifter, rouge unbreakable mirror and double puff. Diameter, about 2⅛ inches.

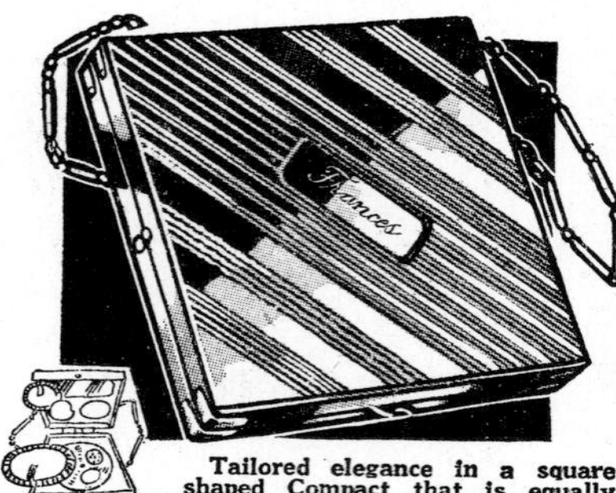

Tailored elegance in a square shaped Compact that is equally at home on the street or at social affairs. Silver plated. About 2x2 inches. Loose powder sifter, rouge, two puffs, mirror. Carrying chain. Print name.

$1.98 Postpaid

4V4631—Postpaid... $1.98

4V4633—With solid silver cover and back, Postpaid......... $3.98

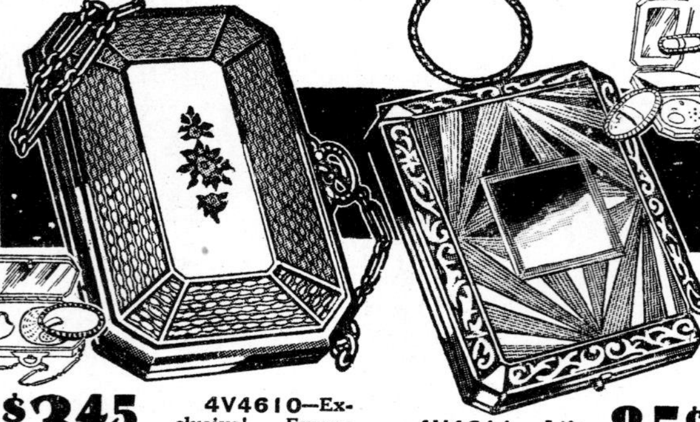

$3.45 Postpaid

4V4610—Exclusive! Expensive looking! Beautiful cloisonne (colored blue enamel) on solid silver top. Carrying chain. About 1⅝x2½ inches. Contains loose powder sifter, rouge, unbreakable mirror and two puffs.

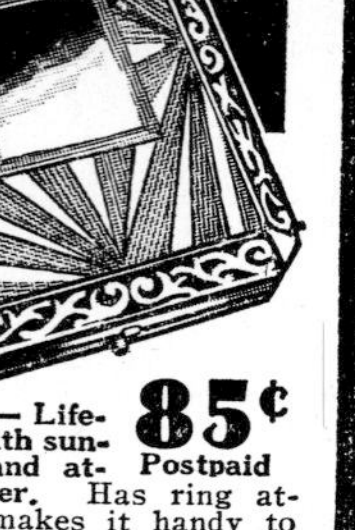

4V4611—Lifetime finish with sunray design and attractive border. Has ring attached that makes it handy to carry. Contains loose powder sifter, rouge, large size mirror and two puffs. Size, about 1¾x2¼ inches. Any initial engraved without extra charge. Print initial wanted.

85¢ Postpaid

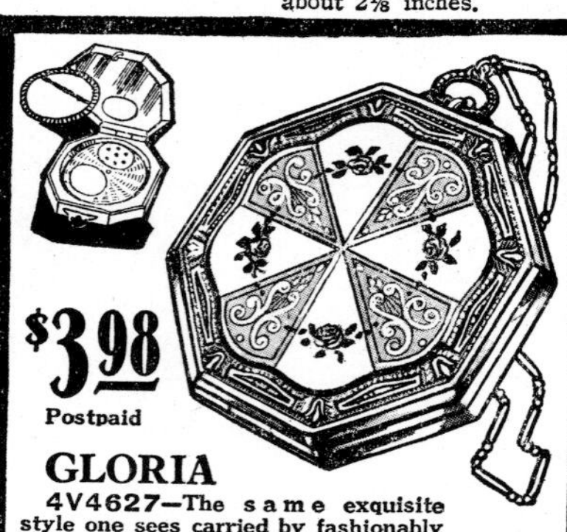

$3.98 Postpaid

GLORIA

4V4627—The same exquisite style one sees carried by fashionably dressed women everywhere. Beautiful cloisonne (green and white enamel) on solid silver top. The low price is another example of our remarkable values. Modish octagon shape. Size, about 2¼x2¼ in. Contains loose powder sifter, rouge, unbreakable mirror and double puff.

Postpaid......................... $3.98

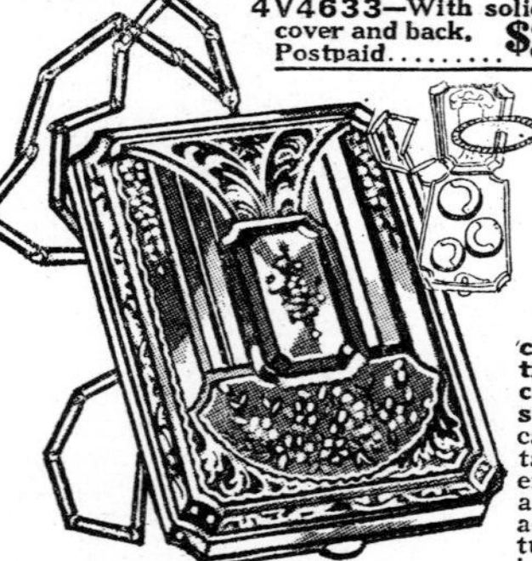

$1.50 Postpaid

4V4622—Dainty chain Purse, attractively decorated with cloisonne enamel on solid silver. Has carrying chain. Contains three coin holders. A very practical as well as attractive accessory to any costume. About 1½x2¼ inches.

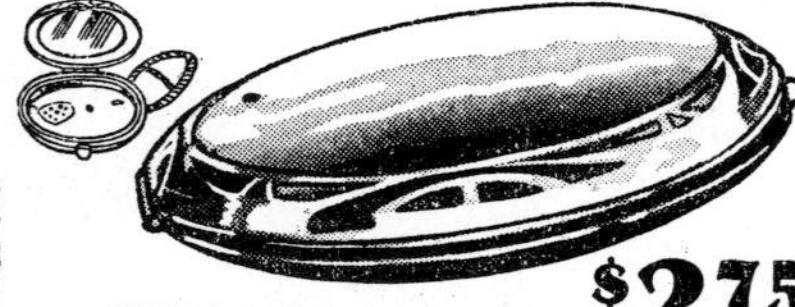

4V4614—Colorful Compacts to match the costume. Slim model. Enameled top and back. Metal trimmed. Colors: Rose, powder blue, jade green or ivory. Loose powder sifter, rouge, large unbreakable mirror and double puff. State color. Diameter, about 2⅛ inches.

$2.75 Postpaid

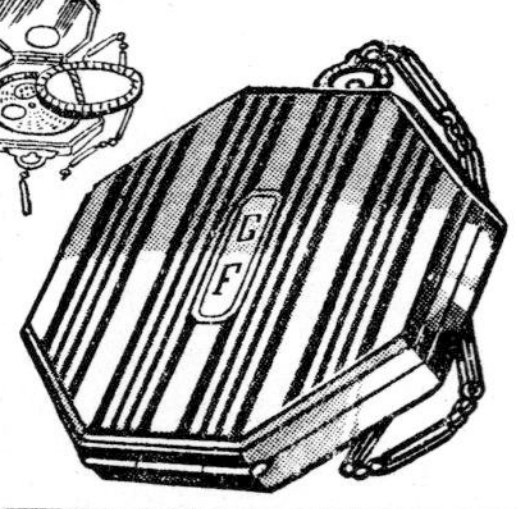

$1.50 Postpaid

4V4606—Neat! Smart Compact! Non-tarnishable finish. In modish octagon shape. Contains loose powder sifter, rouge, unbreakable mirror and double puff. Carrying chain. 2¼x2¼ inches. Initial engraved without extra charge. Print initial.

Mesh Bags Are in Vogue This Spring

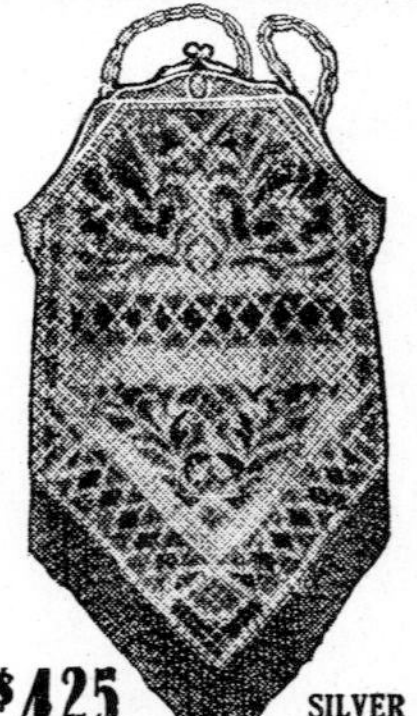

$4.25 Postpaid

SILVER PLATED FRAME

Enameled Mesh Bag. State color: (A) White background with light blue and black; (B) Cream color background with black and reddish brown, or (C) White background with lavender, green and gold. About 4½x8⅜ in. Including fringe. Postpaid.

4V4650 $4.25

$6.98 And Up Postpaid

Clever! Unusual! Beautifully enameled Mesh Bag with Compact attached to top! Compact is silver plated, with colored enameled design on top. Contains powder, rouge, small comb, mirror and two puffs. Measures 3x6½ inches.

4V4653 Postpaid...... $9.98

4V4654—Same style but measures abt. 3x4¾ inches. Postpaid. $6.98

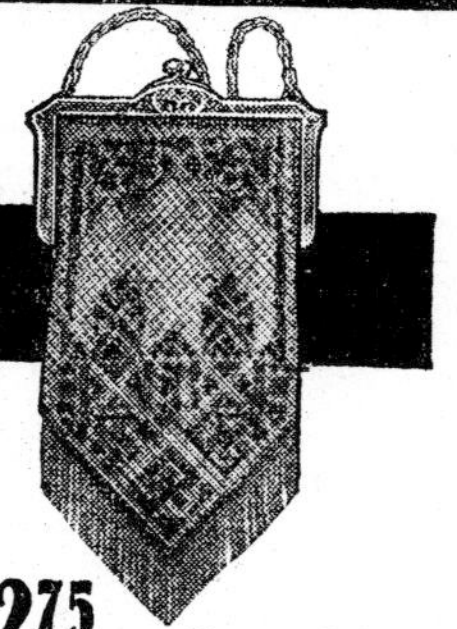

$1.45 Postpaid

For the Little Girl. Dainty enameled Mesh Bag. Size, about 2¾x5 inches (including fringe). Color combinations of: (A) Light blue background with dark blue and gold; (B) Light green background with dark green and gold, or (C) White background with black and gold. State color combination wanted. Silver plated frame and fringe. Enamel guaranteed not to chip. Postpaid.

4V4652..... $1.45

$2.75 Postpaid

Beautifully enameled Mesh Bag. Enamel guaranteed not to chip. Color combinations: (A) White background with black and gold: (B) Light green background with black and gold, or (C) Cream color background with red and blue. State color combination wanted. Gold plated frame and fringe. About 7 inches long including fringe.

4V4644 Postpaid......... $2.75

$3.35 And Up Postpaid

Attractive Mesh Bags. Enameled in colors. Light green background with gold and darker green color design. Gold plated frame and fringe. Enamel guaranteed not to chip. Dampness will not affect gloss.

4V4649—Size, 3½x6½ inches, including fringe. Postpaid............ $3.35

4V4651—Same style. Size, 4½x7 inches, including fringe. Postpaid $4.65

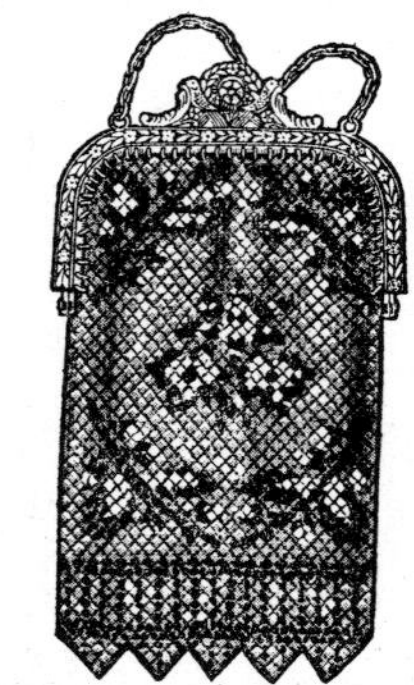

$3.75 And Up Postpaid

Another beautifully styled enameled Mesh Bag in pretty colorings and patterns. Has a light blue background with gold and darker blue color design. Gold plated frame. Enamel guaranteed not to chip. An exceptional value at this price.

4V4645—3½x5¾ in. Postpaid......... $3.75

Pattern similar to above with same colorings.

4V4647—4¼x6 inches Postpaid $4.78

YOUR CHOICE

Francine FOOTWEAR

$4.00 A PAIR POSTPAID $4.00 A PAIR POSTPAID

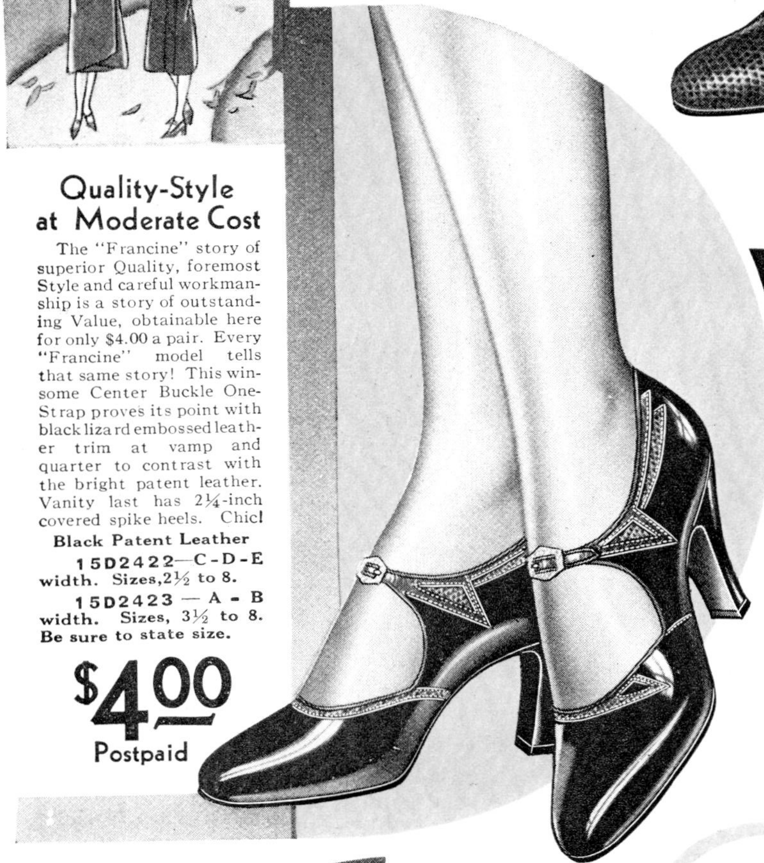

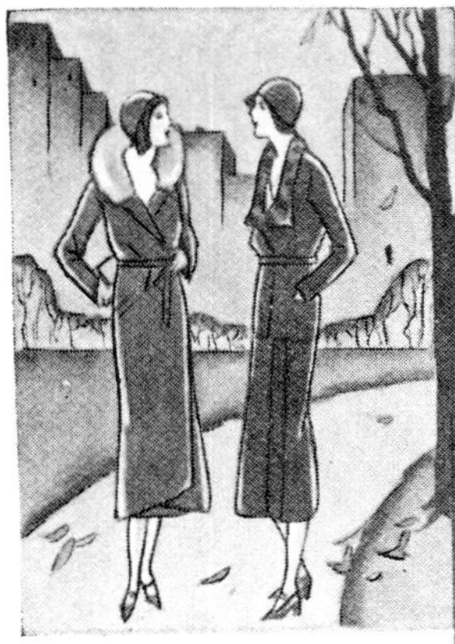

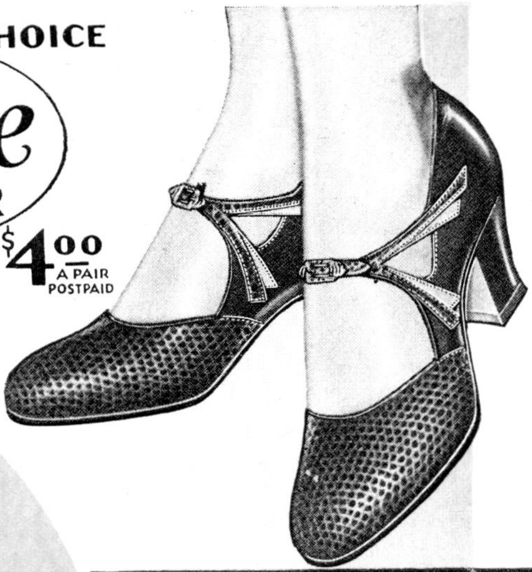

"Browntime"

Brown Lizard embossed leather vamp with Chocolate Drop kid quarter in contrast makes this center buckle one strap a favorite with our Francine line for fall and winter. Vanity last; 1¾-inch covered military heel.

Chocolate Drop Brown
15D2410—C-D-E width. Sizes, 2½ to 8.
15D2411 — A-B width. Sizes, 3½ to 8.
Be sure to state size.

$4.00 Postpaid

Quality-Style at Moderate Cost

The "Francine" story of superior Quality, foremost Style and careful workmanship is a story of outstanding Value, obtainable here for only $4.00 a pair. Every "Francine" model tells that same story! This winsome Center Buckle One-Strap proves its point with black lizard embossed leather trim at vamp and quarter to contrast with the bright patent leather. Vanity last has 2¼-inch covered spike heels. Chic!

Black Patent Leather
15D2422—C-D-E width. Sizes, 2½ to 8.
15D2423 — A-B width. Sizes, 3½ to 8.
Be sure to state size.

$4.00 Postpaid

$4.00 Postpaid

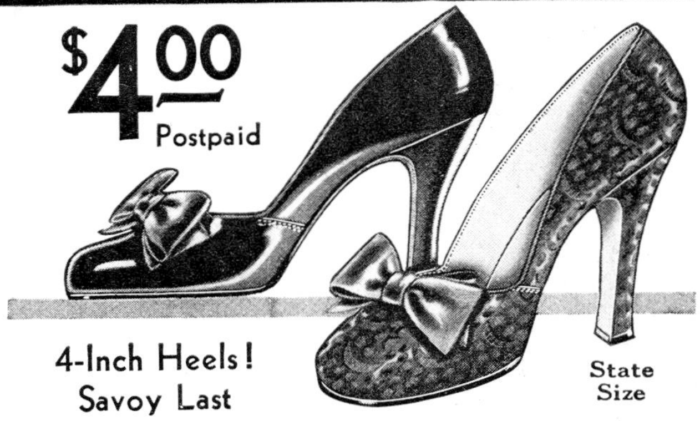

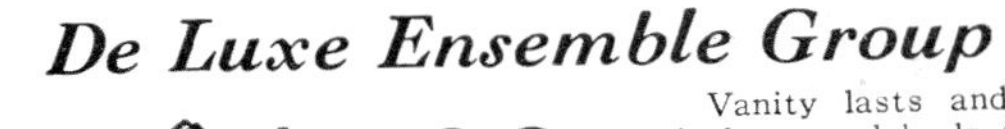

4-Inch Heels! Savoy Last

State Size

Tip top style for the most formal occasions or costume. Black Brocaded Satin or Patent Leather for these regally correct D'Orsay Bow Pumps on perfectly poised 4-inch covered spike heels with short vamp on Ritz "fashion" last. **State size.**

C-D-E width. Sizes, 2½ to 8.
15D2214—Brocaded Satin.
15D2216—Patent Leather. **Postpaid.**

A-B width. Sizes, 3½ to 8.
15D2215—Brocaded Satin.
15D2217—Patent Leather

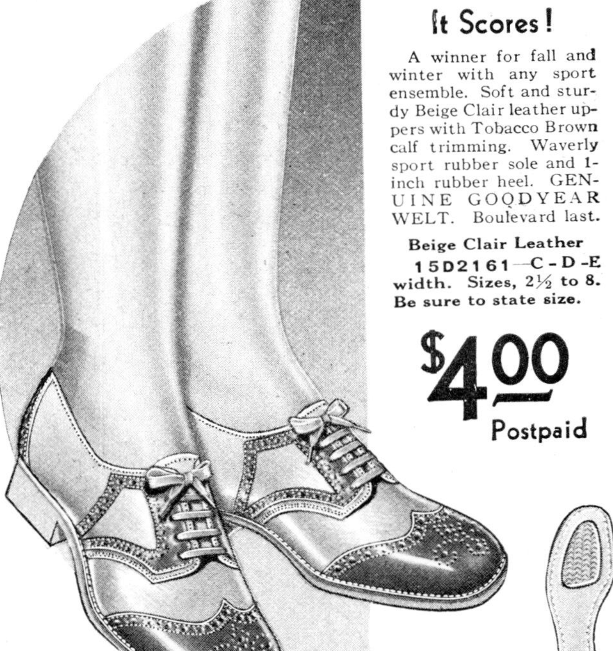

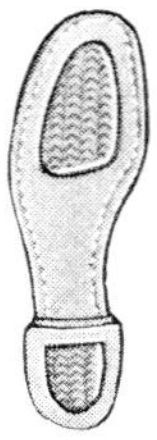

It Scores!

A winner for fall and winter with any sport ensemble. Soft and sturdy Beige Clair leather uppers with Tobacco Brown calf trimming. Waverly sport rubber sole and 1-inch rubber heel. GENUINE GOODYEAR WELT. Boulevard last.

Beige Clair Leather
15D2161—C-D-E width. Sizes, 2½ to 8.
Be sure to state size.

$4.00 Postpaid

De Luxe Ensemble Group

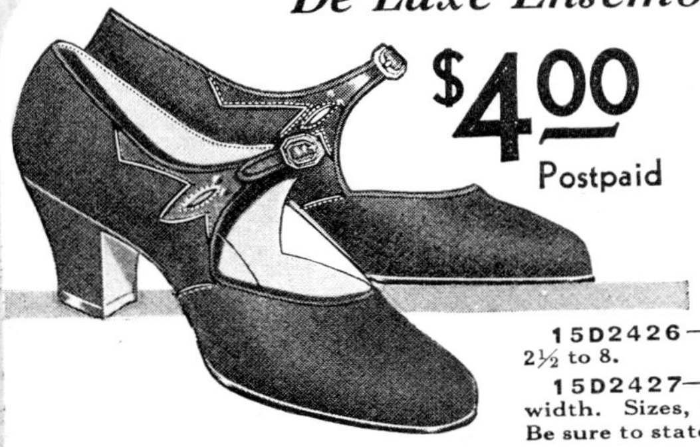

$4.00 Postpaid

Vanity lasts and 1¾ inch covered heels finish this beauty group!

Chocolate Drop Brown Suede, with Deer Tan Kid Trim.
15D2424—C-D-E width. Sizes, 2½ to 8.
15D2425 — A-B width. Sizes, 3½ to 8.
Black Suede, with Black Calf Trim
15D2426—C-D-E width. Sizes, 2½ to 8.
15D2427—A-B width. Sizes, 3½ to 8.
Be sure to state size.

$4.00 Postpaid

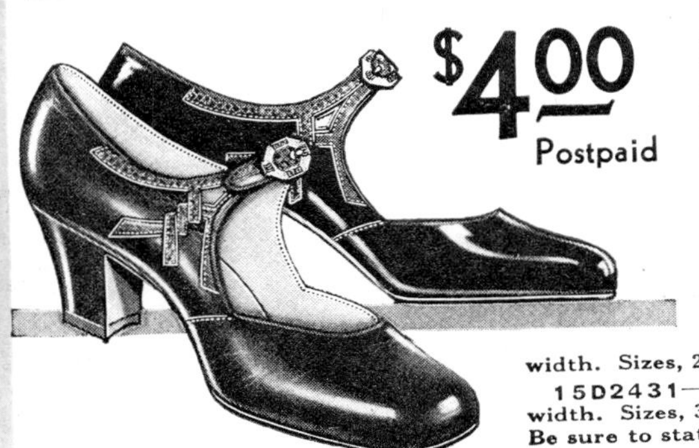

$4.00 Postpaid

Captivating are these Center Buckle One-Strap leaders, both trimmed with black embossed lizard and 1¾-inch covered military heels on Boulevard last.

Black Kid Leather
15D2428—C-D-E width. Sizes, 2½ to 8.
15D2429 — A-B width. Sizes, 3½ to 8.
Black Patent Leather
15D2430—C-D-E width. Sizes, 2½ to 8.
15D2431—A-B width. Sizes, 3½ to 8.
Be sure to state size.

$4.00 Postpaid

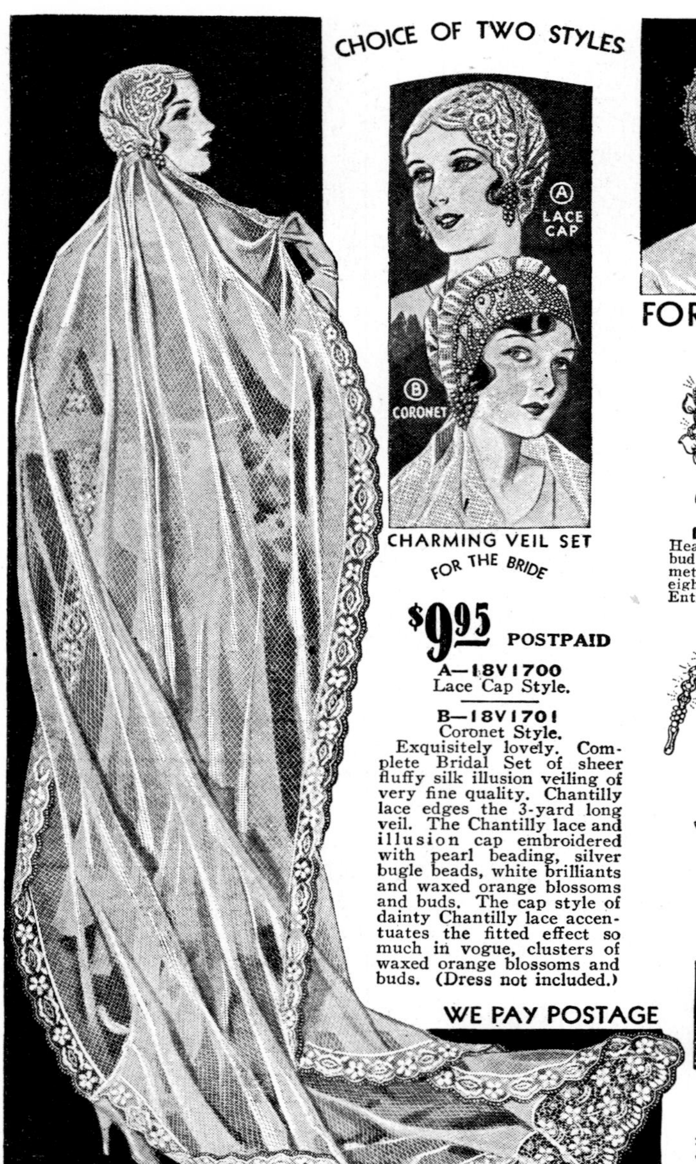

CHOICE OF TWO STYLES

(A) LACE CAP

(B) CORONET

CHARMING VEIL SET FOR THE BRIDE

$9.95 POSTPAID

A—18V1700 Lace Cap Style.

B—18V1701 Coronet Style.

Exquisitely lovely. Complete Bridal Set of sheer fluffy silk illusion veiling of very fine quality. Chantilly lace edges the 3-yard long veil. The Chantilly lace and illusion cap embroidered with pearl beading, silver bugle beads, white brilliants and waxed orange blossoms and buds. The cap style of dainty Chantilly lace accentuates the fitted effect so much in vogue, clusters of waxed orange blossoms and buds. (Dress not included.)

WE PAY POSTAGE

BRIDAL CORONETS

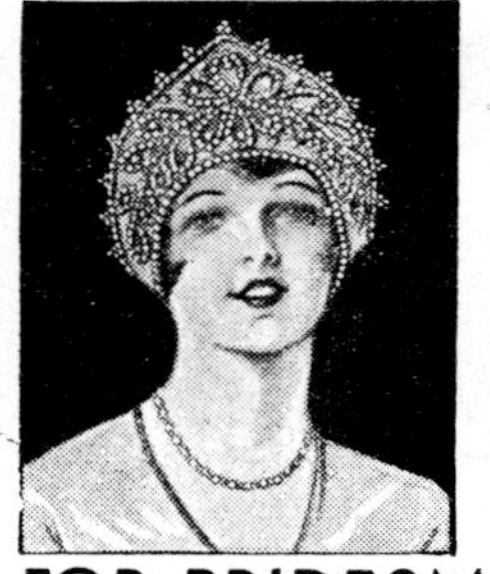

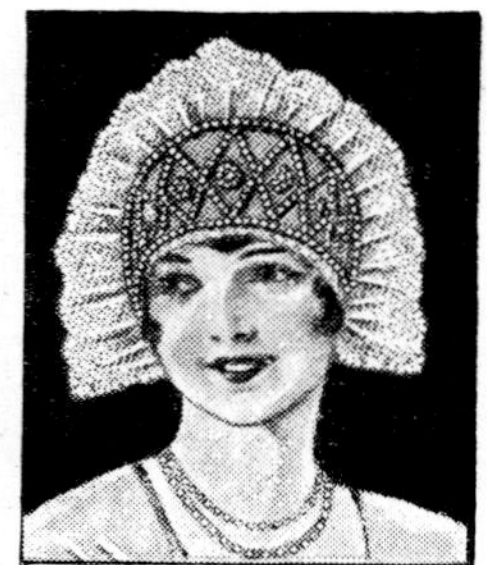

$3.79 POST PAID 18V1703

Coronet of fine illusion veiling (2 layers) over foundation, set with pearl-like beads and sparkling white brilliants. Easily attached.

Wear With Your Own Veil

$3.95 POST-PAID 18V1702

Bridal Coronet of finest quality illusion veiling and Chantilly lace over foundation. Attractive design of pearl-like beads and white brilliants.

FOR BRIDESMAIDS AND FOR SOCIAL EVENTS

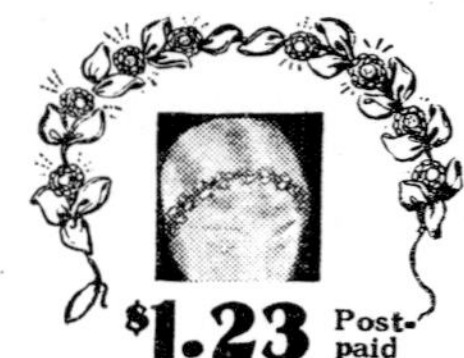

$1.23 Post-paid

18V1707—Attractive Headband in floral and bud design, of silver color metallic cloth set with eight sparkling brilliants. Entire length, 24 inches.

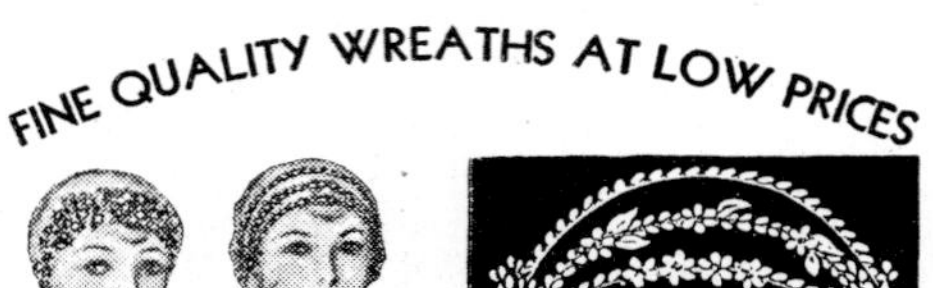

$1.23 Postpaid

18V1708—Lovely Headband of silvered dust sprayed leaves. Entire length, 24 inches. Can be arranged to suit individual dressings.

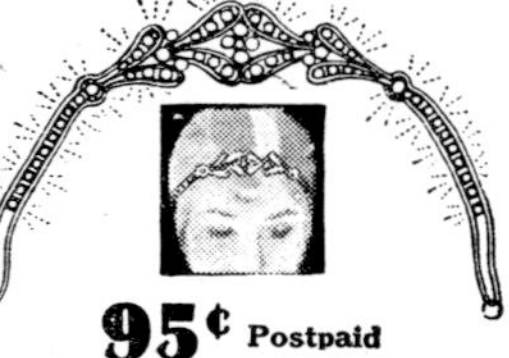

95¢ Postpaid

18V1709—Charming Band, set with 54 white stones. Silver color flexible metallic band, resembles platinum. Length, 12½ inches.

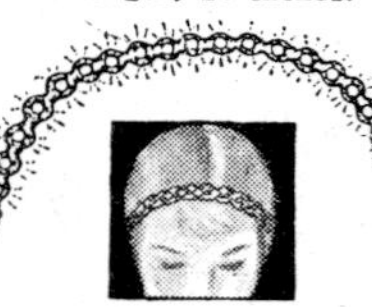

79¢ POSTPAID 18V1720

Silver color flexible metallic Band. Set with 40 white stones. Lgth., 13 inches.

49¢ POSTPAID 18V1721

Silver color, flexible, metallic band, set with 13 white stones. Lgth., 14 inches.

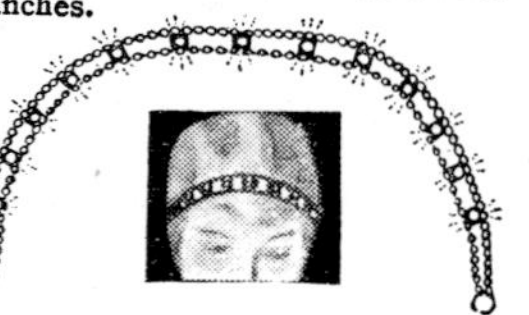

FINE QUALITY WREATHS AT LOW PRICES

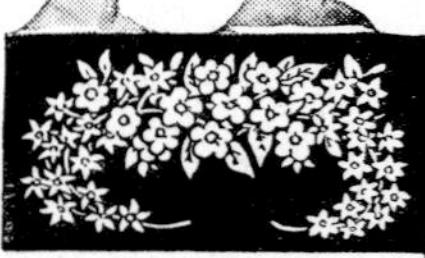

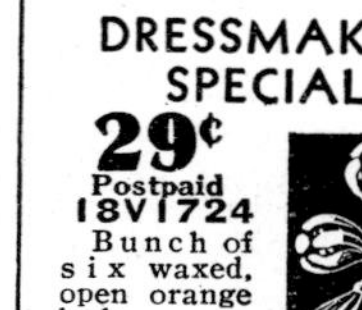

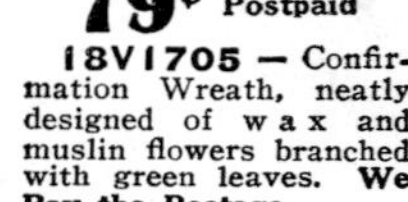

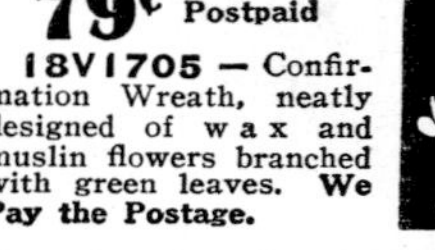

89¢ Post-paid

18V1704—Very attractive Bridal or Confirmation Wreath, made of white wax buds and green leaves.

79¢ Postpaid

18V1705 — Confirmation Wreath, neatly designed of wax and muslin flowers branched with green leaves. We Pay the Postage.

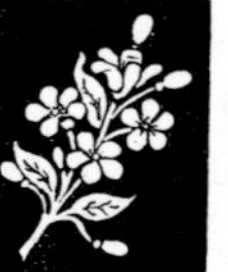

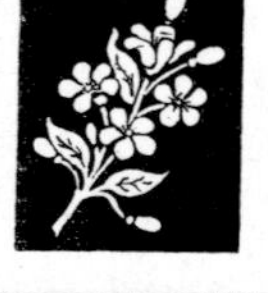

19¢ Post-paid 18V1706

Neat style Bridal or Confirmation Bouquet of tiny wax blossoms and buds, with green leaves. Very dainty.

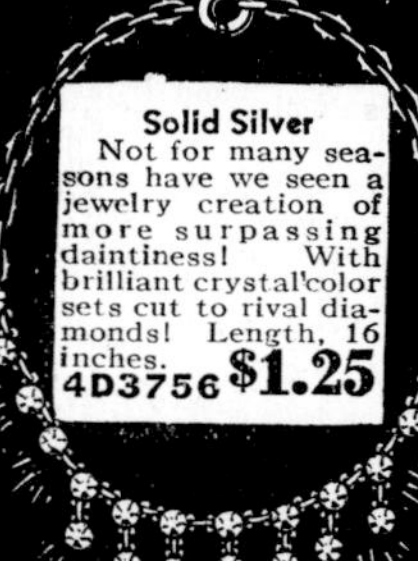

DRESSMAKER'S SPECIALS

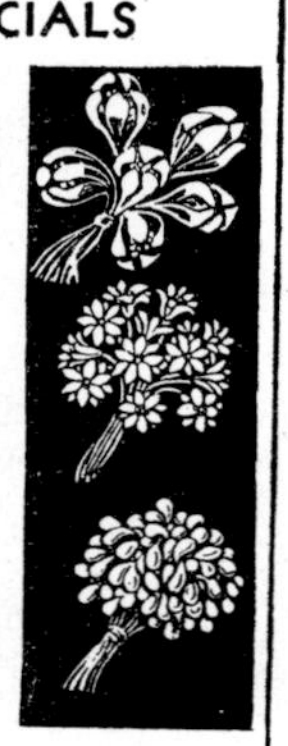

29¢ Postpaid 18V1724

Bunch of six waxed, open orange buds.

29¢ Postpaid 18V1725

Bunch of twelve, small size, waxed orange blossoms.

29¢ Postpaid 18V1723

Bunch of 72 waxed orange buds.

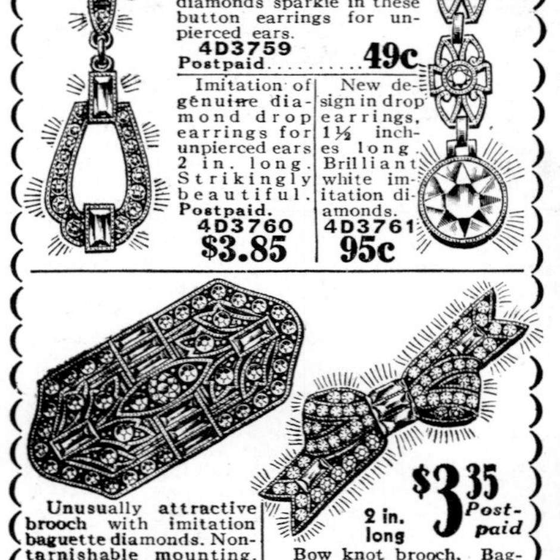

Square cut imitation diamonds sparkle in these button earrings for unpierced ears. 4D3759 Postpaid........ **49c**

Imitation of genuine diamond drop earrings for unpierced ears 2 in. long. Strikingly beautiful. Postpaid. 4D3760 **$3.85**

New design in drop earrings, 1½ inches long Brilliant white imitation diamonds. 4D3761 **95c**

Unusually attractive brooch with imitation baguette diamonds. Non-tarnishable mounting. Safety catch. About ⅞ x1¾ inches. 4D3696... **$2.95**

$3.35 Post-paid

2 in. long

Bow knot brooch. Baguettes and artificial diamonds. 4D3762.... **$3.35**

A charming proof of our up to date jewelry offerings—very modish festoon necklace! The latest style, with fancy motifs and chain links set off by artificial diamonds and crystal color baguettes. Length, about 15 inches. 4D3754 Post-paid...... **$4.35**

A choker style necklace with triangular shaped pendant and chain links set with crystal color baguettes and imitation diamonds. A charming example of how closely the beauty of expensive platinum pieces can be copied. Length, about 16 inches. Postpaid. 4D3755 **$4.85**

Solid Silver

Not for many seasons have we seen a jewelry creation of more surpassing daintiness! With brilliant crystal color sets cut to rival diamonds! Length, 16 inches. 4D3756 **$1.25**

An elaborate pendant necklace. Set with imitation diamonds. Pendant drop has a large solitaire stone Length, 18 in. including drop. 4D3642 **$2.40**

A necklace, brooch and drop earrings for unpierced ears. Imitation diamonds. Chain length, 16 inches. Earrings 1½ in. long. 4D3757—Complete Set. Postpaid.. **$2.98**

Presenting fashion's very last word in a necklace and brooch set! Large square cut crystal color stone in modernistic white metal settings studded with brilliant imitation diamonds. Chain length, about 16 in. Postpaid. 4D3758 **$1.95**

BEAUTY AND STYLE

Margot Set

Popular sweetheart shape neatly embroidered on good quality cotton net with Venise design lace medallion. Light ecru.
25V4014
Per Set, Postpaid. 42c

Attractive Neckwear

Fancy Panel Collar

Neatly tailored. Made of silk Georgette in combination with Venise and Valenciennes pattern lace. Light ecru.
25V4024
Each, Postpaid. 79c

Novel Collar With Jabot

New and stylish. Well made of silk Georgette in combination with Venise pattern and fancy cotton lace. Light ecru.
25V4020
Each, Postpaid..... 89c

Novelty Lace Set

A popular set made of good quality cotton Alencon pattern lace with neat lace insertion. Light ecru.
25V4012
Per Set, Postpaid. $1.10

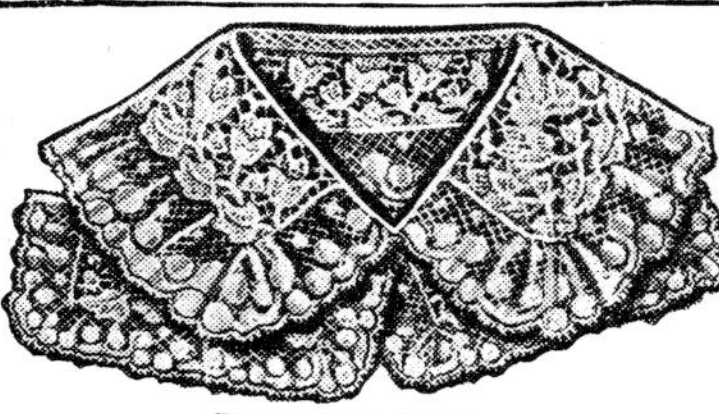

Buster Set

Well made of good quality Venise pattern lace and trimmed with attractive lace edge. Ecrue only.
25V4011—Set, Postpaid........85c

Lace Set

A novelty set much in vogue. Well made of good quality cotton Alencon design lace in combination with imported cotton net in tucked effect and trimmed with black ribbon bow. Light ecru.
25V4022
Per Set, Post paid, $1.89

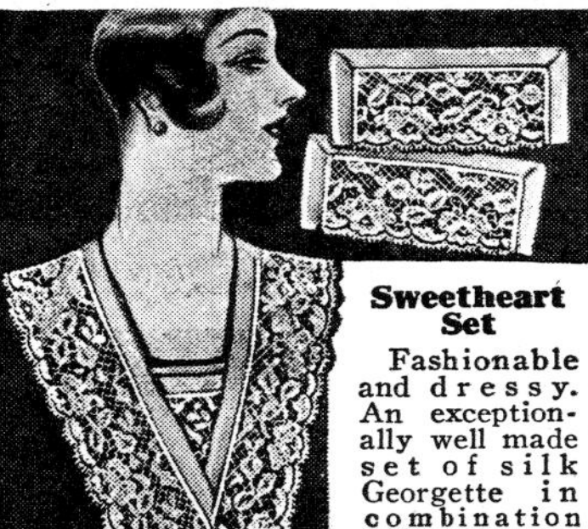

Sweetheart Set

Fashionable and dressy. An exceptionally well made set of silk Georgette in combination with cotton Alencon pattern lace. Of neat design. Light ecru.
25V4015
Per set, Post paid... $1.00

Dus-Tite Cap

Neatly and attractively made of durable quality washable percale in assorted colored floral designs. Has white pull cord for fastening. Easily adjusted.
25V4039—Each, Postpaid..................22c

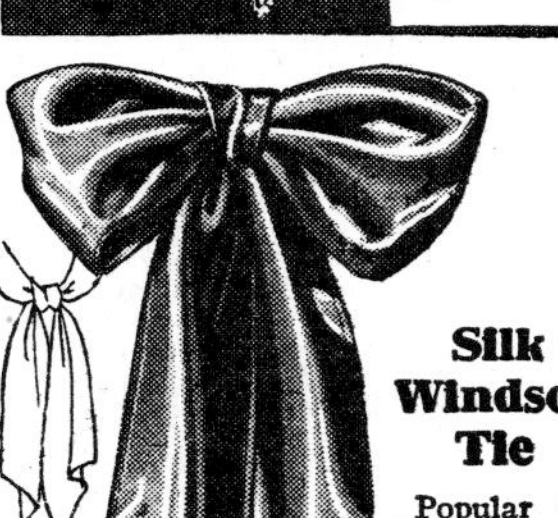

Silk Windsor Tie

Popular for Buster Brown collar and children's wear. Colors: Red, black, navy blue or white. State color. Size, about 4¾x35 inches.
25V4034—Each, Postpaid....................23c

Better quality. Same colors as above. State color. Size, about 6½x 45 inches.
25V4035—Each, Postpaid...42c

Georgette Silk Ruffling

Width, 2½ inches. Colors: White, tan, red or delft. State color.
25V4040
Per yd., Postpaid 49c

Same quality and colors as above. Width, 5 inches.
25V4041
Per yd., Postpaid 75c

Durable quality fancy cotton lace. Width, 3 inches. Light ecru.
25V4042
Per yd., Postpaid 52c

Ruffling

Good quality imported cotton net in tucked effect and is trimmed with durable lace Alencon pattern. Width, about 3 in. Light ecru.
25V4044
Per yard, Postpaid...... 45c

A good quality Point De Esprit net now very much in vogue. 2½-inch. Light ecru.
25V4043
Per yard, Postpaid...... 55c

LOVELY YET INEXPENSIVE

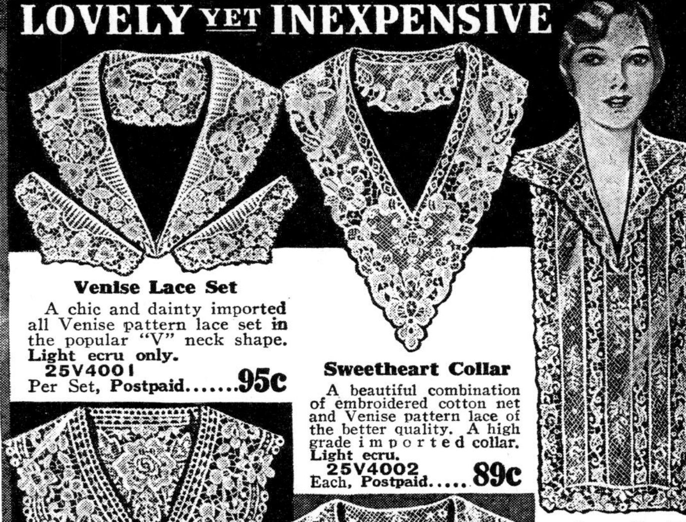

Venise Lace Set

A chic and dainty imported all Venise pattern lace set in the popular "V" neck shape. Light ecru only.
25V4001
Per Set, Postpaid.......95c

Sweetheart Collar

A beautiful combination of embroidered cotton net and Venise pattern lace of the better quality. A high grade imported collar. Light ecru.
25V4002
Each, Postpaid..... 89c

Lace Vestee

Our own importation. An effective combination of Venise and oriental design lace of the better quality. Light ecru.
25V4006—Each, Post-paid...$1.59

Imported Lace Collar

Rich in appearance. Neatly made of embroidered cotton net on good quality Venise pattern lace. A beautiful collar. Ecru only.
25V4004
Each, Postpaid... $1.89

Venise Buster Set

A smart imported set made of oriental and Venise pattern lace. Light ecru.
25V4000
Per set, Postpaid....85c

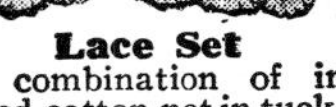

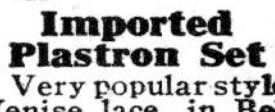

Lace Set

A combination of imported cotton net in tucked effect and Venise pattern lace. Light ecru.
25V4008
Per Set, Postpaid...55c

Imported Bertha Collar

A well balanced and effective pattern, of the better quality Venise lace. Width across shoulders, 22 in. Light ecru.
25V4005—Each, Postpaid. $2.15

Imported Plastron Set

Very popular style. Venise lace, in Belgian design, very effective. Light ecru
25V4003
Per set, Post paid.. $1.95

POPULAR and SMART

Triangle Scarf

Vogue and value. Good quality heavy silk crepe de chine. Attractive design neatly hand painted in multi-color. Ground colors: Blue, red, orange, green, gold or tan. State color. Size, about 18x45 inches.
25V4037
Ea., Postpaid. 98c

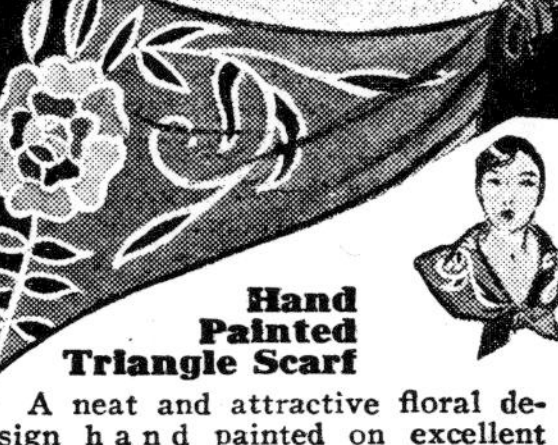

Hand Painted Triangle Scarf

A neat and attractive floral design hand painted on excellent quality heavy silk crepe de chine. Ground colors: Blue, tan, red, orange, green, gold or tan. State color. Size, about 21x48 inches.
25V4038
Each, Postpaid...... $1.59

Lace Triangle

Beautiful combination of Georgette and imported fancy cotton lace in Alencon design. One of the most popular and fashionable articles in neckwear. Light ecru.

We Pay the Postage.

25V4036
Each....... 69c

Silk Georgette Sleeves

More popular than ever. Neatly embroidered in rayon with attractive double cuff hemstitched and shirred. Twenty-four inches long. Colors: Black, tan, navy, red, Copen, white, flesh, medium green or silver gray. State color.
25V4032—Per pair, Postpaid.. $1.69

A slightly lighter weight with single shirred cuff. Same size and colors as above.
25V4033—Per pair, Postpaid........................$1.00

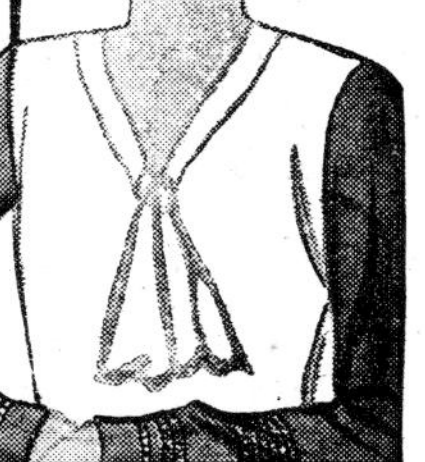

Your Orders Shipped Within 24 Hours!

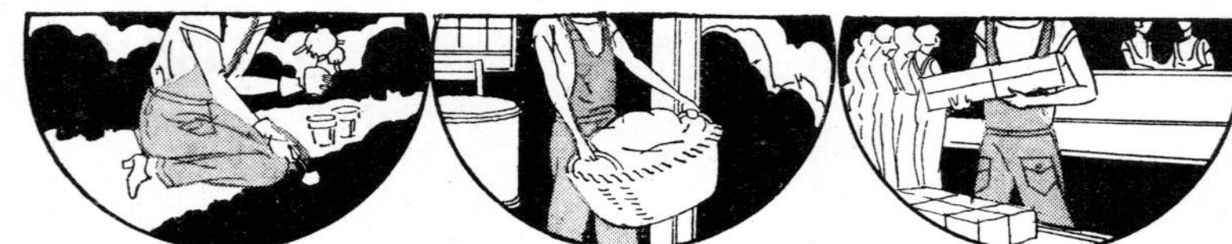

NEW PRACTICAL POPULAR OVERALLS FOR WOMEN-

DAINTY FADEPROOF COLORS

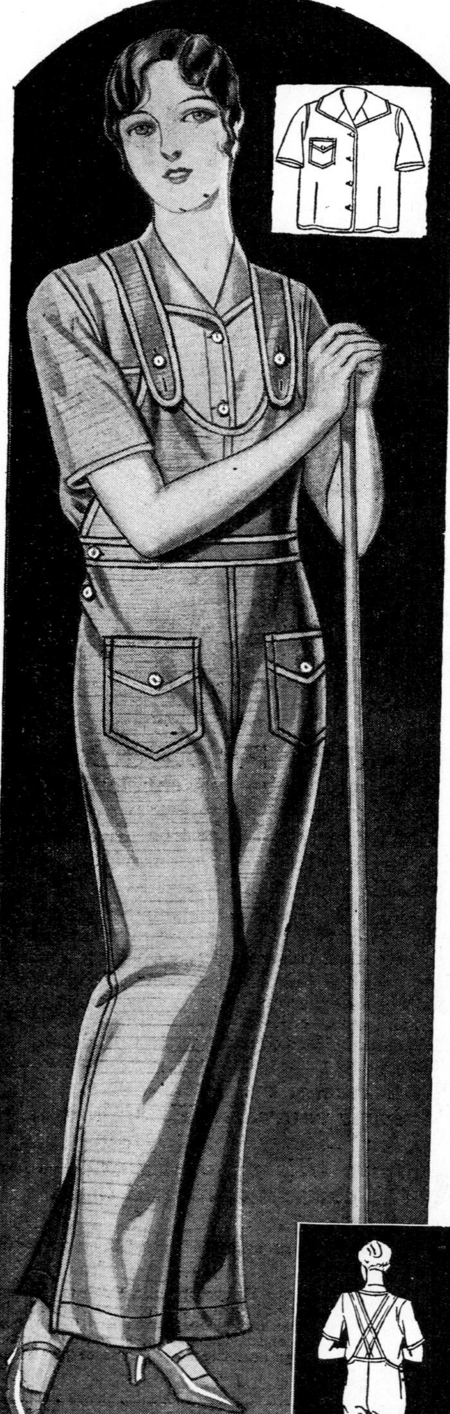

EVERYBODY'S wearing them! Wearing what? Why, wearing overalls, of course! They're all the rage in every fashionable center in the country! The most exclusive shops on Fifth Avenue are selling them! And smart women everywhere are finding them the most sensible, the most comfortable, as well as the most chic style ever! Your wardrobe is incomplete without a pair of them.

And no wonder! For here is a time honored masculine garment, with all its original masculine convenience and masculine comfort, plus a strictly feminine appeal! Here is the charm of six lovely and most becoming colors—FADEPROOF, by the way. At the beach—in the garden or laundry—at house-cleaning—for camping and touring—in stores—industrial work—at a hundred chores or pleasures this garment is ideal and in the smartest mode. Nothing to worry about—nothing to get in the way—and it launders like a charm.

Stylish Blouse to Match

The blouse is especially designed to be worn with the overalls and will give you the ideal combination outfit. It has smart lines, is excellently finished, cool and comfortable. Both garments are dyed with Gregg INDELIBLE colors, **guaranteed fadeproof** against sun, washing, wear or perspiration. Actual laboratory tests, many times more severe than any to which you could possibly subject them, have absolutely proved these colors just what they are called—Indelible! Both we and the manufacturer back them with our unqualified guarantee of **a new garment if they fade!** After repeated washings they come from the tub as fresh and sparkling as new! Easy to iron, too, and just the right weight. Made of a special linen-like cotton fabric as smart as it is long wearing. All well made, neatly piped in white, with bell bottoms on overalls, and godets of contrasting color. Six desirable fast colors: Rose, Orchid, Tan, Blue, Green or Peach. **State color desired; also age size.**

41V50—Overalls. Girls' sizes, 8, 10 and 12 years. Postpaid.......... $1.75
41V40—Blouse to Match. Sizes, 8, 10 and 12 years. Postpaid.......... 1.09
41V51—Overalls. Women's sizes, 14, 16, 18 and 20 years. Postpaid.......... 1.98
41V41—Blouse to Match. Sizes, 14, 16, 18 and 20 years. Postpaid.......... 1.19

Blue Denim or Hickory Stripe, Too!

Also furnished in two standard overall materials; medium weight white back blue denim or hickory stripe, which are now universally worn by girls and women working in factories. **State choice; also age size.** Blouse of Blue Chambray to be worn with either pair overalls.

41V56—Overalls. Girls' sizes, 8, 10 and 12 years. Postpaid.......... $1.39
41V46—Blue Chambray Blouse. Girls' sizes, 8, 10 and 12 years. Postpaid.......... .75
41V58—Overalls. Women's sizes, 14, 16, 18 and 20 years. Postpaid.......... 1.59
41V48—Blue Chambray Blouse. Sizes, 14, 16, 18 and 20 years. Postpaid.......... .85

WE PAY POSTAGE

MEN'S PRE-SHRUNK DUCK JACKETS

For druggists — soda clerks — restaurant and grocery men—barbers—dentists—home entertainment — and for many other professions and occupations these splendid quality white duck coats are almost indispensable. Made from an exceptionally high grade preshrunk 8-ounce duck, bleached to a snowy whiteness, and tailored to neat well fitting patterns. They go far toward symbolizing the purity and cleanliness of your establishment, and impressing it upon the minds of your customers. They save your better clothes from dirt and stain. They are easily laundered, and they wear almost indefinitely. **It's cheaper to buy them here than to rent them from a laundry service! SIZES—36 to 46 inches chest. State chest measure.**

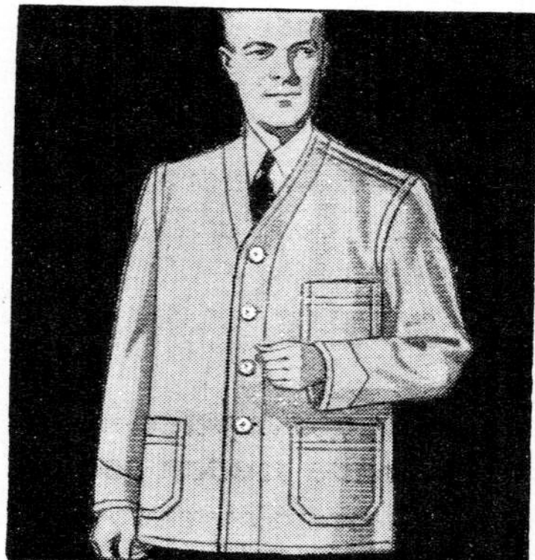

Coat Style With V Neck
41V75—Postpaid....... **$1.89**

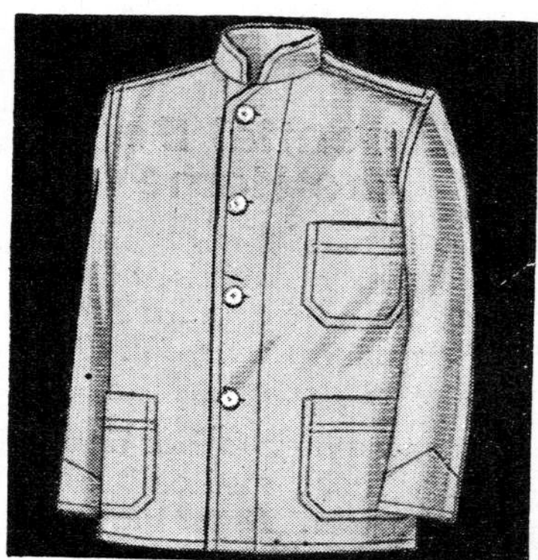

Coat Style With Semi-Military Collar
41V76—Postpaid....... **$1.89**

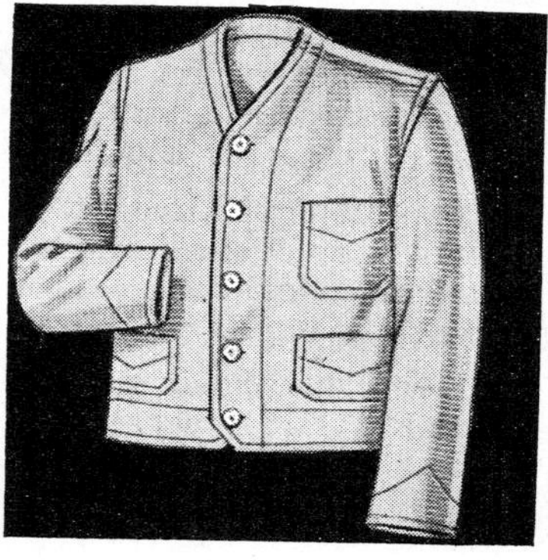

V Neck Vest With Sleeves
41V77—Postpaid....... **$1.69**

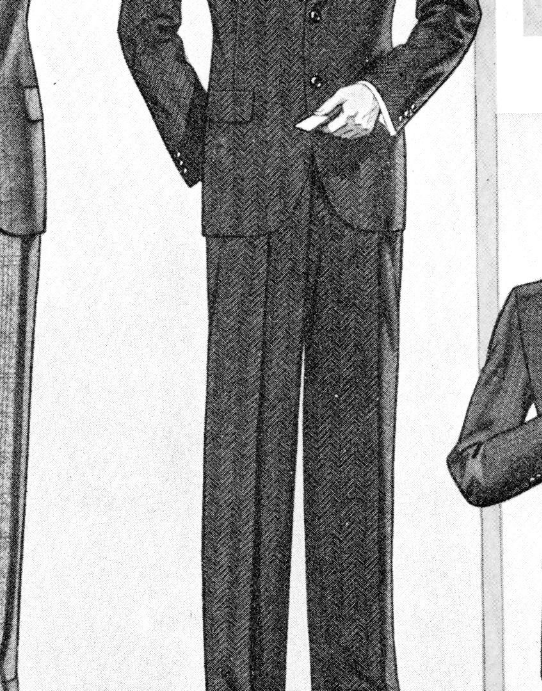

FASHION TAILORED SUITS

WITH ONE PAIR OF TROUSERS $19.85 POSTPAID

WITH TWO PAIR OF TROUSERS $25.00 POSTPAID

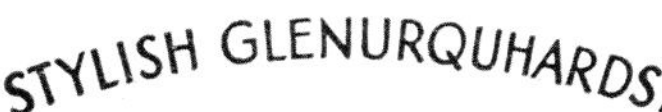

STYLISH GLENURQUHARDS.

Ask the young man who's always just a little bit ahead of the style—he will tell you that Glenurquhard Plaids are "It" this spring! And, of course, for wear, nothing beats an all pure **wool worsted.** Take that combination—FASHION TAILORED—and you have a suit to brag about! An approved model with the snappy new "lifted" sleeves to give it the desirable square shoulder effect. Coat half lined with fine alpaca. **SIZES—34 to 42 inches chest, 29 to 40 inches waist, and 29 to 35 inches inseam. State measurements.**

45V5164—Medium Brown Glen Plaid All Wool Worsted. Postpaid.................... **$19.85**

45V5165—Brown as Above With Two Pairs Trousers. Postpaid.................... **$25.00**

45V5166—Gray Glen Plaid All Wool Worsted. Postpaid.................... **$19.85**

45V5167—Gray as Above With Two Pairs Trousers. Postpaid.................... **$25.00**

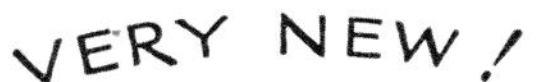

VERY NEW!

Notice the shaped waistline on this peppy style; observe the new "lifted" sleeve, and the notched lapels—all designed to give an athletic square-shouldered appearance. That's the essence of the very latest style—so new that it's still news to many, but already going like brush fire among stylish young men the nation over. As for the fabric, it's an **all wool worsted** shadow stripe, as up to date as television! Coat half lined with fine alpaca. **SIZES—34 to 42 inches chest, 29 to 40 inches waist, and 29 to 35 inches inseam. State measurements.**

45V5156—Dark Oxford Gray. Postpaid............ **$19.85**

45V5157—Dark Oxford Gray With Two Pairs Trousers. Postpaid.................... **$25.00**

45V5160—Dark Oxford Blue. Postpaid............ **19.85**

45V5161—Dark Oxford Blue With Two Pairs Trousers. Postpaid.................... **$25.00**

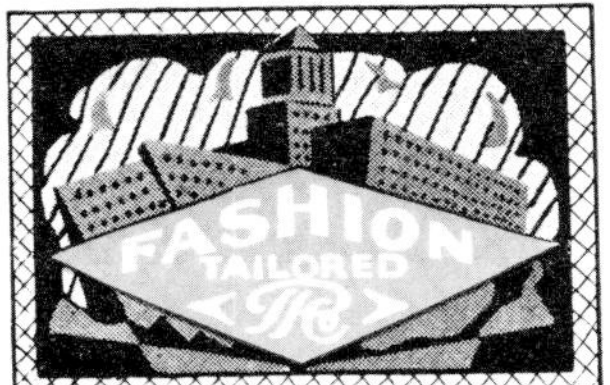

WE PAY THE POSTAGE

A NEW YORK FAVORITE.

Favored for style, and favored for fabric in the style centers of America. A handsome two-button notch lapel coat. There's nothing extreme about this style, yet there's an air about it that tells the world its wearer is right up to the minute. And the fabric in our opinion is one of the best we have ever shown. It's a particularly fine **all wool worsted** with handsome silk stripes. In addition we offer this suit in ever popular blue serge. Regular vest and **two pairs of trousers** with nineteen-inch bottoms. Coat half alpaca lined. **SIZES—34 to 42 inches chest, 29 to 40 inches waist, and 29 to 35 inches inseam. State measurements.**

45V5120—Brown All Wool Fancy Silk Stripe Worsted With Extra Trousers. Postpaid............ **$25.00**

45V5118—Gray All Wool Fancy Silk Stripe Worsted With Extra Trousers. Postpaid............ **25.00**

45V5122—Dark Blue All Wool Silk Stripe Worsted With Extra Trousers. Postpaid............ **25.00**

45V5123—All Wool Blue Serge With Extra Trousers. Postpaid.................................. **25.00**

ONE OF THE SMARTEST!

We could talk a lot about this suit, but we're not going to, because we feel that it will sell itself! In the first place, its style is apparent—a two-button notch lapel coat with a well rounded front, six-button vest, and straight hanging trousers with nineteen-inch cuff bottoms—it commands respect in any style gathering! And the fabric is just as good—**an all pure wool worsted two-ply twist.** The coat is half lined with quality alpaca. **SIZES—34 to 42 inches chest, 29 to 40 inches waist, and 29 to 35 inches inseam. State measurements; also age, weight and height.**

45V5173—Light Brown Stripe All Wool Worsted Twist. One Pair Trousers. Postpaid.......... **$19.85**

45V5174—Light Brown Stripe Twist as Above With Extra Trousers. Postpaid.................... **25.00**

45V5175—Gray All Wool Worsted Twist. One Pair Trousers. Postpaid............................ **19.85**

45V5176—Gray Stripe Twist as Above With Extra Trousers. Postpaid............................ **25.00**

100,000 SPORTSMEN WILL BUY FROM THIS PAGE

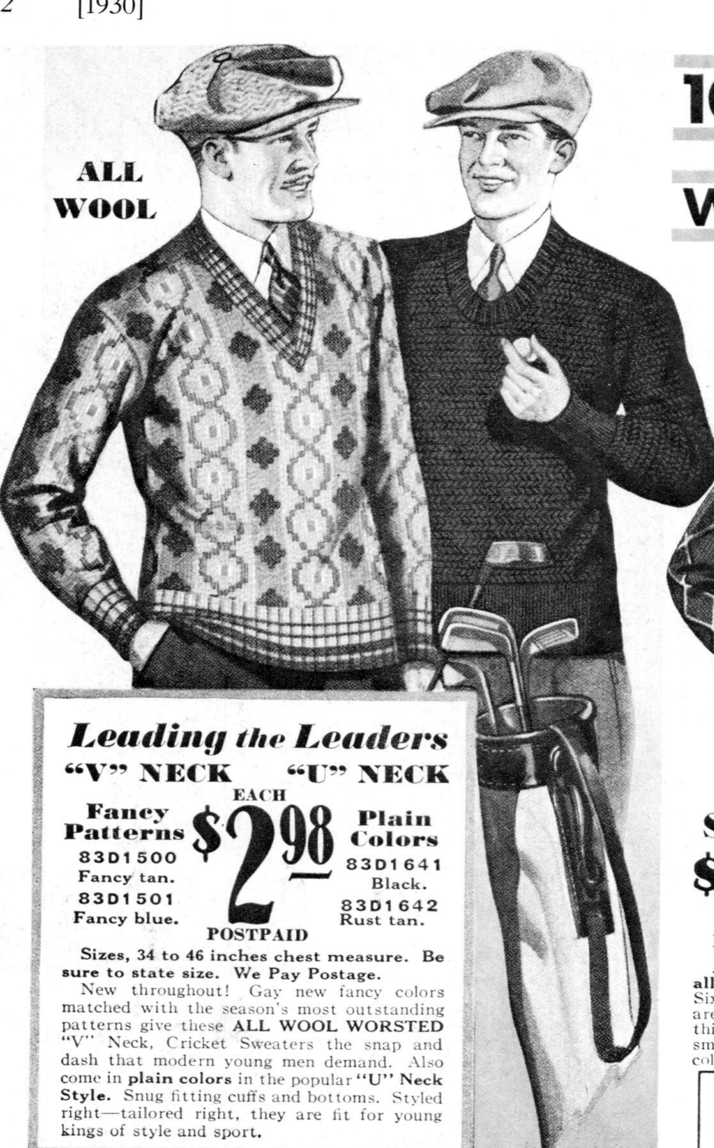

Leading the Leaders

"V" NECK **"U" NECK**

Fancy Patterns — EACH **$2.98** POSTPAID — **Plain Colors**

83D1500 Fancy tan.
83D1501 Fancy blue.

83D1641 Black.
83D1642 Rust tan.

Sizes, 34 to 46 inches chest measure. Be sure to state size. We Pay Postage.

New throughout! Gay new fancy colors matched with the season's most outstanding patterns give these **ALL WOOL WORSTED** "V" Neck, Cricket Sweaters the snap and dash that modern young men demand. Also come in **plain colors** in the popular **"U" Neck Style.** Snug fitting cuffs and bottoms. Styled right—tailored right, they are fit for young kings of style and sport.

For Measuring Instructions Refer to Page 396

ALL WOOL

Style and Warmth — Serviceable All Wool

$3.98 POSTPAID

83D1548 Fancy rust tan.
83D1549 Fancy brown.
Sizes, 34 to 46 inches chest measure. Be sure to state size.

A **"V" Neck Fancy Sport Coat** knit from **all wool worsted** yarns in a neat pattern. Six-button front. Two handy pockets. You are going to have money left to spend for other things when you make the saving on this smart new serviceable sweater in its rich colors. For general wear.

$2.75 POSTPAID

83D1624 Navy Blue
83D1625—Black
83D1626—Maroon
Sizes, 34 to 46 inches chest measure. Be sure to state size.

Another big saving for smart dressers and keen buyers. **All wool yarns** knit into a fine gauge **shaker stitch.** High-fitting **"U" neck** style collar. Snug fitting cuffs and bottom. Of durable medium weight in the popular pullover style. **Remember, too, We Pay Postage.**

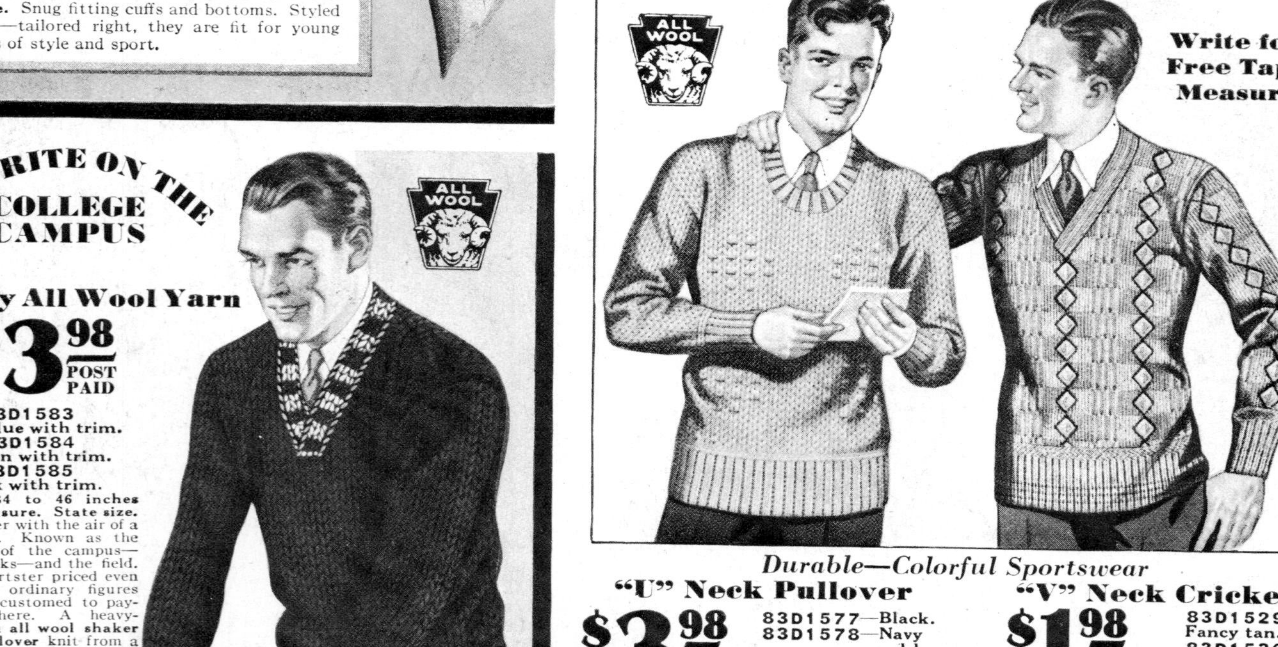

FAVORITE ON THE COLLEGE CAMPUS

Heavy All Wool Yarn

$3.98 POST PAID

83D1583 Navy blue with trim.
83D1584 Maroon with trim.
83D1585 Black with trim.
Sizes, 34 to 46 inches chest measure. State size.

A sweater with the air of a sportsman. Known as the champion of the campus—the golf links—and the field. A real sportster priced even below the ordinary figures you are accustomed to paying elsewhere. A heavy-weight—an **all wool shaker stitch pullover** knit from a high quality yarn. Around the "V" neck, cuffs and bottom is a neat trim of bright contrasting colors. Exceptionally well tailored and trim fitting. Order one today on our guarantee of money back if not satisfied. We believe our sweater prices are the lowest in America. **Remember, too, We Pay the Postage.**

Write for Free Tape Measure

Durable—Colorful Sportswear

"U" Neck Pullover

$3.98 POST PAID

83D1577—Black.
83D1578—Navy blue.
83D1579—Tan beige.

Sizes, 34 to 46 inches chest measure. Be sure to state size.

Slated to be a big favorite this season. Expensive looking colors with new novelty designs patterned right into the knitting; something quite new at our usual savings. Finely knit, narrow gauge **shaker stitch** of **finest all wool worsted yarns** in a suitable weight for Fall and Winter. The "U" Neck style is very popular.

"V" Neck Cricket

$1.98 POST PAID

83D1529 Fancy tan.
83D1530 Fancy blue.
Sizes, 34 to 46 in. chest measure. State size.

Cricket sweaters are identifying smart dressers everywhere. Here is a golden opportunity to have one at low cost. In the **"V" Neck Style.** Knit from worsted wool and cotton yarns in the seasons newest colors and patterns. Knit of about one-half wool, the balance fine cotton yarns. Ribbed bottom and cuffs give neat snugness. Priced low. Sears-Roebuck always lead in Men's furnishing values.

AMERICA'S HANDY GARMENT

It's All Wool
It's Priced Low

$2.98

POSTPAID

83D1620—Navy blue.
83D1621—Maroon.
83D1622—Cardinal.
83D1623—Black.

Sizes 34 to 46 inches. State size. We Pay Postage.

Extravagance couldn't buy you more wool in a sweater—style couldn't bring you more up-to-the-minute, trimly tailored lines, yet the price is one of the most worthwhile savings the sweater market has ever known! It's a good medium weight, just that handy kind that combines rugged warmth with the right thickness for comfort and easy on-and-off. You'd scarcely believe that such an all-around good garment could have the price squeezed down so low. Yet, here it is, a saving in which our sweater buyers take well-deserved pride. Good quality **all wool** yarn is sturdily knit in a cardigan stitch. It has a large shawl collar and two handy pockets. The cuffs are close fitting. This coat will stand up throughout a long period of rough usage.

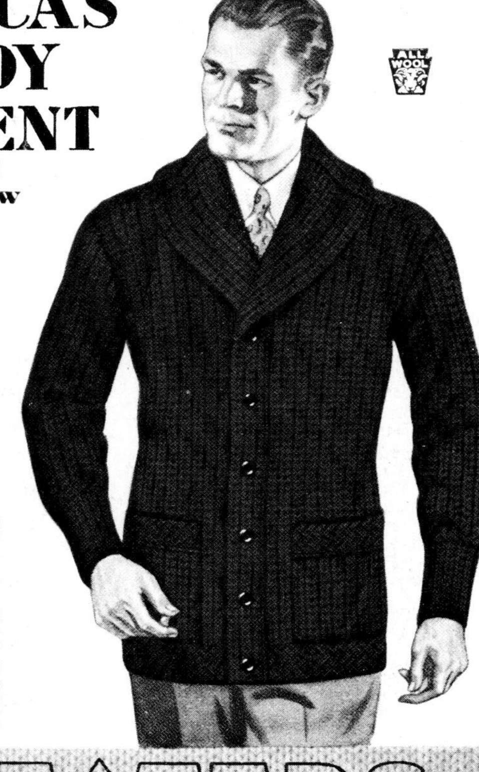

ALL WINTER WARMTH

At a Saving

$4.89

POSTPAID

83D1512—Navy blue.
83D1513—Maroon.
83D1514—Black.

Sizes, 34 to 46 inches chest measure. State size. We Pay Postage.

A new offering that our savings make available at this price, now for the first time. A sturdy, masculine style, big and warm to stand up to the toughest gales that blow. Well tailored in the new trim fitting lines decreed for men this season. It is now brought to you at one of the substantial savings that has made this institution famous. Its heavy **ALL WOOL** yarn is knitted into the popular **shaker stitch.** Coat is made with extra large double shawl collar, two knit-in pockets and six-button front. Fashioned and designed by skilled craftsmen to fit as nearly perfect as a sweater can. It is the kind of big, husky sweater that is worn in rough weather by men who originate sweater styles for the world. For work, for play, for sport, for the boulevard and the campus, everywhere you'll find this wonderful sweater keeping people warm and saving men money. For comfort, class and savings. Try it.

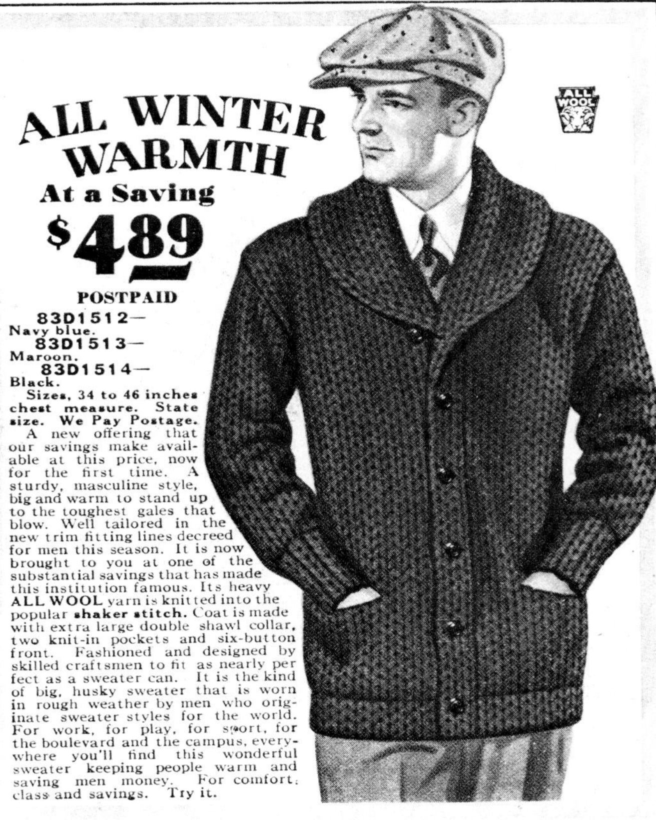

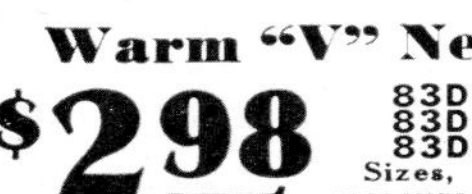

We Pay the Postage

Supreme Brand KNIT WEAR
SEARS, ROEBUCK and CO.

Warm "V" Neck Jacket

$2.98

POSTPAID

83D1587—Seal brown.
83D1588—Black.
83D1589—Navy blue.

Sizes, 34 to 46 inches chest measure. State size. Postpaid.

A general utility garment, heavy enough to provide plenty of extra warmth in tough weather, smart enough to be in any "style picture." Its high grade **All Wool yarn** is knitted in a popular narrow gauge shaker stitch. **"V" Neck** style with a six-button front. Two roomy inverted pockets.

For Measuring Instructions Refer to Page 396. Write for Free Tape Measure.

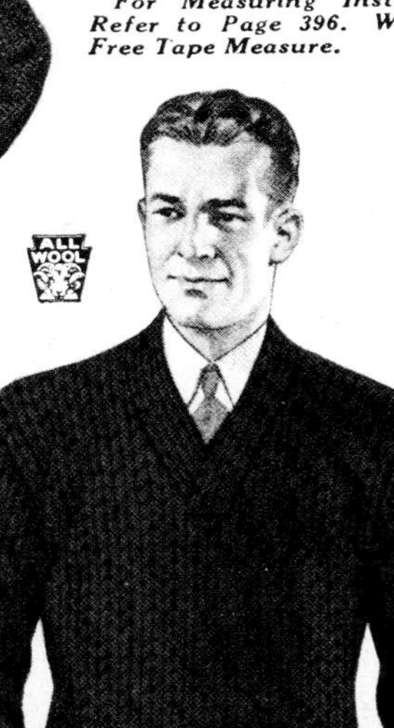

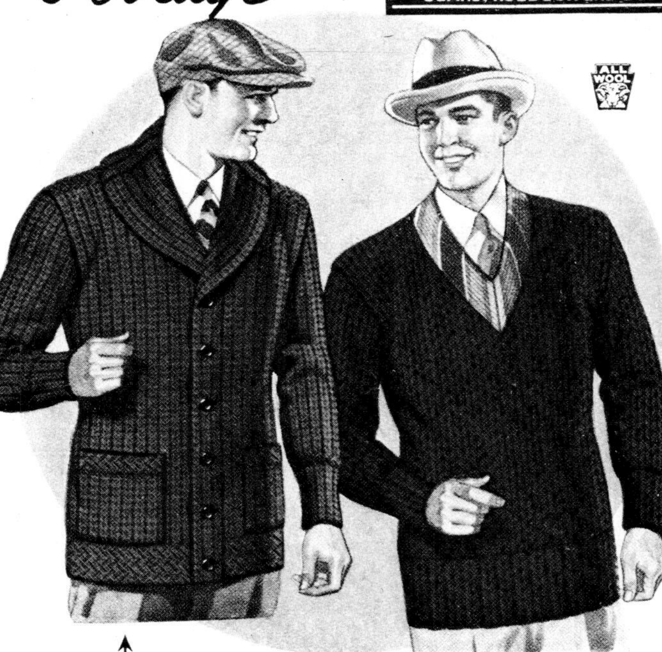

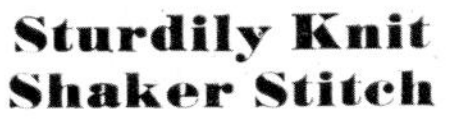

$3.89

Postpaid

83D1506—Navy blue.
83D1507—Black.
83D1508—Maroon.

Sizes, 34 to 46 inches chest measure. Be sure to state size. We Pay the Postage.

You'll begin to know real sweater comfort and style in this natty "V" **Neck Pullover Sweater.** Its price is well within the reach of the keenest buyers. Hard to beat in quality. Knit from **All Wool** yarns in a heavy **shaker stitch.** Well made and fashioned to insure a perfect fit. Snug fitting cuffs and bottom. The ideal garment for every man's wardrobe. Order one today on our usual guarantee of perfect fit and complete satisfaction or your money back.

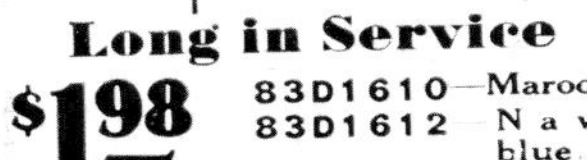

$1.98

Postpaid

83D1610—Maroon.
83D1612—Navy blue
83D1613—Brown.

Sizes, 34 to 46 inches chest measure. Be sure to state size.

The man who has rough, tough wear in store for his sweater will find a rugged model that can "take it" in this sturdy **Mediumweight, Shawl Collar Cotton Sweater** with a small percentage of wool. He can save, too. Strongly knit in the wear resisting cardigan stitch. Has two large pockets and large size double shawl collar.

Heavy All Wool

$2.98

Postpaid

83D1596—Black with trim.
83D1597—Navy blue with trim.
83D1598—Maroon with trim.

Sizes, 34 to 46. State size. Men's "V" Neck Pullover Sweater. Knit of **all wool** yarns in the sturdy **Shaker Stitch.** A neat trim of bright contrasting colors around the "V" neck. For sports or general outdoor wear. We pride ourselves on being able to get the high quality sweaters our customers prefer at prices they are glad to pay. This is an example of our ability to save you money on sweater purchases.

Your Orders Shipped Within 24 Hours!

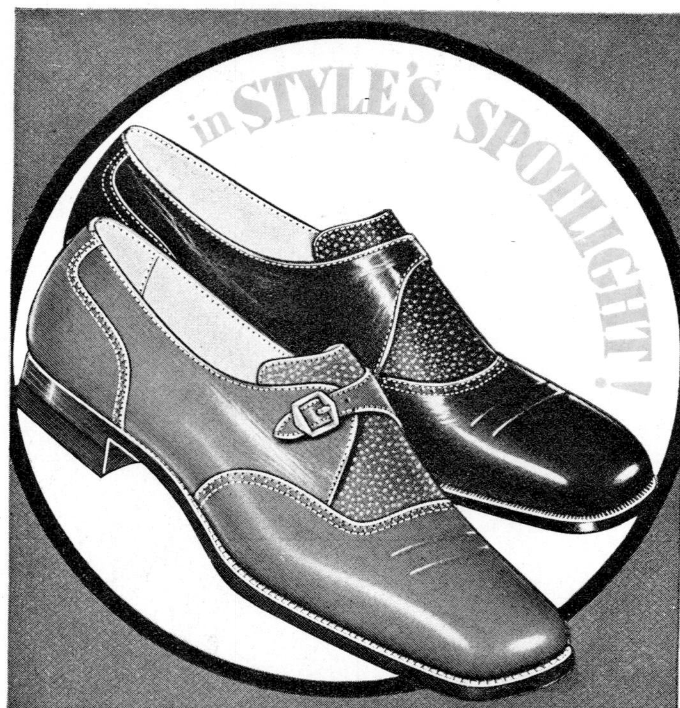

Refinement in dress begins with your Shoes. With that in mind, we selected this particularly fine style as exemplifying all that is new and good this season. We need only to ask you to look at $10.00 shoes elsewhere to prove that this is a most exclusive style. Moreover, it is an exceptional value. Uppers are of soft, carefully graded calfskin with fine pebble grain leather tongue. Soles of selected genuine oak leather; rubber heels. GENUINE GOODYEAR WELT construction adds to the quality.

BROWN
67V4504—D-E width.
67V4505—B-C width.

BLACK
67V4506—D-E width.
67V4507—B-C width.

Sizes, 5 to 11. Be sure to state size and width.

$4.95 POSTPAID

$2.98 POSTPAID

A distinctly young men's style built on the popular balloon last in bal pattern. Grain leather uppers with attractive trim and specially treated genuine leather RESISTOL soles. GENUINE GOODYEAR WELTS. Rubber heels.
67V4354—Brown.
67V4355—Black.
D-E width. Sizes, 5 to 11. State size and width.

A gallant style especially appealing to young men of today. With French toe and slightly creased vamp. Side leather uppers in bal pattern. GENUINE GOODYEAR WELT. Rubber heels.
67V4362—Brown.
67V4363—Black.
D-E width. Sizes, 5 to 11. State size and width.

$3.75 POSTPAID

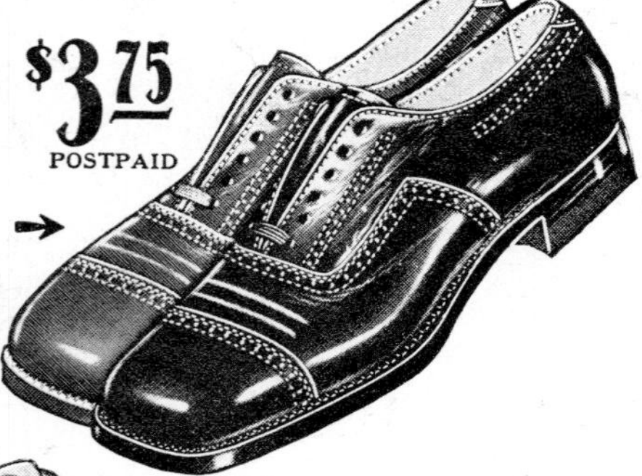

$4.95 POSTPAID

A very high grade two-tone Sport Oxford copied from a stylish imported model. White chrome tanned "elkskin" leather uppers with brown or black calfskin trim. GENUINE GOODYEAR WELT. Rubber heels.
BROWN TRIM
67V4538—D-E width.
67V4539—B-C width.
BLACK TRIM
67V4540 D-E width.
67V4541 B-C width.
Sizes, 5 to 11. POSTPAID

$4.95

Be Sure to State Size and Width

Gold Bond $4.00 A PAIR POSTPAID

This Oxford will be the big thing this season, unless every stylist on our staff is wrong. The wing tip on the broad balloon toe is "right"; the extended oak tanned leather sole is what the young fellows want; the perforations and stitchings add the necessary finish to the calfskin uppers. You'll know it's everything it ought to be in workmanship and value when we tell you it's a GOLD BOND. Attention, men: See the "clatter plug" in the leather heel! GENUINE GOODYEAR WELT.

BROWN
67V4426—D-E width.
67V4427—B-C width.
BLACK
67V4428—D-E width.
67V4429—B-C width.
Sizes, 5 to 11. Be sure to state size and width.

$4.00 POSTPAID

Gold Bond $4.00 A PAIR POST PAID

Hot style! "One, two, three" brass slugs—like a "clatter plate"—in the springy rubber heel. They're GOLD BOND high quality calfskin Oxfords. Bal pattern. GENUINE GOODYEAR WELT.

BROWN
67V4476—D-E width.
67V4477—B-C width.
BLACK
67V4478—D-E width.
67V4479 B-C width.
Sizes, 5 to 11. State size and width.

3 BRASS SLUGS

$4.00 POSTPAID

We Guarantee to Satisfy You and Save You Money

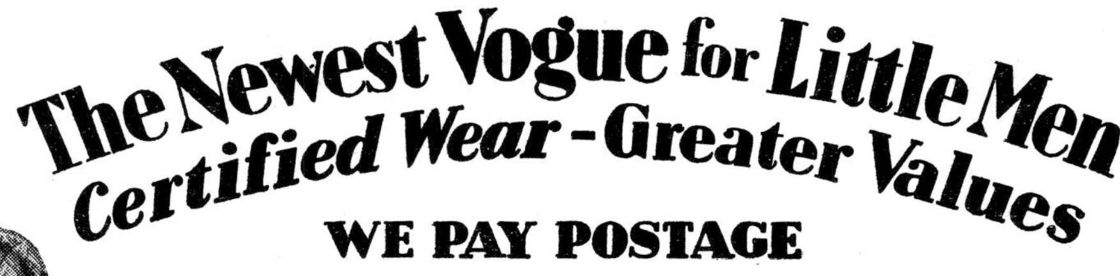

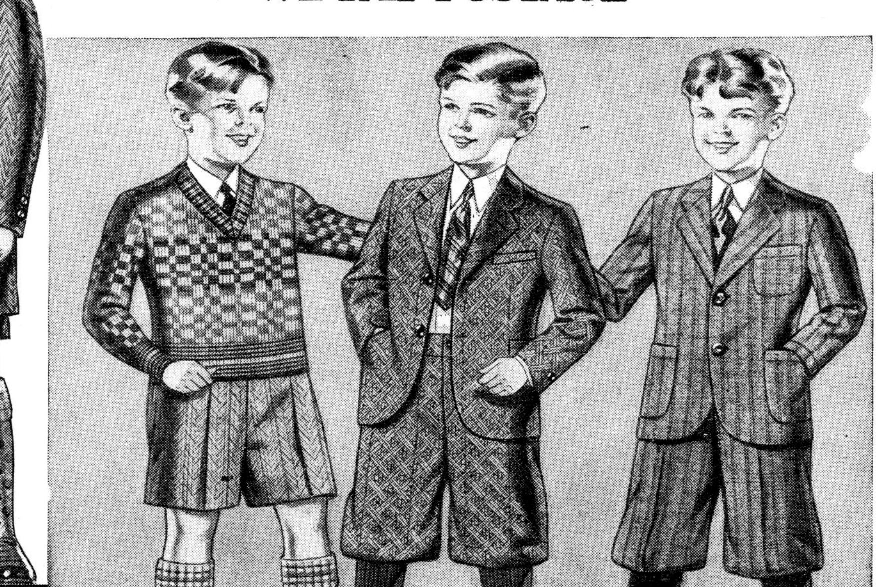

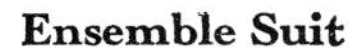

All Wool and Silk

A medium brown all wool and silk cassimere in a neat diamond weave with Rayon decorations. Coat is a two-button model with notched lapels. Lined with fancy durable lining. English shorts style pants are full lined and have self belt with buckle. **SIZES—4 to 9 years. State age size.**

40V3319—Brown All Wool and Silk Cassimere Suit With Extra Pants. Postpaid. $5.45

40V3323—Suit as Above, With Only One Pair of Shorts. Postpaid.......... $3.95

Ensemble Suit

A very attractive suit consisting of English short style pants which button to a figured madras waist. Harmonizing mercerized tie. The full lined pants have self belt with buckle. Coat listed separately. **SIZES—3 to 8 years. State age size.**

40V3326—Suit Consisting of Bluish Gray, All Wool and Silk Cassimere Pants With Rayon Decorations, Figured Waist and Tie. Postpaid............ $1.79

40V3837—Reefer Coat to Match Suit Above. Fully Lined. Sizes, 3 to 8 years. State age size. Postpaid.................. $3.50

Stylish Combination

A new and stylish outfit the boys will like. Mothers, too, will like it because it is really surprisingly low priced. The pants are the popular straight style with self belt and buckle. They are full lined and have two manly side pockets. The pants are made of a medium tan all wool and silk cassimere with attractive and stylish Rayon stripes. The sweater is rib knit of two-ply all wool worsted yarn in a Jacquard weave of tan and blue. **SIZES—3 to 9 years. State age size.**

40V3338—Sweater and Pants. Postpaid.............. $2.98

Handsome Suit

A handsome long wearing suit of all wool and silk gray novelty weave cassimere with Rayon decorations. The coat is an attractive two-button single breasted model, as illustrated, and fully lined with durable fancy lining. Golf knickers are full lined and have buckle bottoms and usual pockets. **SIZES—4 to 9 years. State age size.**

40V3306—Gray All Wool and Silk Cassimere Suit. Postpaid.......... $4.35

40V3310—Same Suit With Extra Golf Knickers. Postpaid. $5.85

Washable Cloth

A marvelously low priced suit that will keep the boy cool and comfortable in trying warm weather. He will like the style of this garment—it is quite mannish in cut. Mother will appreciate the fact that the material is easy to wash and launder. Made of Blue-gray cotton crash suiting with contrasting stripes. Both the coat and the knickers are unlined. The coat is two-button style with three patch pockets. A very attractive value. **SIZES—5 to 10 years. State age size.**

40V3327—Washable Cotton Crash Suit. Postpaid............ $1.98

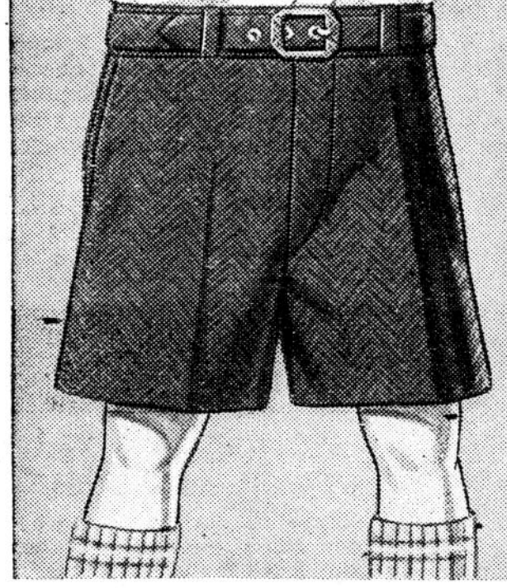

English Shorts

Ideal shorts for active little boys. They are made in the extremely popular English short style, roomy, comfortable and convenient. Will wear well and keep neat through long, hard service. Choice of three handsome, sturdy fabrics. Full lined. Have belt made of self material with a buckle. Sizes, 8, 9 and 10 have fly front, as illustrated. Other sizes have side openings. Two side pockets and one back pocket. **SIZES—4 to 10 years. State age size.**

40V3402—All Wool Blue Cheviot Shorts. Postpaid................ $1.39

40V3405—All Wool and Silk Brown Cassimere With Overplaid Decoration Shorts. Postpaid................ $1.39

40V3454—All Wool and Silk Gray Cassimere With Overplaid Decoration Shorts. Postpaid................ $1.39

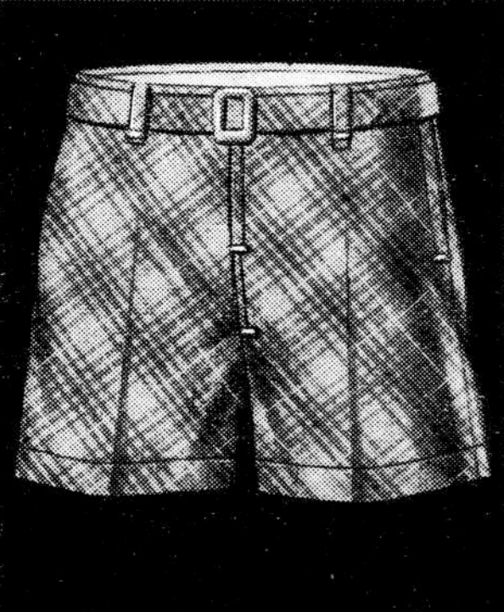

Washable Shorts

The new and very popular English Shorts. All the little fellows are wearing them. Three serviceable materials as listed below. Pants are made to button to waist and have belt loops and belt of same material with attractive belt buckle. Bar tacked. Hip pocket and two side pockets. Sizes, 8, 9 and 10 made with fly front. **SIZES—4 to 10 years. State age size. We Pay the Postage.**

40V3450—Tan Check Washable Cotton Crash. Postpaid................ 69c

40V3409—Assorted Striped Patterns, Imported Linen Shorts. Postpaid........ 79c

40V3421—White Duck Shorts. Postpaid....... 69c

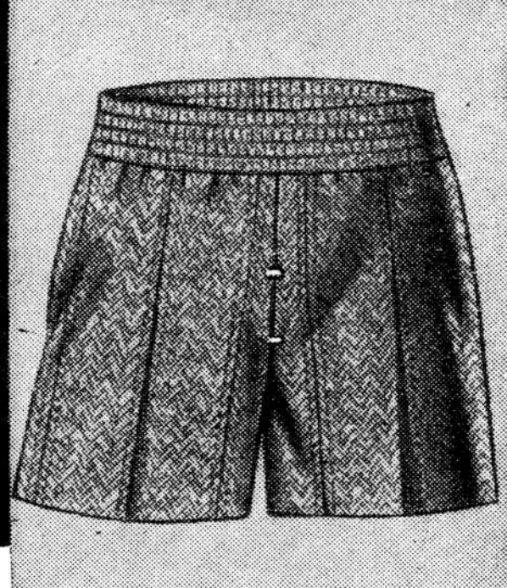

Elastic Waist Band

Attractive, elastic waistband shorts for hard playing youngsters. Practical latest style; popular. The elastic waistband does away with all buckles, belts and buttons and keeps the waist tucked in no matter how strenuous the boy may play. Fully lined. Strongly finished, with bar tacking at all strain points. Has two side pockets and one hip pocket. Either of the fine fabrics will give a world of long wear and satisfaction, and at outstanding values. **SIZES—4 to 9 years. State age size.**

40V3419—Gray Cassimere Elastic Waistband Shorts About Four-Fifths Wool and Silk. Postpaid................ $1.00

40V3420—Brown All Wool and Silk Cassimere Elastic Waistband Shorts With Rayon Decorations. Postpaid........ $1.19

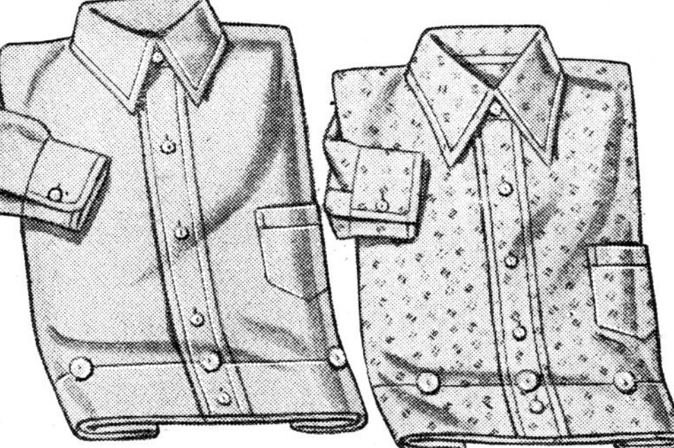

Button-On Style

Very practical waists with large buttons at the bottom to button to the little pants. All fast color cotton broadcloth materials. Lined collars and cuffs, sleeve facings. Open cuffs to button. Long sleeves and regular style collar. Good quality buttons. They launder well. **SIZES—4 to 10 years. State age size.**

40V3524—Tan Pastel Shade Broadcloth. Postpaid.............. 69c

40V3523—Blue Pastel Shade Broadcloth. Postpaid.............. 69c

40V3526—Plain White Broadcloth. Postpaid.............. 69c

Popular Style

An extraordinary opportunity to save on little fellows' waists. Button-on style with large buttons at bottom to button to pants. Will wash and launder well. Open cuffs to button. Lined collar. **SIZES—4 to 10 years. State age size.**

40V3518—Novelty Pattern Doby Weave Cotton Broadcloth. Postpaid.............. 67c

40V3522—Dressy Rayon Stripe Woven Cotton Broadcloth. Postpaid.... 85c

40V3501—Plain Blue Chambray. Postpaid.............. 65c

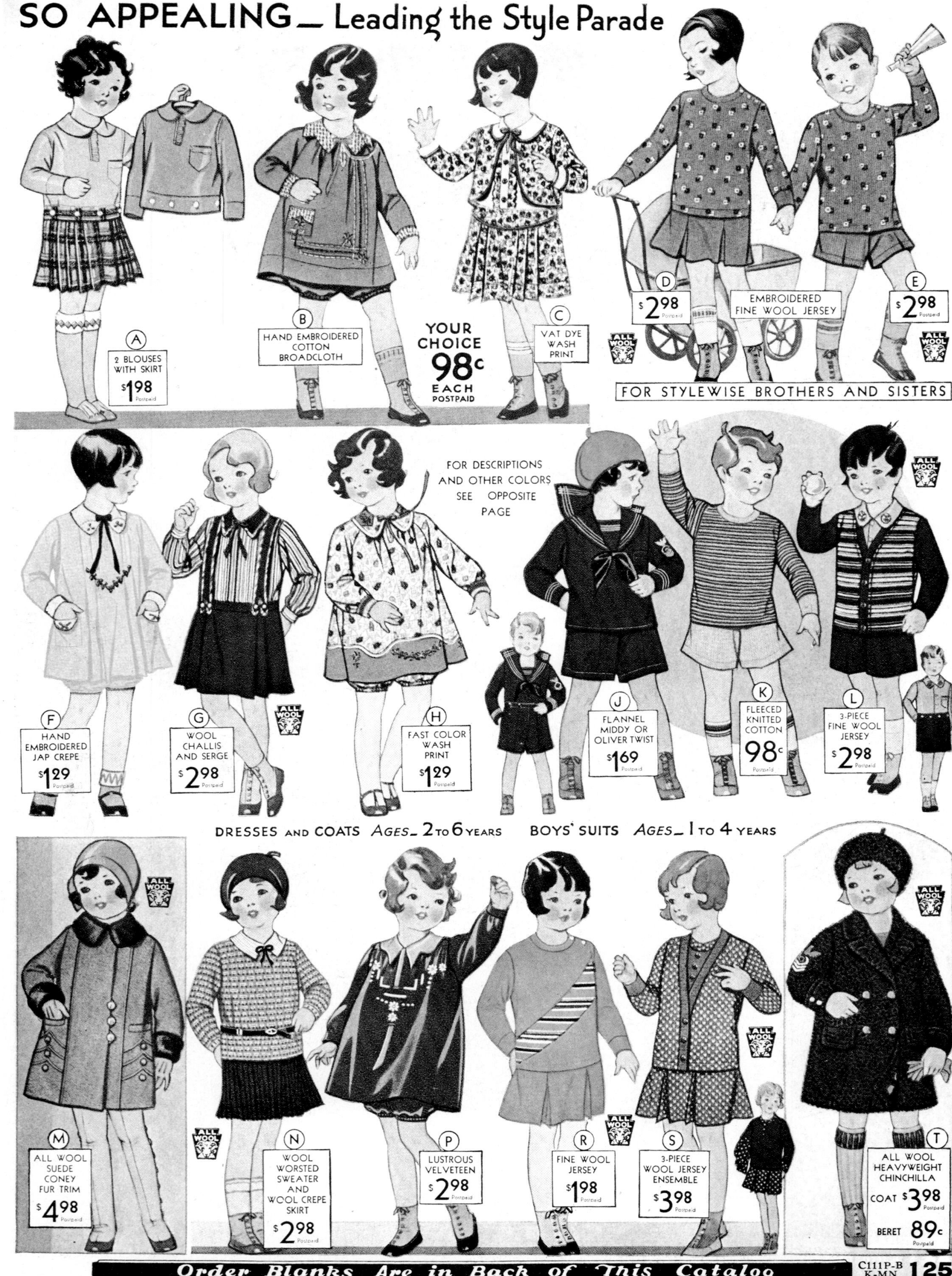
SO APPEALING— Leading the Style Parade
A
2 BLOUSES WITH SKIRT
$1.98 Postpaid
B
HAND EMBROIDERED COTTON BROADCLOTH
YOUR CHOICE 98c EACH POSTPAID
C
VAT DYE WASH PRINT
D
$2.98 Postpaid
EMBROIDERED FINE WOOL JERSEY
E
$2.98 Postpaid
ALL WOOL
FOR STYLEWISE BROTHERS AND SISTERS
FOR DESCRIPTIONS AND OTHER COLORS SEE OPPOSITE PAGE
F
HAND EMBROIDERED JAP CREPE
$1.29 Postpaid
G
WOOL CHALLIS AND SERGE
$2.98 Postpaid
H
FAST COLOR WASH PRINT
$1.29 Postpaid
J
FLANNEL MIDDY OR OLIVER TWIST
$1.69 Postpaid
K
FLEECED KNITTED COTTON
98c Postpaid
L
3-PIECE FINE WOOL JERSEY
$2.98 Postpaid
DRESSES AND COATS AGES—2 TO 6 YEARS
BOYS' SUITS AGES—1 TO 4 YEARS
M
ALL WOOL SUEDE CONEY FUR TRIM
$4.98 Postpaid
N
WOOL WORSTED SWEATER AND WOOL CREPE SKIRT
$2.98 Postpaid
P
LUSTROUS VELVETEEN
$2.98 Postpaid
R
FINE WOOL JERSEY
$1.98 Postpaid
S
3-PIECE WOOL JERSEY ENSEMBLE
$3.98 Postpaid
T
ALL WOOL HEAVYWEIGHT CHINCHILLA
COAT $3.98 Postpaid
BERET 89c Postpaid
Order Blanks Are in Back of This Catalog
C111P-B K-MN 125

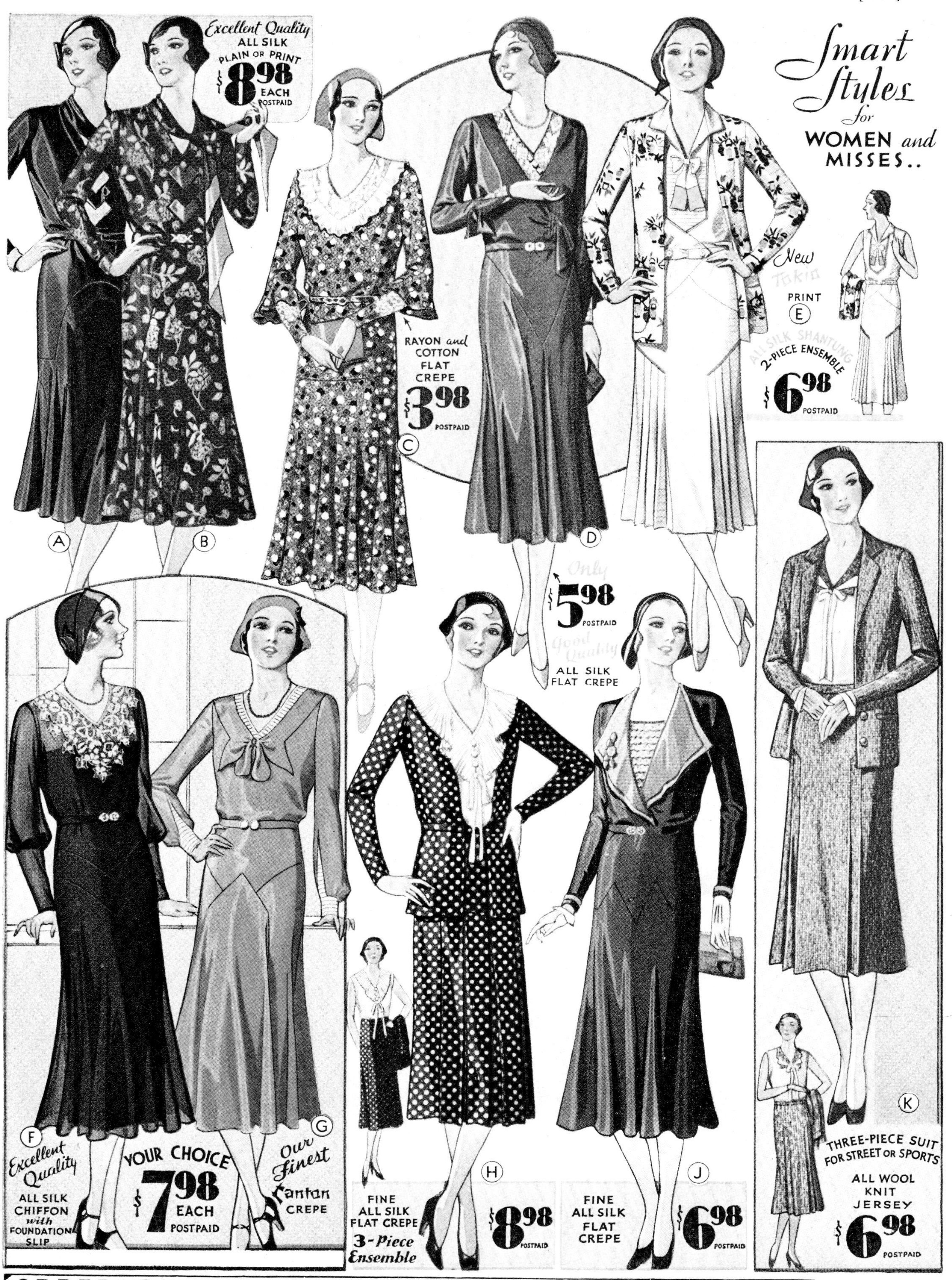

ORDER BLANKS ARE IN BACK OF THIS CATALOG

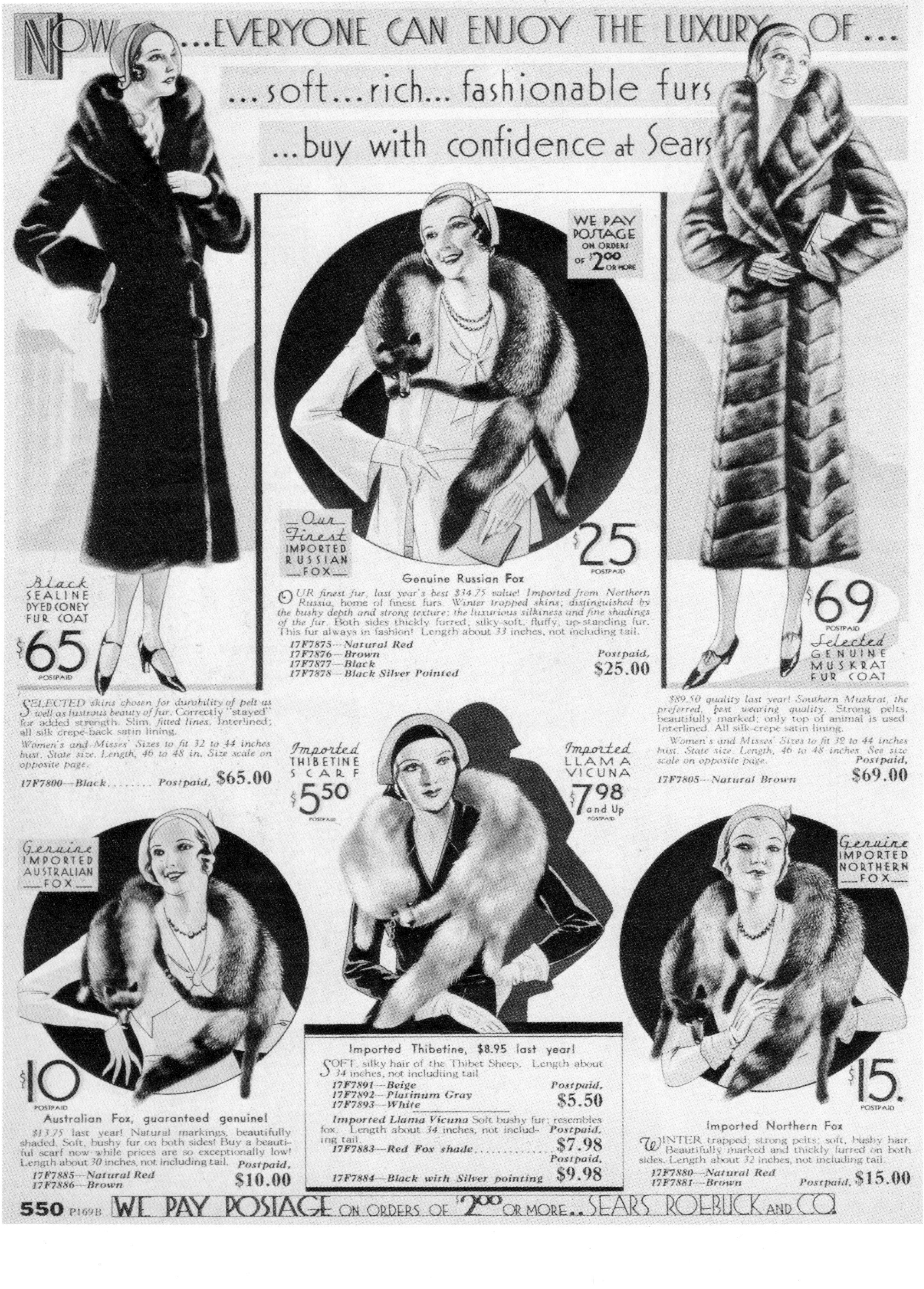

NOW ... EVERYONE CAN ENJOY THE LUXURY OF ...

... soft ... rich ... fashionable furs

... buy with confidence at Sears

WE PAY POSTAGE ON ORDERS OF $2.00 OR MORE

Black SEALINE DYED CONEY FUR COAT

$65 POSTPAID

SELECTED skins chosen for durability of pelt as well as lustrous beauty of fur. Correctly "stayed" for added strength. Slim, *fitted lines.* Interlined; all silk crepe-back satin lining.

Women's and Misses' Sizes to fit 32 to 44 inches bust. State size. Length, 46 to 48 in. Size scale on opposite page.

17F7800—Black .... ***Postpaid,*** **$65.00**

Our Finest IMPORTED RUSSIAN FOX

$25 POSTPAID

Genuine Russian Fox

OUR finest fur, last year's best $34.75 value! Imported from Northern Russia, home of finest furs. *Winter trapped skins; distinguished by the bushy depth and strong texture; the luxurious silkiness and fine shadings of the fur.* Both sides thickly furred; silky-soft, fluffy, up-standing fur. This fur always in fashion! Length about *33* inches, not including tail.

17F7875—Natural Red
17F7876—Brown
17F7877—Black
17F7878—Black Silver Pointed

Postpaid, **$25.00**

$69 POSTPAID

Selected GENUINE MUSKRAT FUR COAT

$89.50 quality last year! Southern Muskrat, the preferred, best wearing quality. Strong pelts, beautifully marked; only top of animal is used Interlined. All silk-crepe satin lining.

Women's and Misses' Sizes to fit 32 to 44 inches bust. State size. Length, 46 to 48 inches. See size scale on opposite page.

17F7805—Natural Brown ***Postpaid,*** **$69.00**

Imported THIBETINE SCARF

$5.50 POSTPAID

Imported LLAMA VICUNA

$7.98 and Up POSTPAID

Genuine IMPORTED AUSTRALIAN FOX

$10 POSTPAID

Australian Fox, guaranteed genuine!

$13.75 last year! Natural markings, beautifully shaded. Soft, bushy fur on both sides! Buy a beautiful scarf now while prices are so exceptionally low! Length about *30* inches, not including tail.

17F7885—Natural Red
17F7886—Brown

Postpaid, **$10.00**

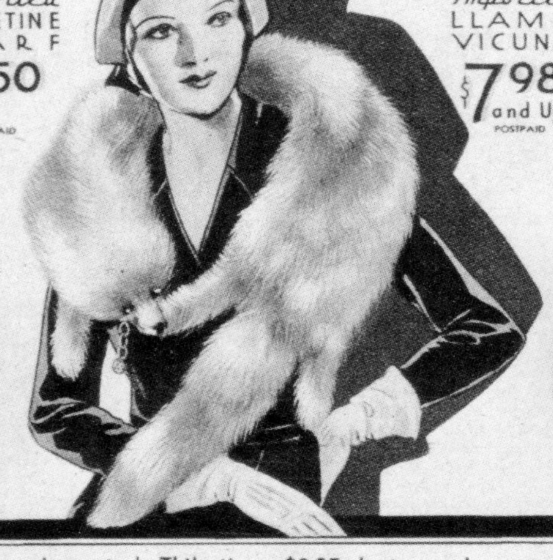

Imported Thibetine, $8.95 last year!

SOFT, silky hair of the Thibet Sheep. Length about *34* inches, not includiing tail

17F7891—Beige
17F7892—Platinum Gray
17F7893—White

Postpaid, **$5.50**

Imported Llama Vicuna Soft bushy fur; resembles fox. Length about *34* inches, not including tail.

17F7883—Red Fox shade .... ***Postpaid,*** **$7.98**

17F7884—Black with Silver pointing ***Postpaid,*** **$9.98**

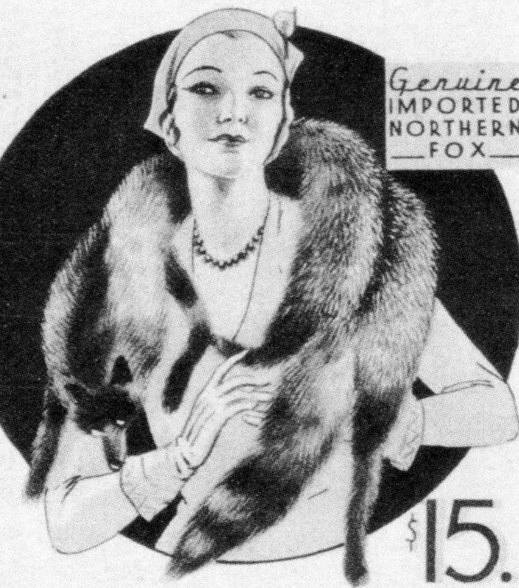

Genuine IMPORTED NORTHERN FOX

$15. POSTPAID

Imported Northern Fox

WINTER trapped; strong pelts; soft, bushy hair. Beautifully marked and thickly furred on both sides. Length about *32* inches, not including tail.

17F7880—Natural Red
17F7881—Brown

Postpaid, **$15.00**

 WE PAY POSTAGE ON ORDERS OF $2.00 OR MORE .. SEARS ROEBUCK AND CO.

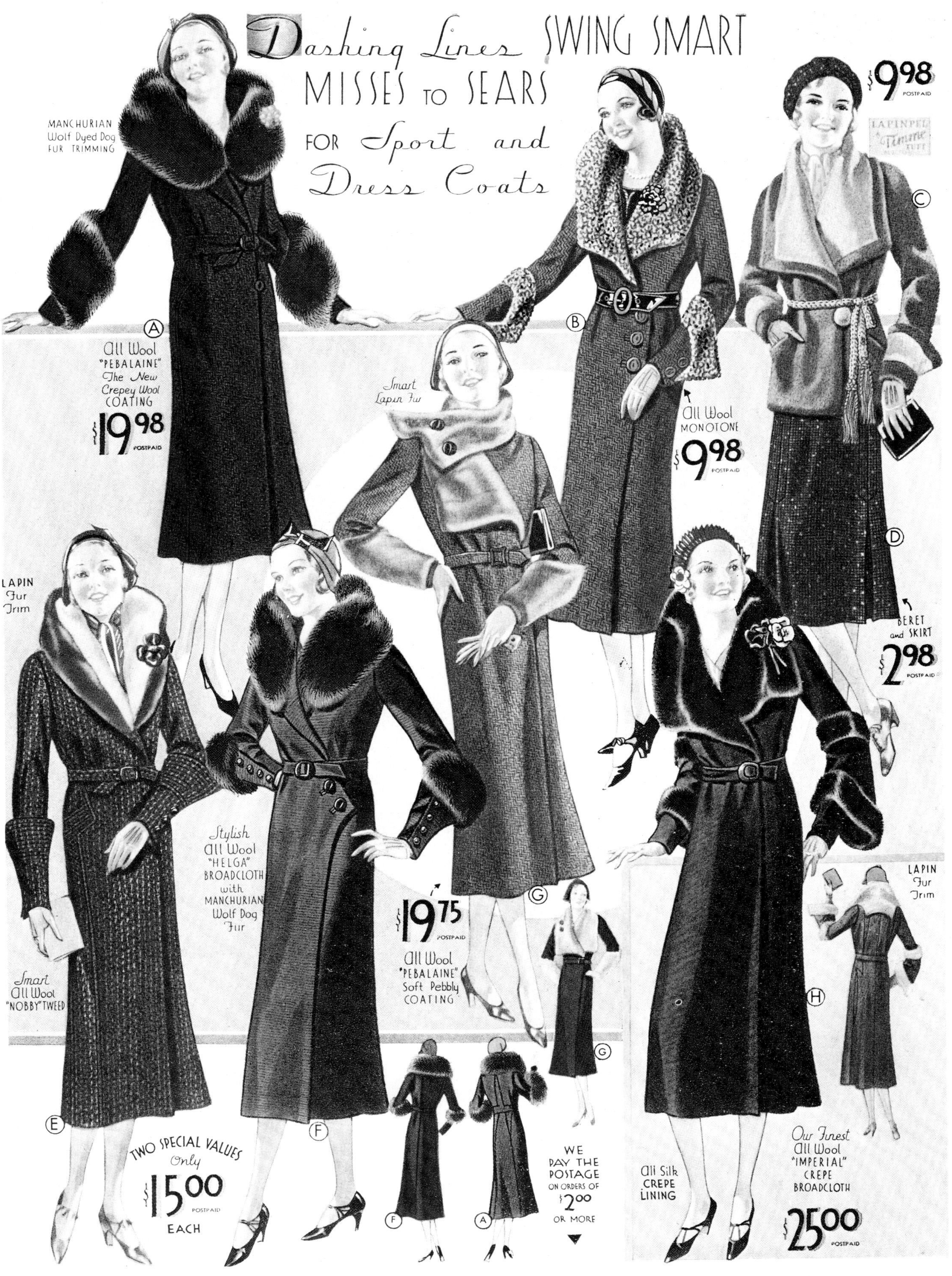
Dashing Lines SWING SMART MISSES TO SEARS FOR Sport and Dress Coats
MANCHURIAN Wolf Dyed Dog FUR TRIMMING
A
All Wool "PEBALAINE" The New Crepey Wool COATING
$19.98 POSTPAID
B
All Wool MONOTONE
$9.98 POSTPAID
$9.98 POSTPAID
C
D
BERET and SKIRT
$2.98 POSTPAID
Smart Lapin Fur
LAPIN Fur Trim
Stylish All Wool "HELGA" BROADCLOTH with MANCHURIAN Wolf Dog Fur
$19.75 POSTPAID
All Wool "PEBALAINE" Soft Pebbly COATING
G
Smart All Wool "NOBBY" TWEED
E
F
TWO SPECIAL VALUES Only
$15.00 POSTPAID
EACH
WE PAY THE POSTAGE ON ORDERS OF $2.00 OR MORE
LAPIN Fur Trim
H
All Silk CREPE LINING
Our Finest All Wool "IMPERIAL" CREPE BROADCLOTH
$25.00 POSTPAID

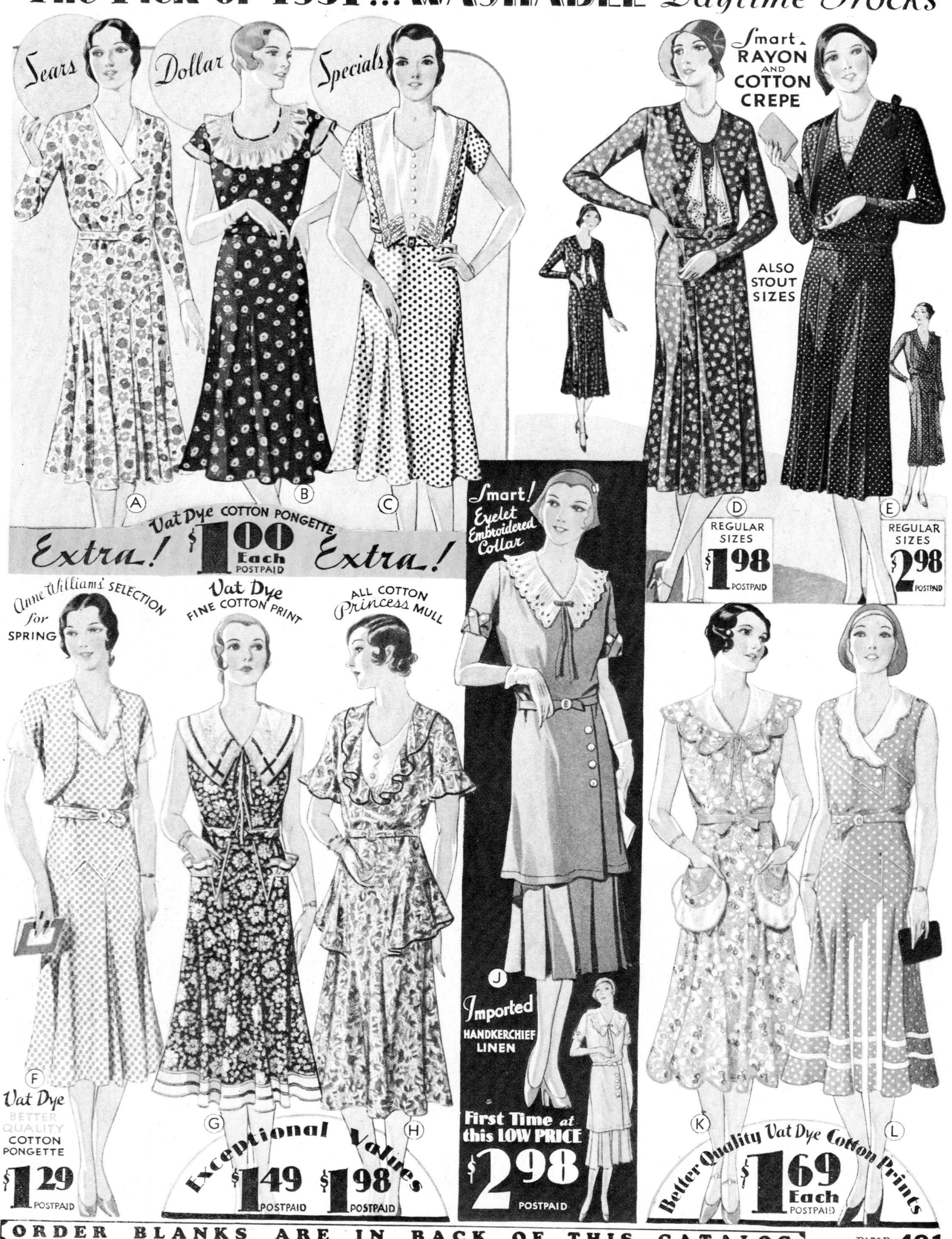

ORDER BLANKS ARE IN BACK OF THIS CATALOG

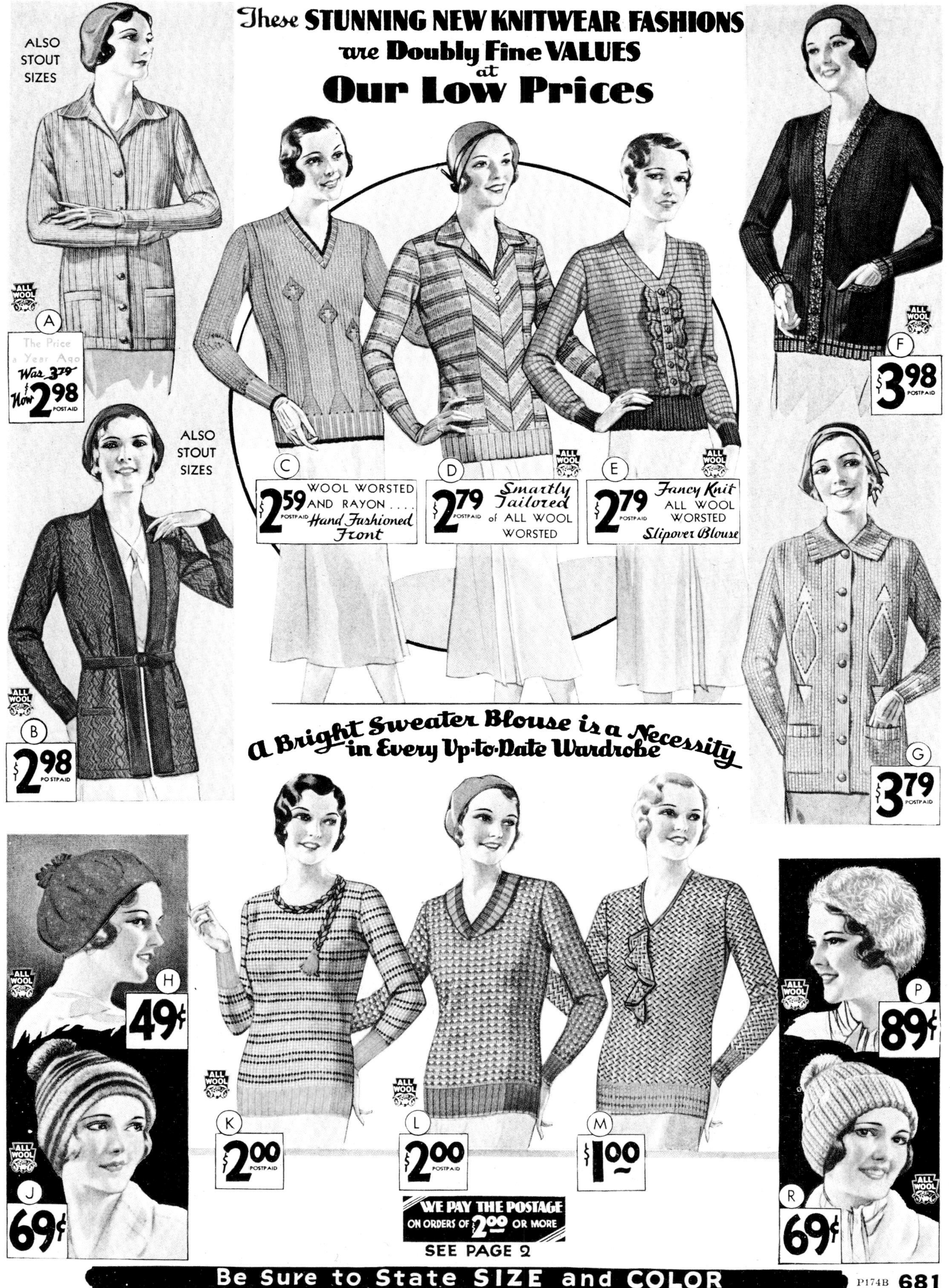

These STUNNING NEW KNITWEAR FASHIONS are Doubly Fine VALUES at Our Low Prices
ALSO STOUT SIZES
ALL WOOL
A
The Price a Year Ago Was 3.79 Now 2.98 POSTPAID
ALSO STOUT SIZES
B
2.98 POSTPAID
C
2.59 POSTPAID WOOL WORSTED AND RAYON.... Hand Fashioned Front
D
2.79 POSTPAID Smartly Tailored of ALL WOOL WORSTED
E
2.79 POSTPAID Fancy Knit ALL WOOL WORSTED Slipover Blouse
F
3.98 POSTPAID
G
3.79 POSTPAID
A Bright Sweater Blouse is a Necessity in Every Up-to-Date Wardrobe
H
49¢
J
69¢
K
2.00 POSTPAID
L
2.00 POSTPAID
M
1.00
P
89¢
R
69¢
WE PAY THE POSTAGE ON ORDERS OF 2.00 OR MORE
SEE PAGE 2
Be Sure to State SIZE and COLOR

Extraordinary BARGAINS

OVERALLS!
At the BEACH! On the FARM!
EVERYBODY IS WEARING THEM
$1.59 Postpaid
$2.98 TERRY CLOTH POSTPAID
COTTON BROADCLOTH BLOUSE 98¢ POSTPAID
Blouse PLAIN OR STRIPED
BLAZER STRIPED BEACH ROBE $1.98 POSTPAID
KNICKERS 98¢ and Up POSTPAID
STRONG as IRON
and Oh! So Cool!
MIDDIES and KNICKERS
BLOUSE or PLAY SHORTS 98¢ EACH POSTPAID

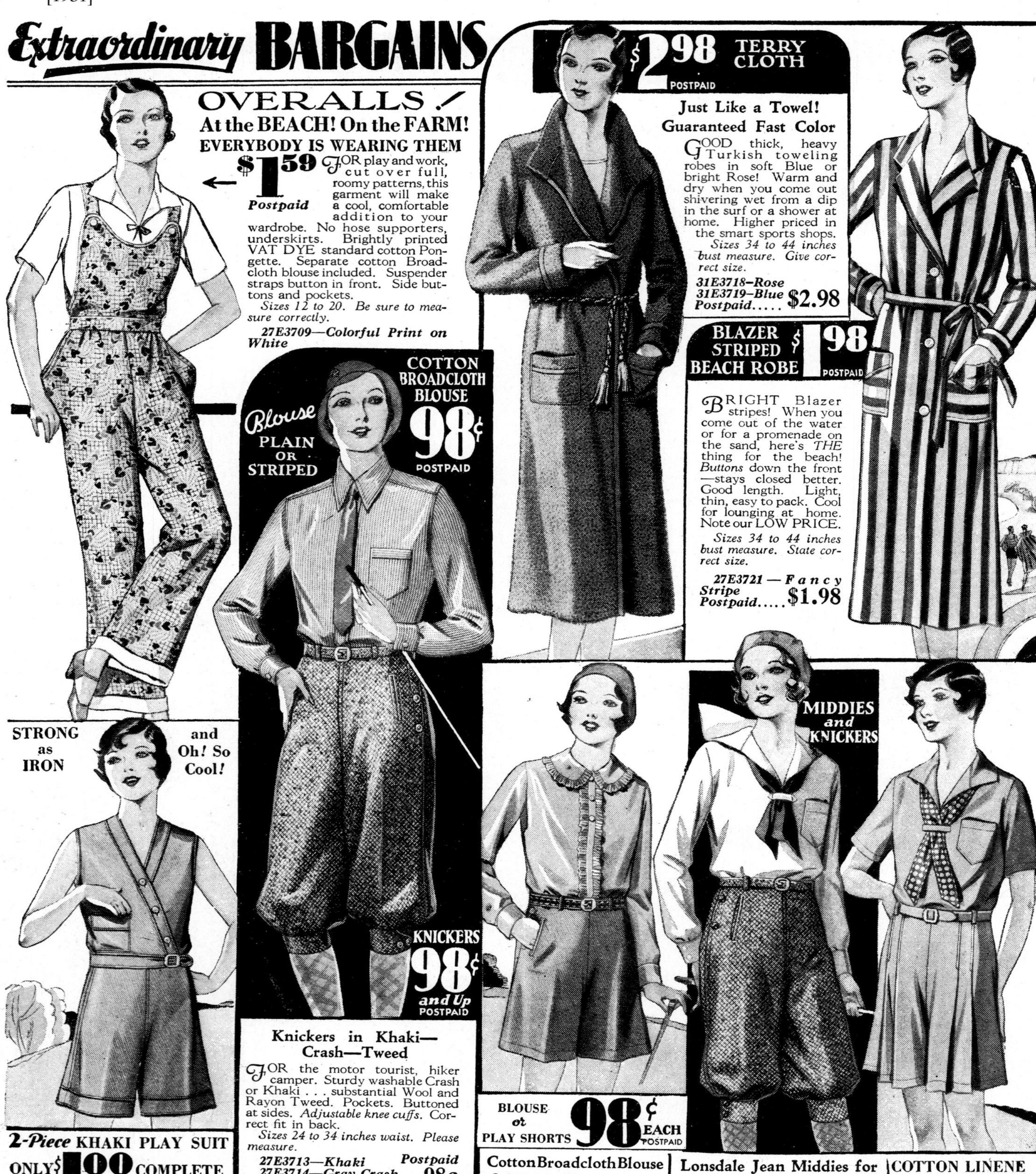

FOR play and work, cut over full, roomy patterns, this garment will make a cool, comfortable addition to your wardrobe. No hose supporters, underskirts. Brightly printed VAT DYE standard cotton Pongette. Separate cotton Broadcloth blouse included. Suspender straps button in front. Side buttons and pockets.
Sizes 12 to 20. Be sure to measure correctly.
27E3709—Colorful Print on White

Just Like a Towel! Guaranteed Fast Color

GOOD thick, heavy Turkish toweling robes in soft Blue or bright Rose! Warm and dry when you come out shivering wet from a dip in the surf or a shower at home. Higher priced in the smart sports shops.
Sizes 34 to 44 inches bust measure. Give correct size.
31E3718–Rose
31E3719–Blue
***Postpaid*..... $2.98**

BRIGHT Blazer stripes! When you come out of the water or for a promenade on the sand, here's *THE* thing for the beach! *Buttons* down the front —stays closed better. Good length. Light, thin, easy to pack. Cool for lounging at home. Note our LOW PRICE.
Sizes 34 to 44 inches bust measure. State correct size.
27E3721 — Fancy Stripe
***Postpaid*..... $1.98**

2-Piece KHAKI PLAY SUIT
ONLY $1.00 COMPLETE
POSTPAID

SAVES far more on other clothes than it costs! No skirts! Let her climb, race, tumble all she pleases! Into *everything*—she can't hurt these togs! They save mending worries! Save laundering—Khaki doesn't soil easily! Gay red pipings to brighten it! Cool sleeveless slipover blouse lets in healthful sunshine. Buttoned side openings. All around belt with sliding metal buckle!
Sizes 7 to 14. State age size. See size scale, page 494.
27E3760—Khaki with Red
***Postpaid*..................$1.00**

Knickers in Khaki—Crash—Tweed

FOR the motor tourist, hiker camper. Sturdy washable Crash or Khaki . . . substantial Wool and Rayon Tweed. Pockets. Buttoned at sides. *Adjustable knee cuffs.* Correct fit in back.
Sizes 24 to 34 inches waist. Please measure.
27E3713—Khaki *Postpaid*
27E3714—Gray Crash **98c**
27E3715—Tan Crash

Wool and Rayon Tweed
27E3716—Gray
27E3717—Tan **$2.69**

TAILORED BLOUSE
Pin Striped or Plain

OF good cotton *Broadcloth*. Gathered on a shoulder yoke in back. Double cuffs. Full length front opening. Checkered cotton tie.
Sizes 34 to 44 in. bust. State size.
27E3710—Blue Stripe
27E3711—All White **98c**
27E3712—All Tan *Postpaid*

Cotton Broadcloth Blouse

LOW PRICED for style so *smart!* Band bottom is tucked in or worn outside. Good cotton Broadcloth, pleated frill. Pearl buttons.
Sizes 8 to 16. State age size.
27E3763—White
27E3764—Tan **98c**

Play Shorts

WASHABLE, sturdy cotton. Buttons at side openings.
Sizes 8 to 16. State age size.
27E3766—Khaki
27E3767—Gray Crash **98c** *Postpaid*

Lonsdale Jean Middies for Girls and Women

REGULATION style. All white.
27E3769*—Sizes 7 to 14 years.*
27E3770*—Sizes 34 to 44 in. bust measure.* **$1.00**

Girls' KNICKERS

BUTTONS at side openings fit them to waist.
Sizes 7 to 14 yrs.—25 to 29 inches waist. State size.
27E3771—Khaki
27E3772—Gray Crash
27E3773—Tan Crash
***Postpaid*...............98c**

Wool and Rayon Tweed
27E3774—Gray
27E3775—Tan **$2.49**

COTTON LINENE TWO-PIECE SUIT

LOOKS expensive, but see the *LOW PRICE!* Our smartest suit for *Tennis, Basketball* or the Playground. Firm *fast* color all cotton Linene. Shorts are pleated in front; slightly gathered in back, and buttoned to waist. Cotton tie.
Sizes 10 to 18 years.
27E3776—Med. Blue
27E3777—Tan
***Postpaid*.....$1.39**

Items on These Pages Shipped Postage Paid by SEARS, ROEBUCK AND CO.

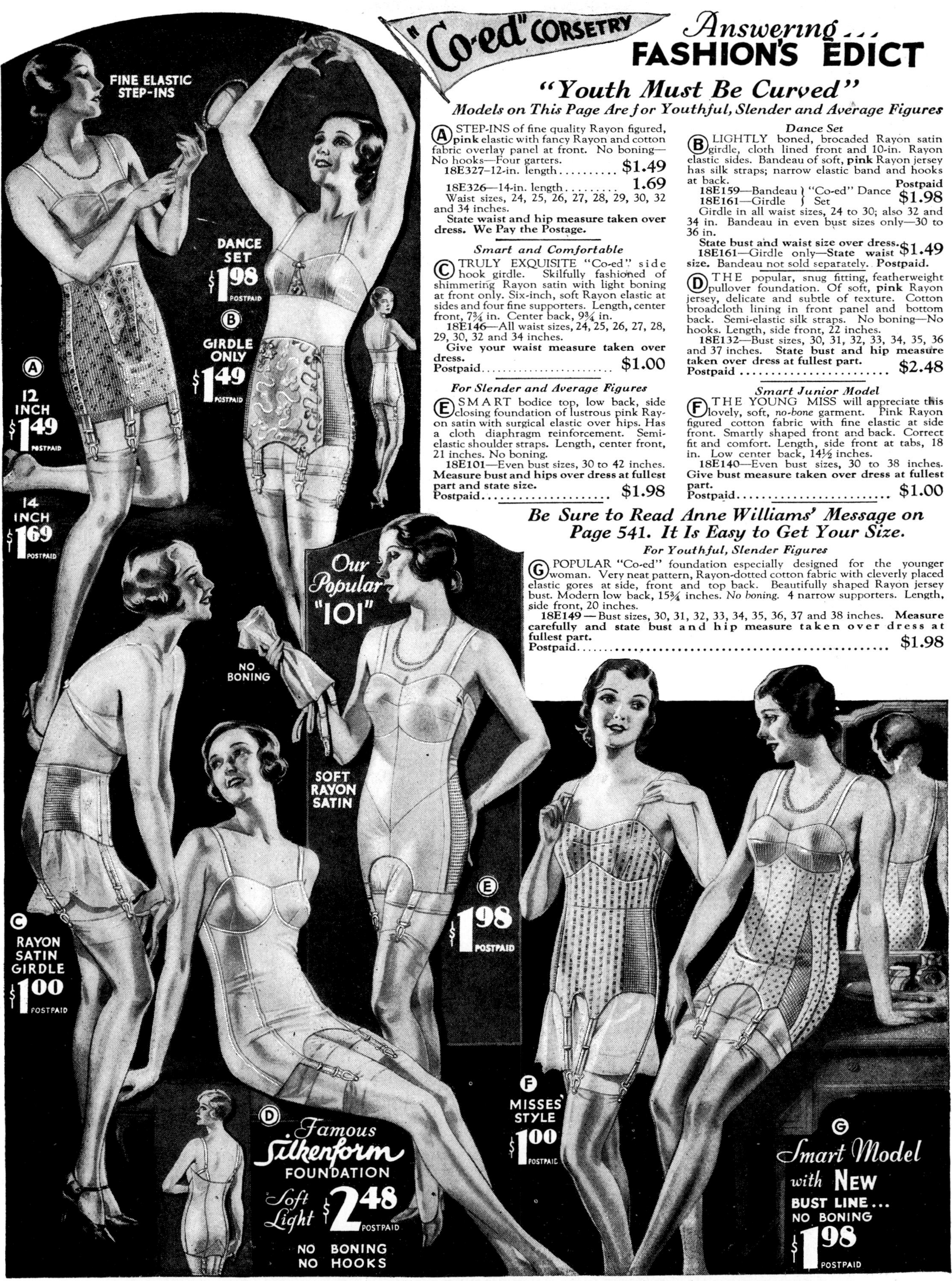
"Co-ed" CORSETRY
Answering . . .
FASHION'S EDICT
"Youth Must Be Curved"
Models on This Page Are for Youthful, Slender and Average Figures
(A) STEP-INS of fine quality Rayon figured, pink elastic with fancy Rayon and cotton fabric overlay panel at front. No boning—No hooks—Four garters.
18E327—12-in. length $1.49
18E326—14-in. length 1.69
Waist sizes, 24, 25, 26, 27, 28, 29, 30, 32 and 34 inches.
State waist and hip measure taken over dress. We Pay the Postage.
Smart and Comfortable
(C) TRULY EXQUISITE "Co-ed" side hook girdle. Skilfully fashioned of shimmering Rayon satin with light boning at front only. Six-inch, soft Rayon elastic at sides and four fine supporters. Length, center front, 7¾ in. Center back, 9¾ in.
18E146—All waist sizes, 24, 25, 26, 27, 28, 29, 30, 32 and 34 inches.
Give your waist measure taken over dress.
Postpaid $1.00
For Slender and Average Figures
(E) SMART bodice top, low back, side closing foundation of lustrous pink Rayon satin with surgical elastic over hips. Has a cloth diaphragm reinforcement. Semi-elastic shoulder straps. Length, center front, 21 inches. No boning.
18E101—Even bust sizes, 30 to 42 inches.
Measure bust and hips over dress at fullest part and state size.
Postpaid $1.98
Dance Set
(B) LIGHTLY boned, brocaded Rayon satin girdle, cloth lined front and 10-in. Rayon elastic sides. Bandeau of soft, pink Rayon jersey has silk straps; narrow elastic band and hooks at back.
18E159—Bandeau } "Co-ed" Dance Postpaid
18E161—Girdle } Set $1.98
Girdle in all waist sizes, 24 to 30; also 32 and 34 in. Bandeau in even bust sizes only—30 to 36 in.
State bust and waist size over dress.
18E161—Girdle only—State waist size. Bandeau not sold separately. Postpaid. $1.49
(D) THE popular, snug fitting, featherweight pullover foundation. Of soft, pink Rayon jersey, delicate and subtle of texture. Cotton broadcloth lining in front panel and bottom back. Semi-elastic silk straps. No boning—No hooks. Length, side front, 22 inches.
18E132—Bust sizes, 30, 31, 32, 33, 34, 35, 36 and 37 inches. State bust and hip measure taken over dress at fullest part.
Postpaid $2.48
Smart Junior Model
(F) THE YOUNG MISS will appreciate this lovely, soft, no-bone garment. Pink Rayon figured cotton fabric with fine elastic at side front. Smartly shaped front and back. Correct fit and comfort. Length, side front at tabs, 18 in. Low center back, 14½ inches.
18E140—Even bust sizes, 30 to 38 inches. Give bust measure taken over dress at fullest part.
Postpaid $1.00
Be Sure to Read Anne Williams' Message on Page 541. It Is Easy to Get Your Size.
For Youthful, Slender Figures
(G) POPULAR "Co-ed" foundation especially designed for the younger woman. Very neat pattern, Rayon-dotted cotton fabric with cleverly placed elastic gores at side, front and top back. Beautifully shaped Rayon jersey bust. Modern low back, 15¾ inches. No boning. 4 narrow supporters. Length, side front, 20 inches.
18E149—Bust sizes, 30, 31, 32, 33, 34, 35, 36, 37 and 38 inches. Measure carefully and state bust and hip measure taken over dress at fullest part.
Postpaid $1.98
FINE ELASTIC STEP-INS
DANCE SET $1.98 POSTPAID
(B) GIRDLE ONLY $1.49 POSTPAID
(A) 12 INCH $1.49 POSTPAID
14 INCH $1.69 POSTPAID
Our Popular "101"
NO BONING
SOFT RAYON SATIN
(E) $1.98 POSTPAID
(C) RAYON SATIN GIRDLE $1.00 POSTPAID
(D) Famous Silkenform FOUNDATION
Soft Light $2.48 POSTPAID
NO BONING NO HOOKS
(F) MISSES' STYLE $1.00 POSTPAID
(G) Smart Model with NEW BUST LINE . . . NO BONING $1.98 POSTPAID

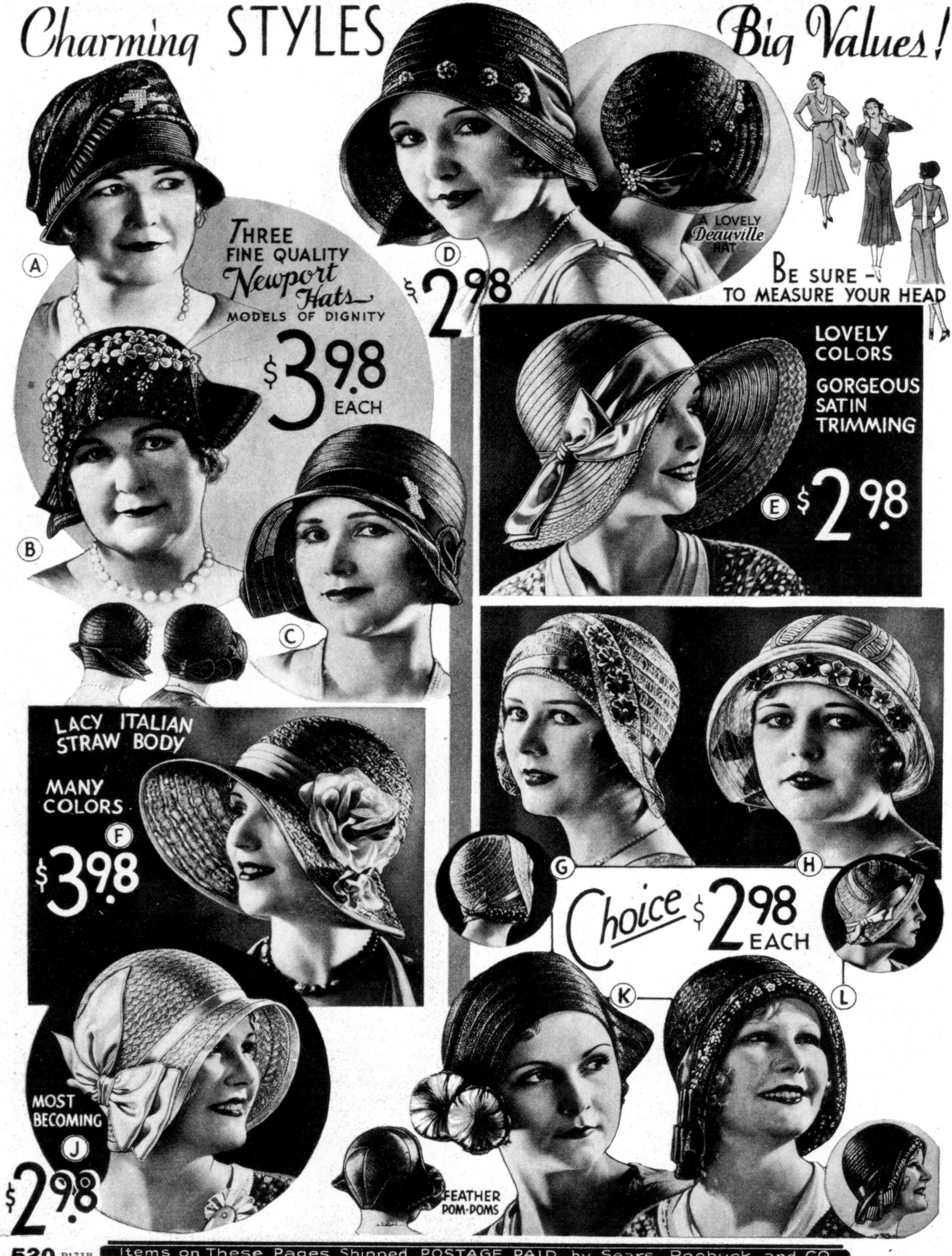

Charming STYLES Big Values!
THREE FINE QUALITY Newport Hats
MODELS OF DIGNITY
$3.98 EACH
A
B
C
D
$2.98
A LOVELY Deauville HAT
BE SURE – TO MEASURE YOUR HEAD
LOVELY COLORS
GORGEOUS SATIN TRIMMING
E $2.98
LACY ITALIAN STRAW BODY
MANY COLORS
F
$3.98
G
H
Choice $2.98 EACH
K
L
MOST BECOMING
J
$2.98
FEATHER POM-POMS

YOU MUST HAVE A PAIR OF SPORTS TROUSERS

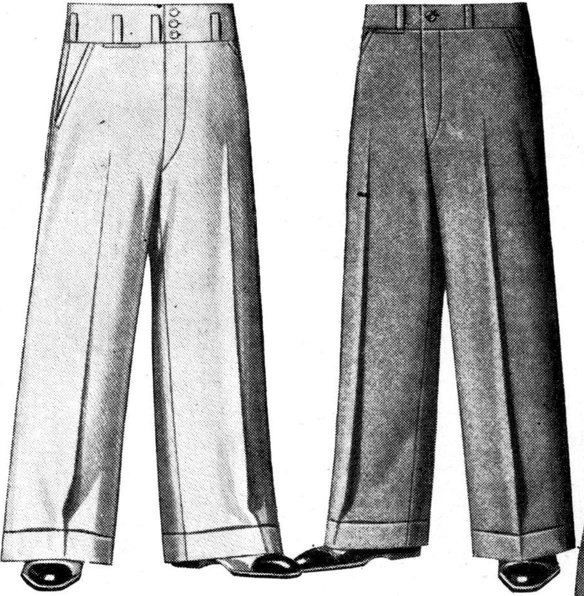

Right Up to Date!

You need white twill trousers for tennis, the beach, and all sorts of summer occasions. The slant pockets, wide waist band, set-down belt loops, and **22-inch cuff bottoms** are right up to the minute, as are the flaps on the two back pockets. The cotton twill is heavy 8-ounce and PRE-SHRUNK! **SIZES—28 to 36 inches waist and 28 to 34 inches inseam. State measurements.**

45E7673—High Quality White Twill Trousers. Postpaid............... **$1.75**

Flannels Are Style

Style critics agree that plain tan and gray flannel trousers are fast replacing knickers for sport wear. These are of high quality all wool flannel and are cut with the up to date slant pockets and twenty-inch bottoms. Others will ask $6 or $7 a pair for this quality! **Sizes—28 to 36 inches waist and 28 to 34 inches inseam. State measurements.**

45E7641—Plain Light Tan All Wool Flannel. Postpaid............. **$3.98**

45E7642—Plain Light Gray All Wool Flannel. Postpaid............. **$3.98**

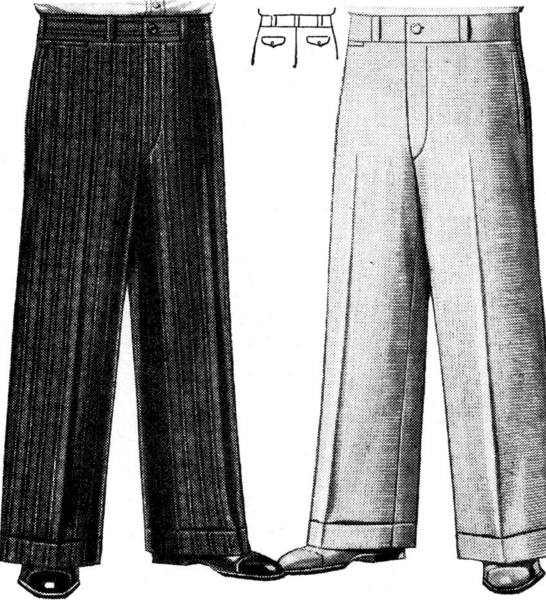

Genuine Palm Beach

In case of heat—keep cool!— You know—Genuine Palm Beach—cool, crisp, comfortable, and washable. The tropical worsteds are over one-third wool, and very light and cool—A hard finished cloth that keeps a crease well. **SIZES—30 to 42 inches waist and 29 to 34 inches inseam. State measurements.**

45E7563—Medium Dark Gray Striped Genuine Palm Beach. Postpaid. **$3.75**

45E7566—Light Gray, Striped Tropical Worsted. Postpaid................ **$2.85**

45E7567—Medium Tan Striped Tropical Worsted. Postpaid.................. **$2.85**

Pre-Shrunk White Duck or Linen

No wonder we lead the field! And now—PRE-SHRUNK! Order the size you need, and it will stay that size no matter how often you wash it! Flaps on two hip pockets. Made just like our regular dress trousers. **SIZES—28 to 42 inches waist and 28 to 36 inches inseam. State measurements.**

45E7562—Standard Quality White Duck. Postpaid............ **$1.19**

45E7565—Higher Quality Heavyweight White Duck. Postpaid..... **$1.49**

45E7523—Genuine White Linen. Postpaid............ **$2.25**

For the Good Old Summertime

YES! THEY'RE COOL!

Stylish Summer Combination

(Sold Separately)

Here is the combination you can't beat for sports wear or for the most dressed up summer occasion! The handsome, well tailored, **tan** or **blue** sport jacket is made of fine quality all wool flannel, ¼ lined for coolness. The three patch pockets and the four pinch pleats in back give it just the swagger that summer style demands. The trousers are carefully tailored of fine quality all wool **white** serge with fancy neat black stripes. The stripings are beautiful, and pure worsted means long wear and shape keeping qualities. You can order either of the coats or the trousers separately. **SIZES—Coat, 34 to 42 inches chest; Trousers, 28 to 42 inches waist and 28 to 34 inches inseam. State measurements.**

45E7320—Medium Light Brown All Wool Flannel Coat. Postpaid...................... **$9.95**

45E7321—Blue All Wool Flannel Coat. Postpaid........ **9.95**

45E7596—White All Wool Worsted Serge Trousers with Fancy Black Stripes. Postpaid......................... **$4.95**

Sport Outfit De Luxe!

(Sold Separately)

Here's a stylish combination of double breasted blue serge coat and plain white flannel trousers. Every man should have at least one such outfit. Now you can save a lot of money. The coat is of excellent quality fine twill blue serge, one-fourth lined, and beautifully tailored—the kind usually sold at $15.00. The trousers are of a standard, nationally known, all wool white flannel, beautifully tailored and really worth $7.50. You can buy either the coat or trousers separately.

SIZES—Coat, 34 to 42 inches chest; Trousers, 28 to 42 inches waist and 28 to 34 inches inseam. State measurements.

45E7313—All Wool Navy Blue Serge Coat. Postpaid...................... **$9.45**

45E7595—All Wool White Flannel Trousers. Postpaid.... **5.50**

Measuring Instructions Are on Back of Order Blanks in Back of Catalog

WARMTH QUALITY and GOOD VALUES...

Here are Overcoats for Every Purpose . . . All at Bargain Prices . . . .

WE PAY THE POSTAGE ON ORDERS OF $2.00 OR MORE

GENUINE GALLOWAY FUR NON-SHEDDING

ALL WOOL $16.85 Postpaid

$11.85 Postpaid

$37.50 Postpaid

Regular and EXTRA Large Sizes

Conservative Chesterfields

Absolutely correct—style, tailoring and price!! So carefully made that it has all the appearance of a custom tailored coat. Good quality **all wool melton.** Plenty of warmth and extra long wear. Hand felled silk faced velvet collar. Body and sleeves full lined with good weight Farr-Ray rayon serge. Length about 45 inches. **REGULAR SIZES—34 to 44 inches chest. EXTRA LARGE SIZES—46 to 50 inches chest. State measure taken over vest. Postpaid.**

45F8312—Black Regular Sizes........**$16.85**
45F8314—Oxford Gray. Regular Sizes. **16.85**
45F8313—Black Extra Large Sizes... **18.50**
45F8315 — Oxford Gray. Extra Large Sizes **$18.50**

A Big Bargain

Here's a coat, men, that's got everything! Style, warmth good looks, quality and a low price that we guarantee to have no equal. Try and wear out this rugged **thru-and-thru all wool plaid 32-ounce fabric.** Note the style—s w a g g e r double breasted box model with wide French facing, deep lapels and b r o a d comfortable collar. Deep yoke and sleeve lining of genuine F a r r-R a y guaranteed rayon satin. Length, 46 inches. **SIZES, 34 to 44 inches chest. State chest measure, also height, weight and age.**

45F8338—Medium Gray. Postpaid.......**$11.85**
45F8340—Medium Brown. Postpaid.... **11.85**

A REAL $22.50 VALUE ELSEWHERE

Mighty good looking and mighty low priced! That's what you men will say when you see this snappy, trimly tailored overcoat of **all wool** worsted finish fabric. The material is the product of the famous La Porte Mills, which is enough to guarantee its unusual quality. You'll be amazed that such an inexpensive coat will give you so much wear. Popular model with plain half belt to slightly shape the back. Tailored big and roomy. Generous yoke and sleeves lined with genuine Farr-Ray guaranteed rayon satin—the kind that will last as long as the coat. Length, 46 inches. **SIZES—34 to 44 inches chest. State chest measure taken over vest, also height, weight and age.**

45F8332—Dark Brown Herringbone All Wool. Postpaid. **$13.85**
45F8333—Dark Gray Herringbone All Wool. Postpaid

$13.85 Postpaid

REAL GALLOWAY Priced at a Saving

Finest Cow Hides

Men, you can beat old man winter at his own game when you wear one of these big, burly Galloways. Not only are they popular among college men, but men who have to buck tough, shivering zero weather find them unequalled for warmth. And this season we've hammered the price down a couple more notches to make it a real bargain! Just note the long hair! That's because we use only first quality hides. The hide is vegetable bark tanned especially treated to make it soft and pliable, non-shedding and odorless even when wet. Made with a huge collar which can be fastened snugly around neck. Sturdy loops and fasteners, body lining of quilted Venetian. Windproof, double knit wristlets. 50-inches long to give added protection. **SIZES—36 to 48 inches chest. State chest measure taken over vest, also height, weight and age.**

45F8350—Black Galloway Fur Coat. Postpaid...........**$37.50**

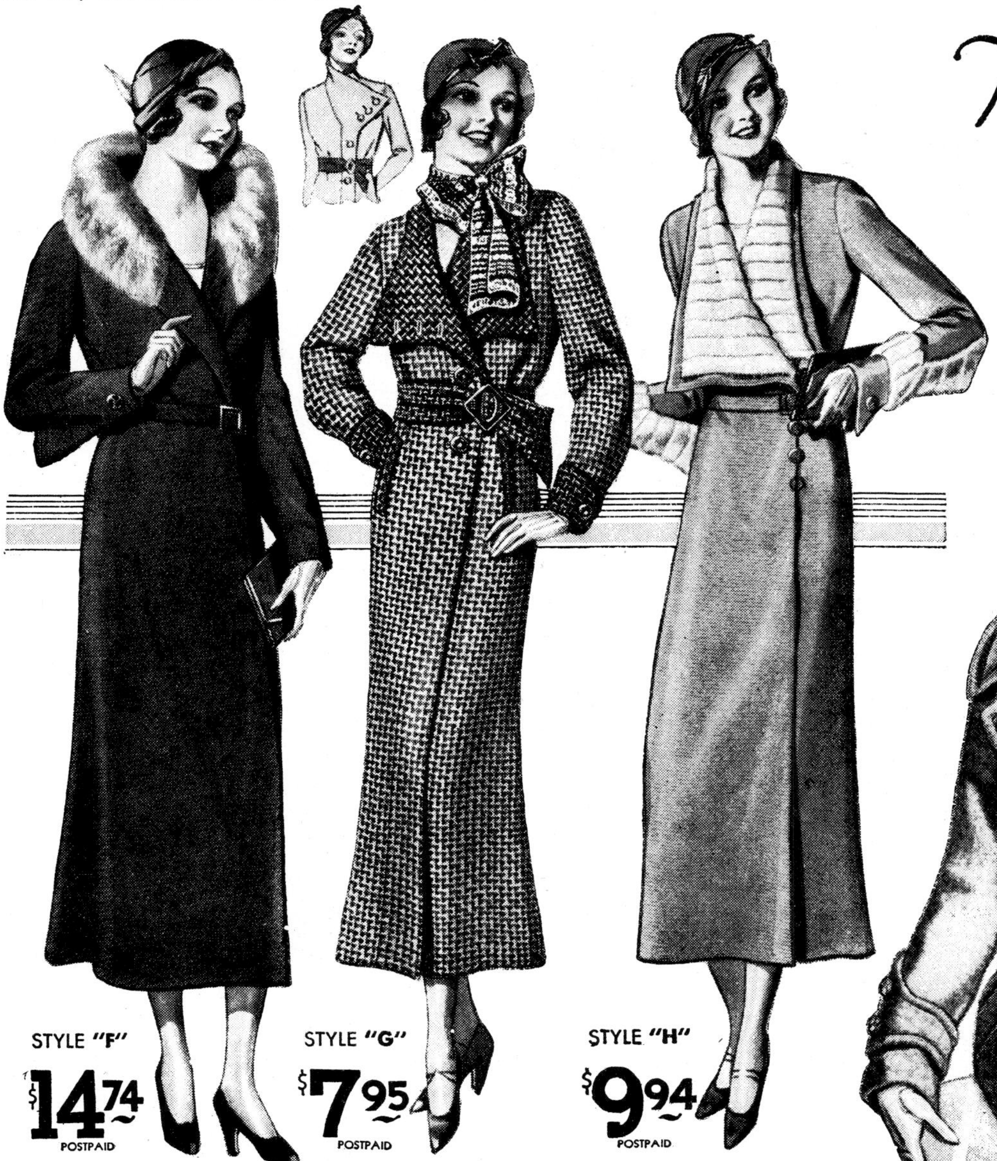

The Hit of the Season ... A POLO COAT

$6.97 POSTPAID

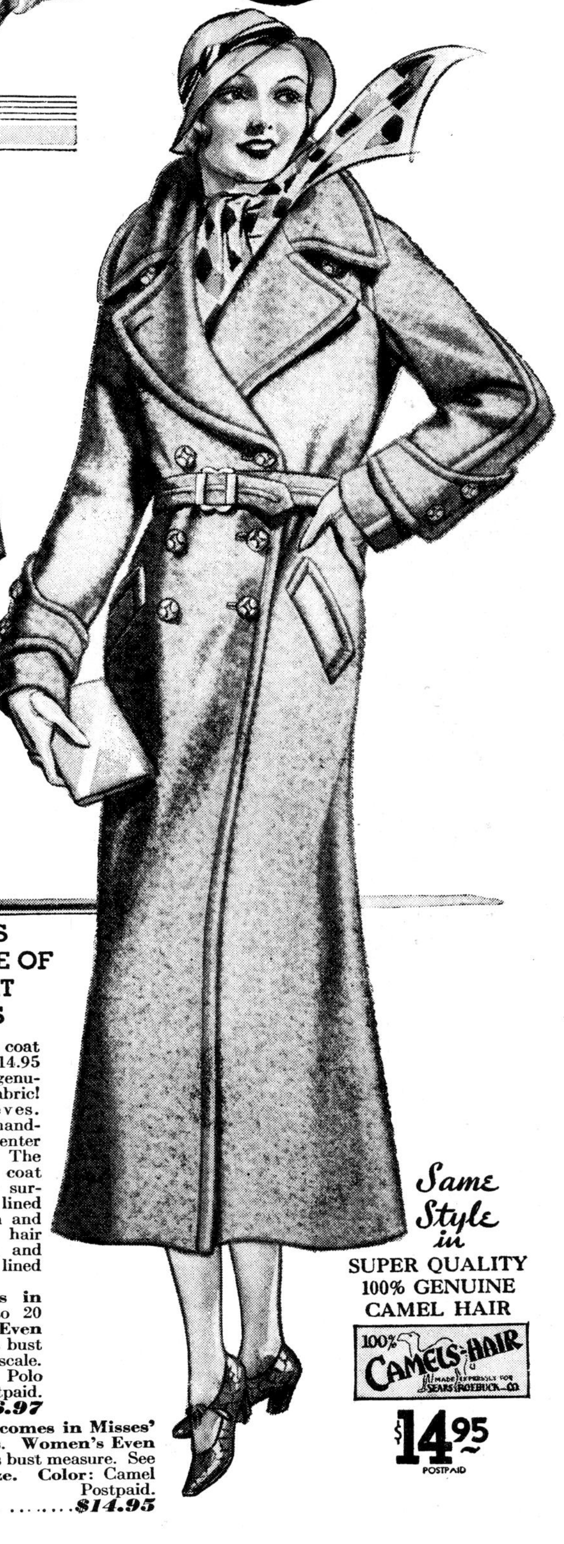

STYLE "F" $14.74 POSTPAID

STYLE "G" $7.95 POSTPAID

STYLE "H" $9.94 POSTPAID

DOWN GO COAT PRICES TO LOWEST LEVELS . . . .

STYLE **"F"** Nobody will deny that an All Wool coat, flatteringly collared with Genuine Pieced Squirrel is a thrilling "find" for only $14.74. The fabric is crisp, firm, smooth-finished All Wool Poiret Twill. Flaring tabs at the wrist give the effect of a gauntlet cuff. The belt alone breaks the seamless smoothness of the back. All Silk Crepe lining adds a bit of luxury. **Misses' Sizes**— 14 to 20 years; **Women's Sizes**—32 to 46 inches bust measure. See size scale. **Color:** Navy Blue with Blonde fur. **State actual bust measure.**
17H2365....................................Postpaid, ***$14.74***

STYLE **"G"** No matter how smart you consider this button-over collar . . . . you'll have to agree that the material is even more striking. Thick wool yarns twisted with a tiny strand of bright, glinting Rayon give a bold, vigorous character to this Tweed coat (three-fourths Wool, one-fourth Rayon) . . . and they are so decorative that we simply reversed the fabric for trimming. The back is shaped and fitted by side seamings, and the inside is lined with sparkling Rayon and Cotton. Scarf is not included. **Misses' Sizes**—14 to 20 years; **Women's Even Sizes**—32 to 44 inches bust measure. See size scale. **Colors:** Tan with Brown, or Medium Green with Dark Green. **State actual bust measure and color.**
17H2370....................................Postpaid, ***$7.95***

STYLE **"H"** Why spend a lot of money for real Lapin fur when this soft close-clipped Cotton Fur fabric gives the same effect—both to your eye and hand! . . . When it comes to you on this coat of fine, warm, All Wool Crepeolaine, a handsome new woolen! . . . When the coat is lined richly with this All Silk Crepe! Fine full length seamings give graceful fitted lines to the back. **Misses' Sizes**—14 to 20 years; **Women's Even Sizes**—32 to 46 inches bust measure. See size scale. **Colors:** Tan, or Black; both with Beige trimming. **State actual bust measure and color.**
17H2375....................................Postpaid, ***$9.94***

BE SURE TO STATE ACTUAL BUST MEASURE AND COLOR.

POLO COATS IN YOUR CHOICE OF TWO SMART 1932 FABRICS

Only $6.97 for a Polo coat that's All Wool! Only $14.95 for a Polo Coat that's genuine Camel Hair fabric! Roomy raglan sleeves. Loose fitted back with handsome over-topped center and side seams . . . The material in our $6.97 coat is soft, light, downy surfaced All Wool fabric, lined with sparkling Rayon and Cotton. The Camel hair cloth is thick, light and warm, and is richly lined with All Silk Crepe.

Wool coat comes in Misses' Sizes: 14 to 20 years. **Women's Even Sizes:** 32 to 42 inches bust measure. See size scale. **State size. Color:** Polo Tan. Postpaid.
17H2380......... ***$6.97***

Camel Hair coat comes in Misses' Sizes—14 to 20 years. **Women's Even Sizes**—32 to 40 inches bust measure. See size scale. **State size. Color:** Camel Tan. Postpaid.
17H2383.................. ***$14.95***

Same Style in SUPER QUALITY 100% GENUINE CAMEL HAIR

100% CAMEL'S-HAIR MADE EXPRESSLY FOR SEARS, ROEBUCK AND CO.

$14.95 POSTPAID

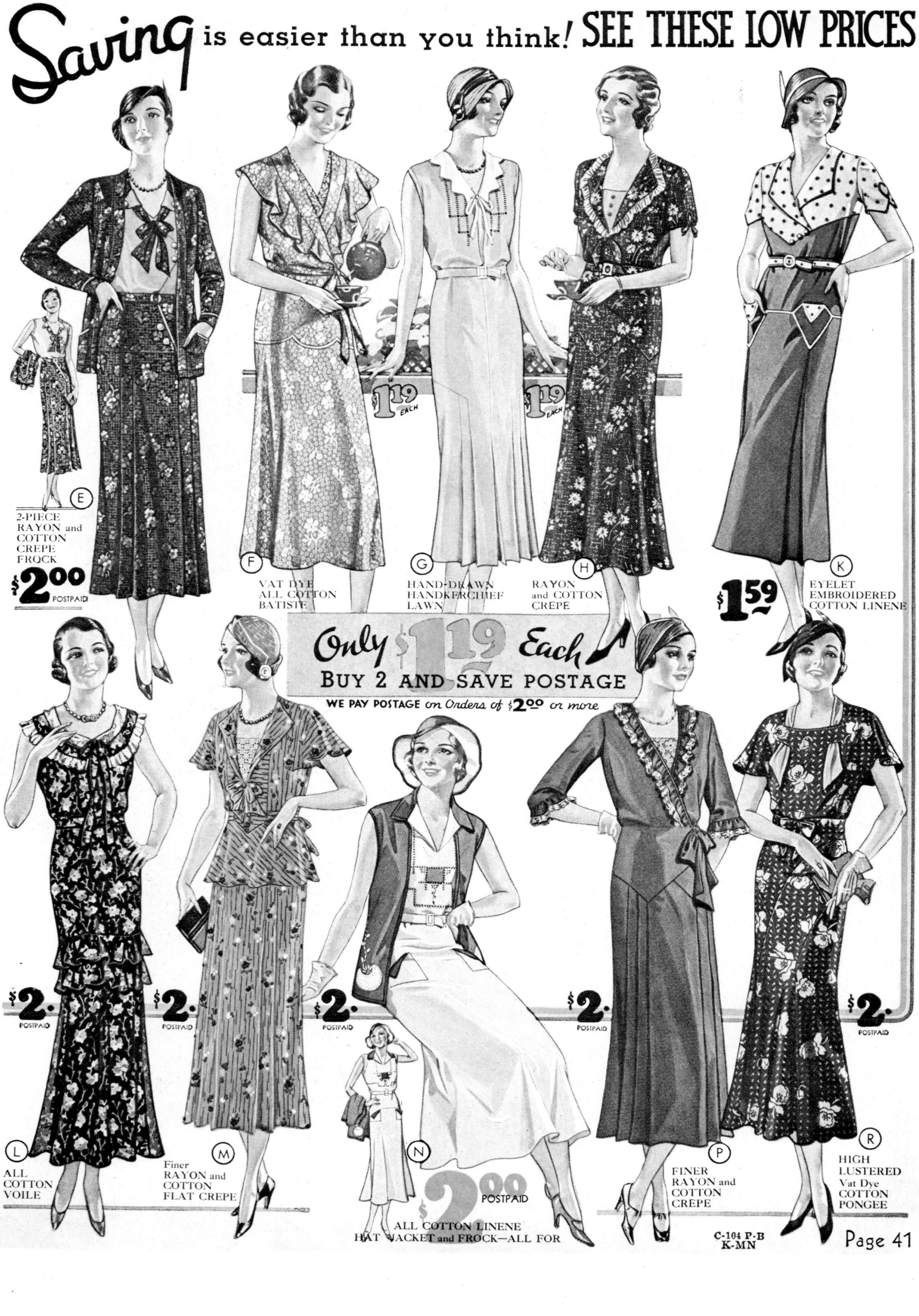

Saving is easier than you think! SEE THESE LOW PRICES

(E) 2-PIECE RAYON and COTTON CREPE FROCK $2.00 POSTPAID

(F) VAT DYE ALL COTTON BATISTE

(G) HAND-DRAWN HANDKERCHIEF LAWN

(H) RAYON and COTTON CREPE

$1.19 EACH

$1.19 EACH

(K) EYELET EMBROIDERED COTTON LINENE $1.59

Only $1.19 Each
BUY 2 AND SAVE POSTAGE
WE PAY POSTAGE on Orders of $2.00 or more

(L) ALL COTTON VOILE $2. POSTPAID

(M) Finer RAYON and COTTON FLAT CREPE $2. POSTPAID

(N) ALL COTTON LINENE HAT JACKET and FROCK—ALL FOR $2.00 POSTPAID

$2. POSTPAID

(P) FINER RAYON and COTTON CREPE $2. POSTPAID

(R) HIGH LUSTERED Vat Dye COTTON PONGEE $2. POSTPAID

C-104 P-B
K-MN

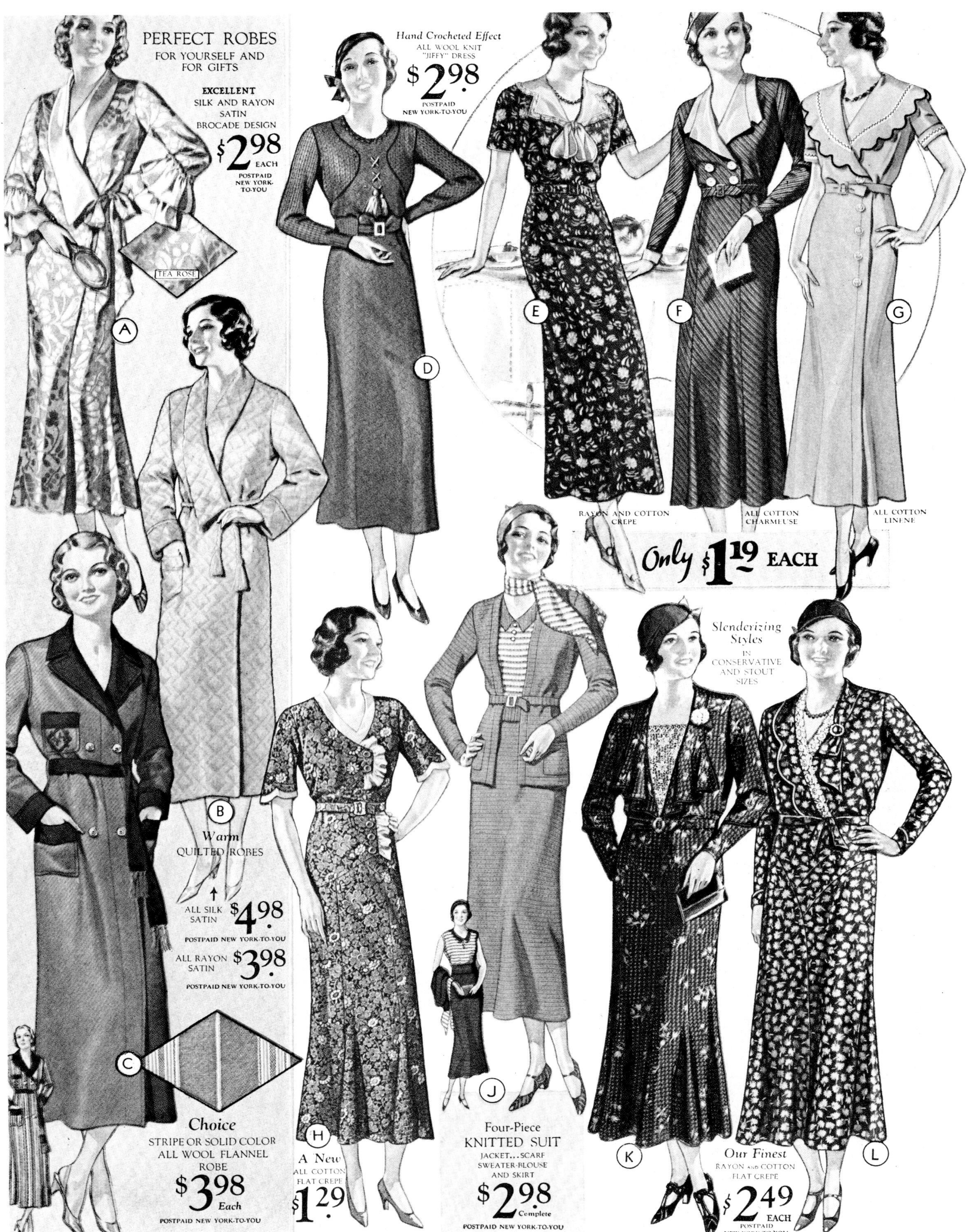
PERFECT ROBES
FOR YOURSELF AND FOR GIFTS
EXCELLENT
SILK AND RAYON SATIN
BROCADE DESIGN
$2.98 EACH
POSTPAID NEW YORK-TO-YOU
TEA ROSE
A
Hand Crocheted Effect
ALL WOOL KNIT "JIFFY" DRESS
$2.98
POSTPAID NEW YORK-TO-YOU
D
E
F
G
RAYON AND COTTON CREPE
ALL COTTON CHARMEUSE
ALL COTTON LINENE
Only $1.19 EACH
B
Warm
QUILTED ROBES
ALL SILK SATIN $4.98
POSTPAID NEW YORK-TO-YOU
ALL RAYON SATIN $3.98
POSTPAID NEW YORK-TO-YOU
C
Choice
STRIPE OR SOLID COLOR
ALL WOOL FLANNEL ROBE
$3.98 Each
POSTPAID NEW YORK-TO-YOU
H
A New
ALL COTTON FLAT CREPE
$1.29
J
Four-Piece
KNITTED SUIT
JACKET... SCARF
SWEATER-BLOUSE AND SKIRT
$2.98 Complete
POSTPAID NEW YORK-TO-YOU
Slenderizing Styles
IN CONSERVATIVE AND STOUT SIZES
K
L
Our Finest
RAYON AND COTTON FLAT CREPE
$2.49 EACH
POSTPAID NEW YORK-TO-YOU

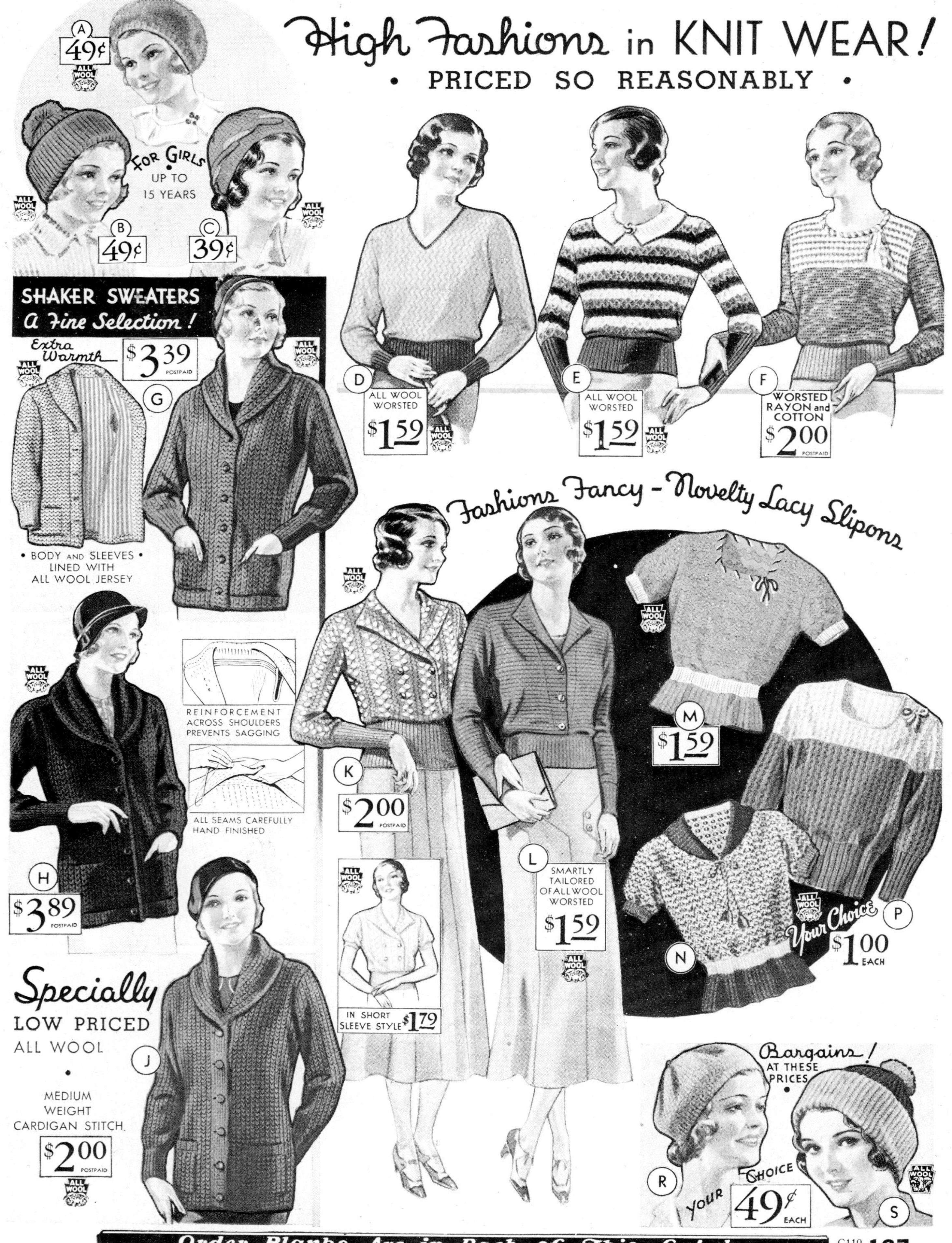
High Fashions in KNIT WEAR!
• PRICED SO REASONABLY •
A 49¢
FOR GIRLS UP TO 15 YEARS
B 49¢
C 39¢
SHAKER SWEATERS
A Fine Selection!
Extra Warmth
$3.39 POSTPAID
G
• BODY AND SLEEVES • LINED WITH ALL WOOL JERSEY
D ALL WOOL WORSTED $1.59
E ALL WOOL WORSTED $1.59
F WORSTED RAYON and COTTON $2.00 POSTPAID
Fashions Fancy - Novelty Lacy Slipons
REINFORCEMENT ACROSS SHOULDERS PREVENTS SAGGING
ALL SEAMS CAREFULLY HAND FINISHED
H $3.89 POSTPAID
K $2.00 POSTPAID
IN SHORT SLEEVE STYLE $1.79
L SMARTLY TAILORED OF ALL WOOL WORSTED $1.59
M $1.59
N
P
Your Choice $1.00 EACH
Specially LOW PRICED ALL WOOL
• MEDIUM WEIGHT CARDIGAN STITCH
$2.00 POSTPAID
J
Bargains! AT THESE PRICES •
R
S
YOUR CHOICE 49¢ EACH
ALL WOOL

FAMOUS
California Style Hats!
WIDELY ADVERTISED
Choice at Sensational Low Price
$1.95 Each

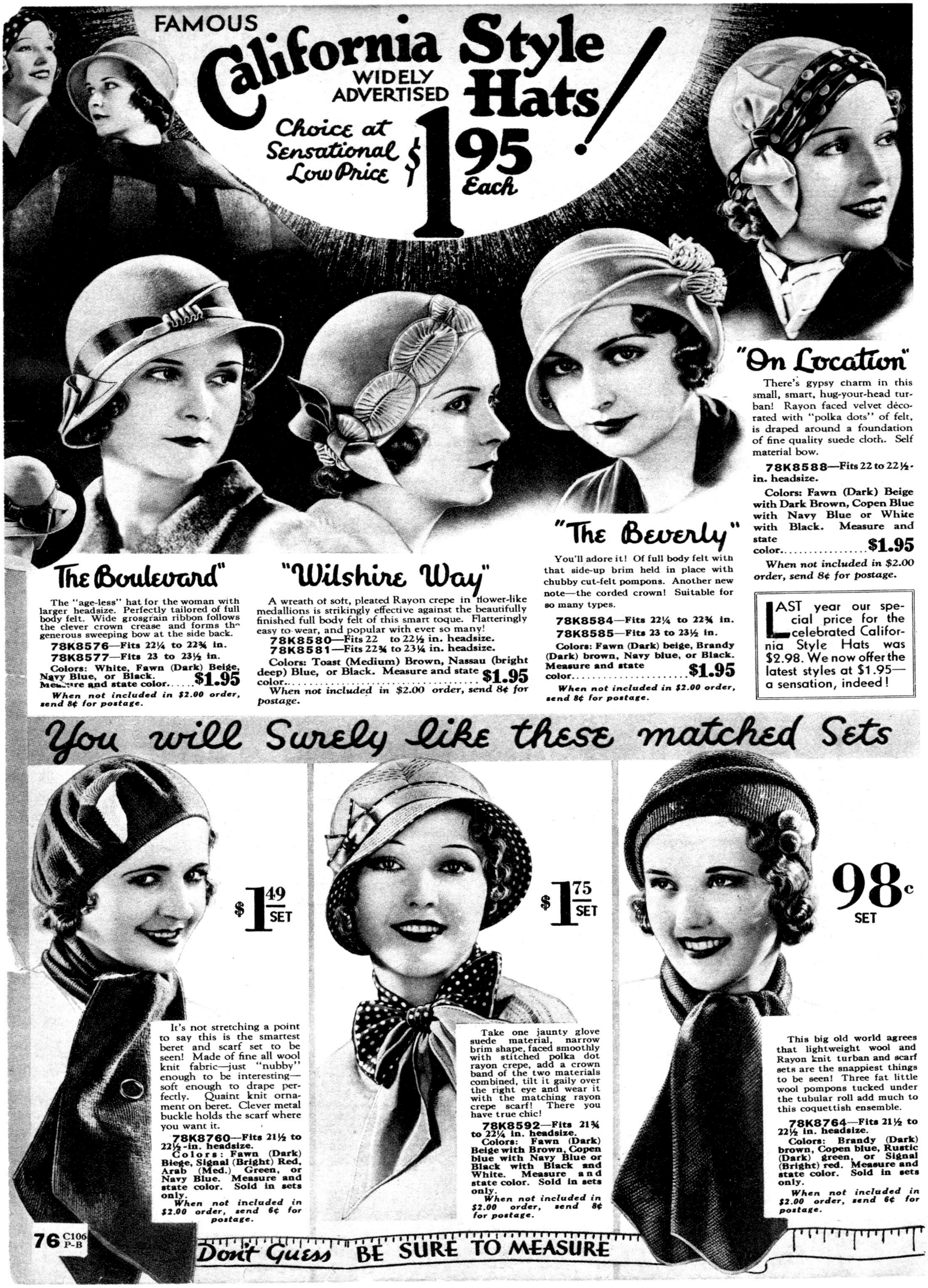

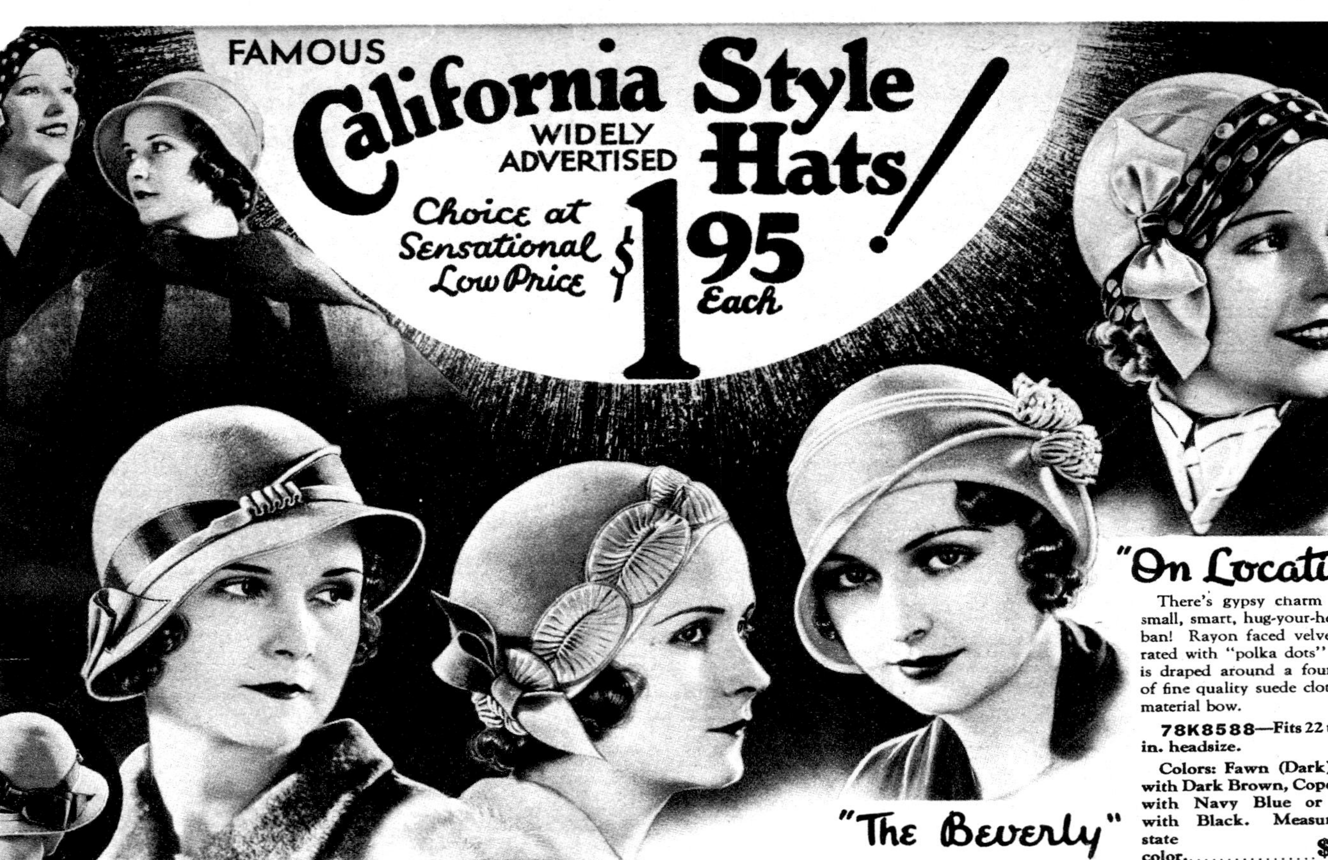

"On Location"

There's gypsy charm in this small, smart, hug-your-head turban! Rayon faced velvet déco-rated with "polka dots" of felt, is draped around a foundation of fine quality suede cloth. Self material bow.

78K8588—Fits 22 to 22½-in. headsize.

Colors: Fawn (Dark) Beige with Dark Brown, Copen Blue with Navy Blue or White with Black. Measure and state color.................$1.95

When not included in $2.00 order, send 8¢ for postage.

"The Beverly"

You'll adore it! Of full body felt with that side-up brim held in place with chubby cut-felt pompons. Another new note—the corded crown! Suitable for so many types.

78K8584—Fits 22¼ to 22¾ in.
78K8585—Fits 23 to 23½ in.

Colors: Fawn (Dark) beige, Brandy (Dark) brown, Navy blue, or Black. Measure and state color......................$1.95

When not included in $2.00 order, send 8¢ for postage.

"The Boulevard"

The "age-less" hat for the woman with larger headsize. Perfectly tailored of full body felt. Wide grosgrain ribbon follows the clever crown crease and forms the generous sweeping bow at the side back.

78K8576—Fits 22¼ to 22¾ in.
78K8577—Fits 23 to 23½ in.

Colors: White, Fawn (Dark) Beige, Navy Blue, or Black. Measure and state color.....$1.95

When not included in $2.00 order, send 8¢ for postage.

"Wilshire Way"

A wreath of soft, pleated Rayon crepe in flower-like medallions is strikingly effective against the beautifully finished full body felt of this smart toque. Flatteringly easy to wear, and popular with ever so many!

78K8580—Fits 22 to 22½ in. headsize.
78K8581—Fits 22¾ to 23¼ in. headsize.

Colors: Toast (Medium) Brown, Nassau (bright deep) Blue, or Black. Measure and state color....................................**$1.95**

When not included in $2.00 order, send 8¢ for postage.

LAST year our special price for the celebrated California Style Hats was $2.98. We now offer the latest styles at $1.95—a sensation, indeed!

You will Surely like these matched Sets

$1.49 SET

It's not stretching a point to say this is the smartest beret and scarf set to be seen! Made of fine all wool knit fabric—just "nubby" enough to be interesting—soft enough to drape perfectly. Quaint knit ornament on beret. Clever metal buckle holds the scarf where you want it.

78K8760—Fits 21½ to 22½-in. headsize.

Colors: Fawn (Dark) Biege, Signal (Bright) Red, Arab (Med.) Green, or Navy Blue. Measure and state color. Sold in sets only.

When not included in $2.00 order, send 6¢ for postage.

$1.75 SET

Take one jaunty glove suede material, narrow brim shape, faced smoothly with stitched polka dot rayon crepe, add a crown band of the two materials combined, tilt it gaily over the right eye and wear it with the matching rayon crepe scarf! There you have true chic!

78K8592—Fits 21¾ to 22¼ in. headsize.

Colors: Fawn (Dark) Beige with Brown, Copen blue with Navy Blue or Black with Black and White. Measure and state color. Sold in sets only.

When not included in $2.00 order, send 8¢ for postage.

98c SET

This big old world agrees that lightweight wool and Rayon knit turban and scarf sets are the snappiest things to be seen! Three fat little wool pompons tucked under the tubular roll add much to this coquettish ensemble.

78K8764—Fits 21½ to 22½ in. headsize.

Colors: Brandy (Dark) brown, Copen blue, Rustic (Dark) green, or Signal (Bright) red. Measure and state color. Sold in sets only.

When not included in $2.00 order, send 6¢ for postage.

Don't Guess BE SURE TO MEASURE

"Chassis-Bilt" Gives These Unusual Durability....

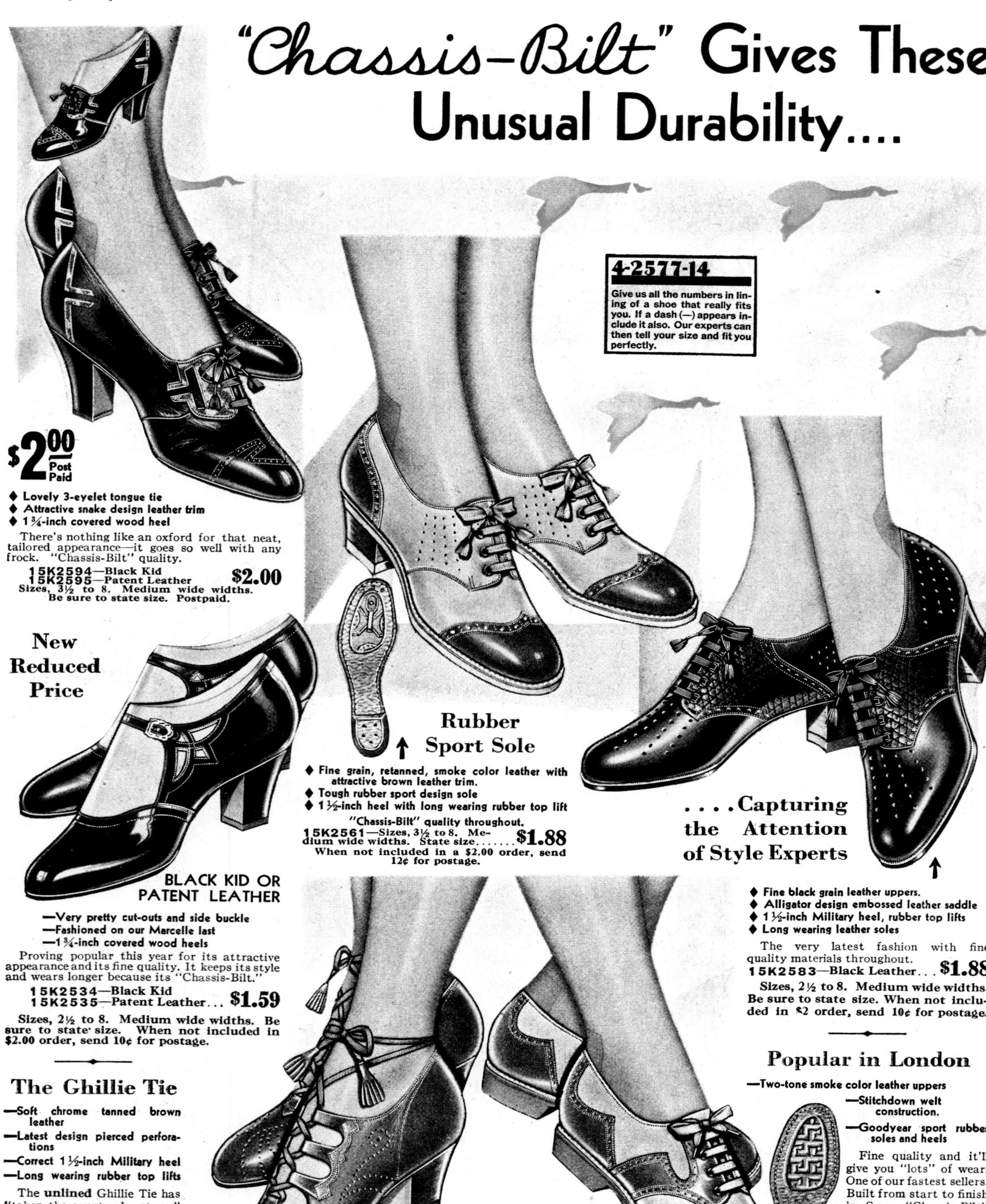

$2.00 Post Paid

- Lovely 3-eyelet tongue tie
- Attractive snake design leather trim
- 1¾-inch covered wood heel

There's nothing like an oxford for that neat, tailored appearance—it goes so well with any frock. "Chassis-Bilt" quality.

15K2594—Black Kid
15K2595—Patent Leather $2.00
Sizes, 3½ to 8. Medium wide widths. Be sure to state size. Postpaid.

New Reduced Price

BLACK KID OR PATENT LEATHER

—Very pretty cut-outs and side buckle
—Fashioned on our Marcelle last
—1¾-inch covered wood heels

Proving popular this year for its attractive appearance and its fine quality. It keeps its style and wears longer because its "Chassis-Bilt."

15K2534—Black Kid
15K2535—Patent Leather... $1.59
Sizes, 2½ to 8. Medium wide widths. Be sure to state size. When not included in $2.00 order, send 10¢ for postage.

The Ghillie Tie

—Soft chrome tanned brown leather
—Latest design pierced perforations
—Correct 1½-inch Military heel
—Long wearing rubber top lifts

The unlined Ghillie Tie has "taken the country by storm"—it's so popular. Suitable for all kinds of wear, and all occasions, they'll give service, too.

15K2562—Women's. Sizes, 2½ to 8. Medium wide widths. $1.49
State size. When not included in $2 order send 10¢ for postage.

Rubber Sport Sole

- Fine grain, retanned, smoke color leather with attractive brown leather trim.
- Tough rubber sport design sole
- 1½-inch heel with long wearing rubber top lift

"Chassis-Bilt" quality throughout.

15K2561—Sizes, 3½ to 8. Medium wide widths. State size....... $1.88
When not included in a $2.00 order, send 12¢ for postage.

....Capturing the Attention of Style Experts

- Fine black grain leather uppers.
- Alligator design embossed leather saddle
- 1½-inch Military heel, rubber top lifts
- Long wearing leather soles

The very latest fashion with fine quality materials throughout.

15K2583—Black Leather... $1.88
Sizes, 2½ to 8. Medium wide widths. Be sure to state size. When not included in $2 order, send 10¢ for postage.

Popular in London

—Two-tone smoke color leather uppers
—Stitchdown welt construction.
—Goodyear sport rubber soles and heels

Fine quality and it'll give you "lots" of wear. One of our fastest sellers. Built from start to finish in Sears "Chassis-Bilt" way. Read Page 270.

15K2559 Smoke color. $1.49
Sizes, 2½ to 8. Medium Wide Width. State size. When not included in a $2 order, send 10¢ for postage.

BRIDGE SLIPPER

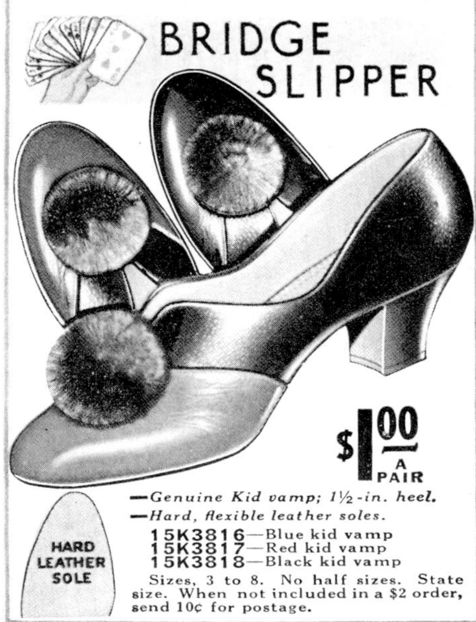

$1.00 A PAIR

HARD LEATHER SOLE

—*Genuine Kid vamp; 1½-in. heel.*
—*Hard, flexible leather soles.*
15K3816—Blue kid vamp
15K3817—Red kid vamp
15K3818—Black kid vamp
Sizes, 3 to 8. No half sizes. State size. When not included in a $2 order, send 10¢ for postage.

UTILITY SLIPPER

If in Doubt About Size Give All Numbers in Old Shoe

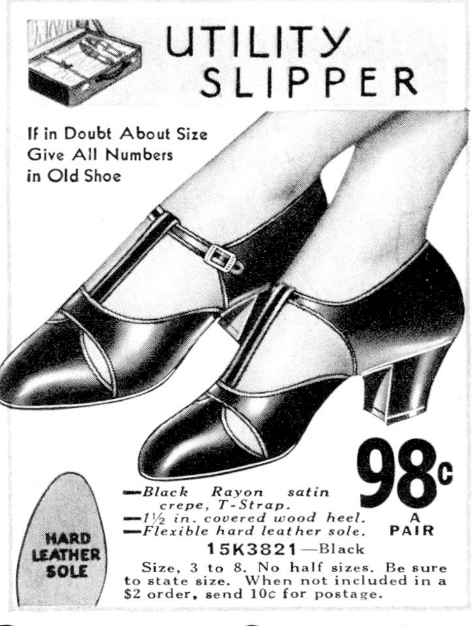

98c A PAIR

HARD LEATHER SOLE

—*Black Rayon satin crepe, T-Strap.*
—*1½ in. covered wood heel.*
—*Flexible hard leather sole.*
15K3821—Black
Size, 3 to 8. No half sizes. Be sure to state size. When not included in a $2 order, send 10¢ for postage.

STYLISH COMFORT

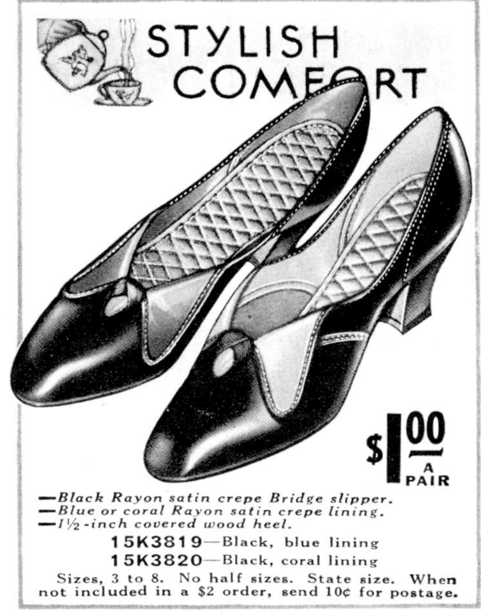

$1.00 A PAIR

—*Black Rayon satin crepe Bridge slipper.*
—*Blue or coral Rayon satin crepe lining.*
—*1½-inch covered wood heel.*
15K3819—Black, blue lining
15K3820—Black, coral lining
Sizes, 3 to 8. No half sizes. State size. When not included in a $2 order, send 10¢ for postage.

for GIFTS or for YOURSELF

All Slippers on This Page in Gift Box, on Request. See First Index Page.

The secret of long wear in Felt slippers is the weight of the felt. Sears use only heavyweight felts in the construction of their slippers. Heavyweight means longer life and more lasting beauty. When you compare prices be sure to compare the thickness and quality of the felt.

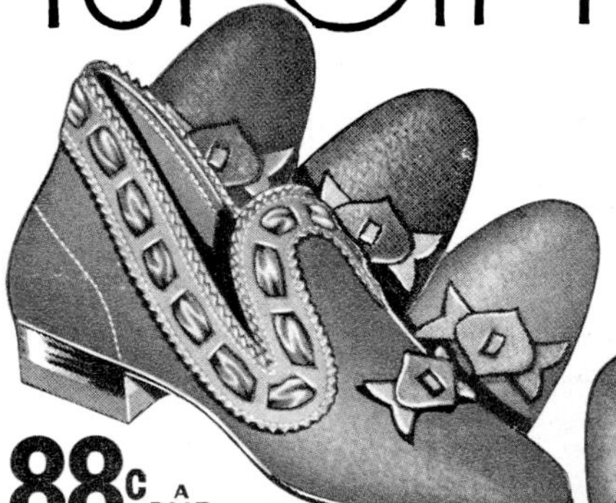

88c A PAIR

—*Good warm felt uppers.*
—*Neatly trimmed with ribbon and vamp ornament.*
—*Low heels with rubber top lifts and flexible hard leather soles.*
15K3736—Wine
15K3738—Blue
15K3739—Gray
15K3764—Buff
Per Pair 88c
Sizes, 3 to 9. No half sizes. Wide widths only. State size. When not included in a $2 order, send 10¢ for postage.

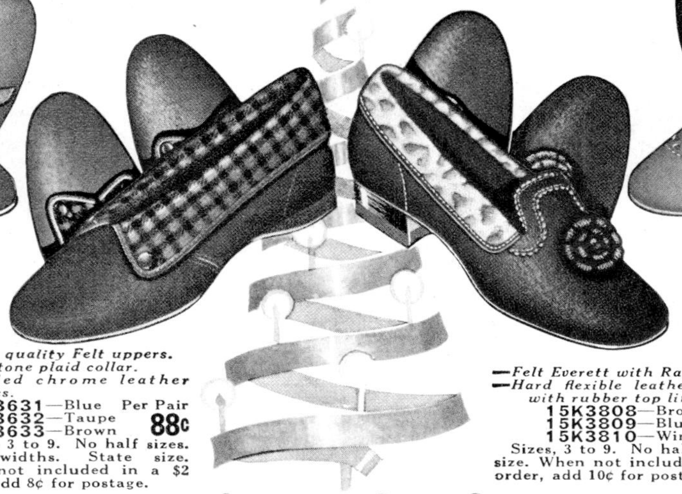

—*Extra quality Felt uppers.*
—*Two-tone plaid collar.*
—*Padded chrome leather soles.*
15K3631—Blue
15K3632—Taupe
15K3633—Brown
Per Pair 88c
Sizes, 3 to 9. No half sizes. Wide widths. State size. When not included in a $2 order, add 8¢ for postage.

—*Felt Everett with Rayon velvet collar.*
—*Hard flexible leather soles; low heels with rubber top lift.*
15K3808—Brown
15K3809—Blue
15K3810—Wine
95c
Sizes, 3 to 9. No half sizes. State size. When not included in a $2 order, add 10¢ for postage.

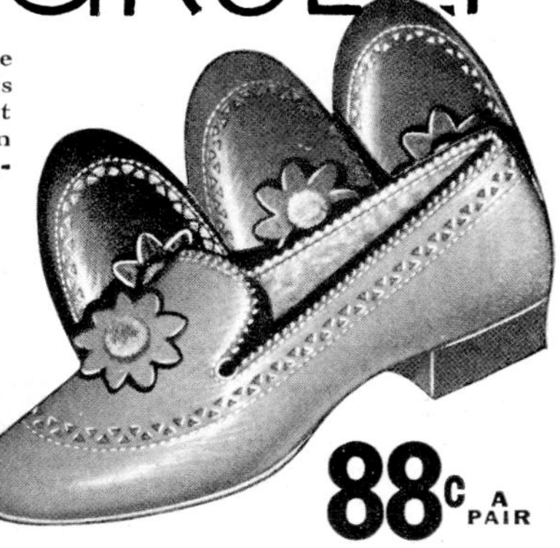

88c A PAIR

—*Genuine leather Everett slippers.*
—*Soft padded chrome leather soles.*
—*Medium round toe, low rubber heels.*
15K3800—Red 15K3801—Blue
15K3802—Black 15K3803—Brown
Sizes, 3 to 9. No half sizes. Wide widths only. State size. When not included in a $2 order, send 10¢ for postage.

SAVE AT SEARS

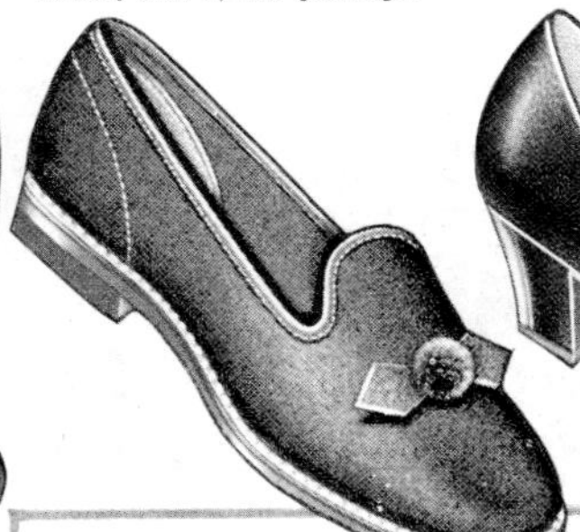

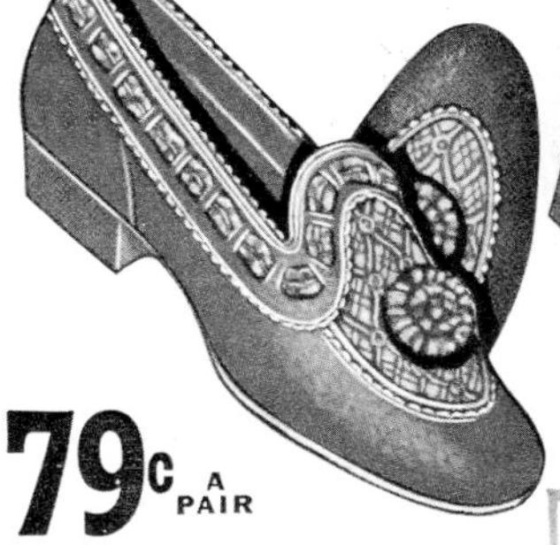

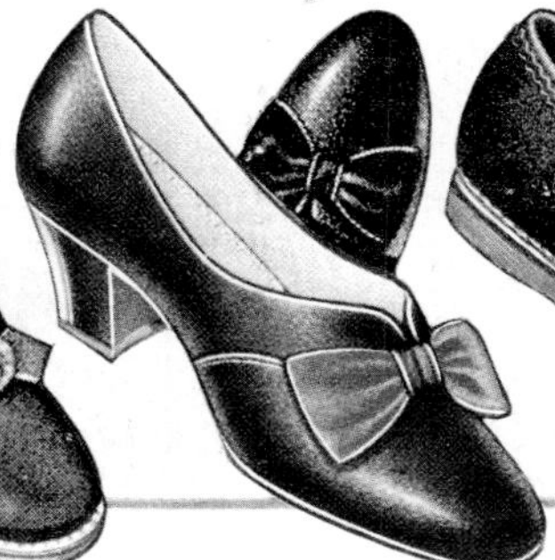

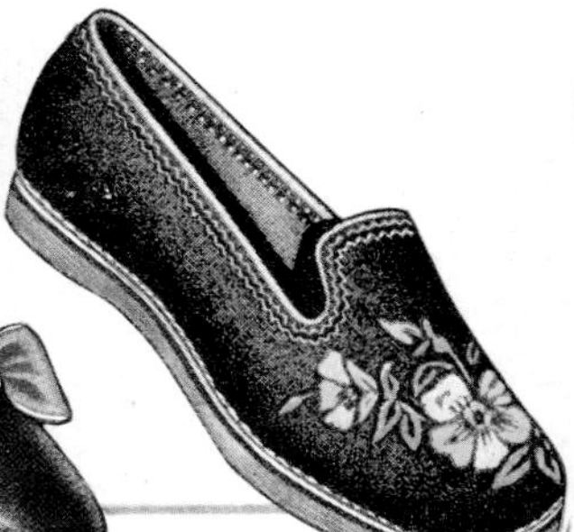

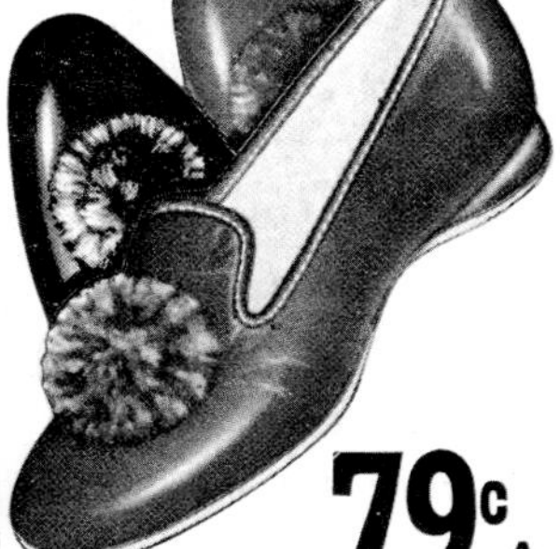

79c A PAIR

Very New

—*Felt slippers with Rayon trimmed moccasin effect.*
—*Padded chrome leather soles.*
—*Long wearing rubber heels.*
15K3709—Wine
15K3710—Blue.......... 79c
Sizes, 3 to 9. No half sizes. Wide widths only. State size. When not included in a $2 order, add 10¢ for postage.

Warmth

—*Gray felt Everett style.*
—*Good quality hard leather soles of flexible stitch-down construction.*
—*Well made throughout.*
15K3606—Women's Sizes, 3 to 9............ 79c
No half sizes. Wide widths only. Be sure to state size. When not included in a $2 order, add 10¢ for postage.

A Beauty

—*Bridge style slipper of "Shuskin" fabric.*
—*Rayon velvet bow.*
—*Soft padded chrome leather soles.*
—*1½-inch heel.*
15K3806—Blue.
15K3807—Black. 79c
Sizes, 3 to 8. No half sizes. State size. Wide widths. When not included in a $2 order, add 10c for postage.

Comfort

—*Black felt Everetts.*
—*Durable and long wearing hair felt soles.*
—*Floral pattern on vamp.*
The ideal comfortable House Slipper at a price within the reach of all.
15K3629—Black. Women's. Sizes 3 to 9. No half sizes......... 65c
State size. Wide widths. When not included in a $2 order, send 8¢ for postage.

79c A PAIR

Durable

—*Fine quality, good looking Genuine Kid uppers.*
—*Padded chrome leather soles, so comfortable.*
—*Very flexible throughout.*
15K3725—Black
15K3726—Brown
15K3727—Blue...... 79c
Sizes, 3 to 9. No half sizes. Be sure to state size. Wide widths. When not included in a $2.00 order, send 10¢ for postage.

Practical Dress Raincoats . . .

- Nationally Advertised Doubleweight Buckskein
- 100% WATERPROOF
- Guaranteed Fadeproof and Windproof
- WASHABLE

Handsome Plaid Lining

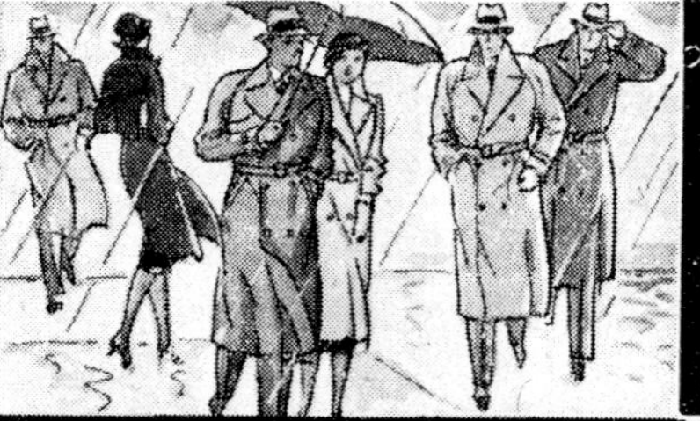

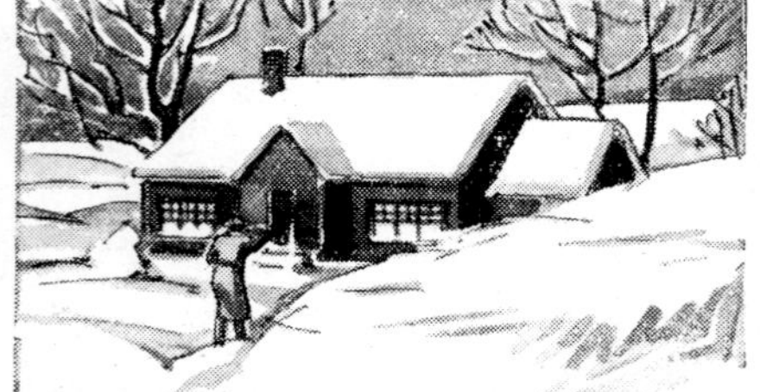

DURABLE TRENCH MODEL

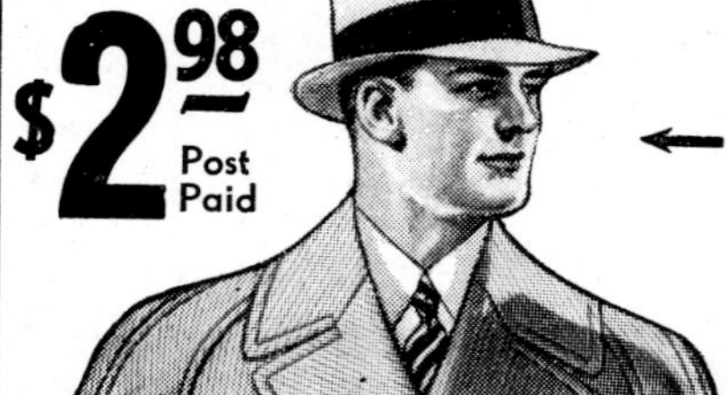

$2.98 Post Paid

—Light tan cotton twill trench coat.
—Rainproof and windproof throughout.
—Twill vulcanized with live rubber to a fast color plaid lining.
—Genuine leather buckles and buttons.
—Large convertible collar with storm tab.
—Extra 48 inches long, giving complete protection.

King of the style parade! Its dressy, well-tailored lines fairly sparkle with style. A Trench Coat whose sturdy, weather-defying fabric is just as practical as a top coat or a raincoat. Raglan sleeves and large convertible collar. Roomy slash pockets and all-around belt. Adjustable straps with leather buckles on sleeves. SIZES, 34 to 48 inches chest. State chest measurements taken over vest; also age, weight and height.

45K6457—Twill Weave Tan Gabardine. Postpaid................ $2.98

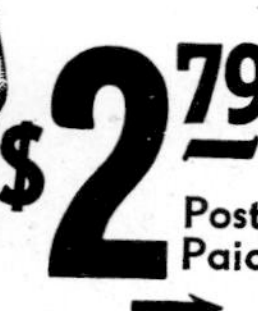

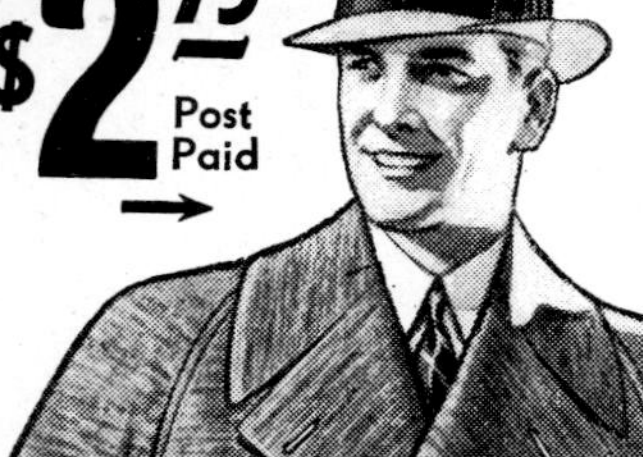

$2.79 Post Paid

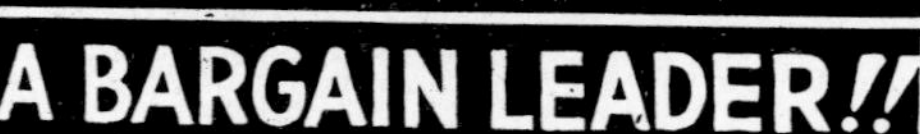

A BARGAIN LEADER!!

—Serviceable Cotton Jersey Knit fabrics.
—Rainproof and windproof.
—Jersey Vulcanized with live rubber to a fast color plaid lining.
—Leak proof, double stitched seams.
—Large convertible collar.

A coat that gives service 52 weeks out of the year—a topcoat in chilly weather—a raincoat in the wet season, a style leader on any day. An all-around serviceable coat at a big saving. Raglan sleeves, all around belt with buckle, adjustable sleeve straps with buckles to match. Patch pockets with flaps. 46 inches long. SIZES—34 to 48 inches chest. State measurements taken over vest, also age, weight and height.

45K6463—Medium Dark Gray Cotton Jersey Knit. Postpaid.................. $2.79

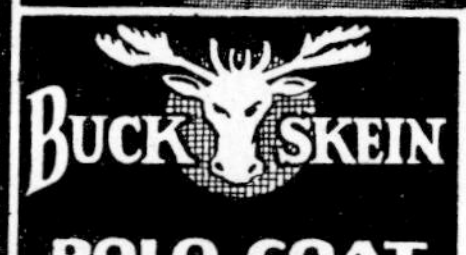

POLO COAT

$4.95 Postpaid

- Soft, sturdy leather-like cotton suede.
- Withstands 40 lbs. water pressure.
- Double-stitched seams, absolutely leak-proof.
- Fast color handsome plaid lining.
- New Polo Model . . . belt all around.
- Genuine leather buttons and buckle.
- Adjustable storm tabs on sleeves.

The greatest top coat and rain coat combination ever offered. Nationally advertised "Buckskein" fabric, 100% waterproofed by special Du Pont process. You could play a firehose on it and not a drop of water could seep through. Wears like saddle leather. Washes as easily clean as a handkerchief. 48 in. long.

SIZES—34 to 46 in. chest. State chest measurement, taken over vest; also age, height and weight.

45K6450—Medium Brown Buckskein Coat. Postpaid...................................... $4.95

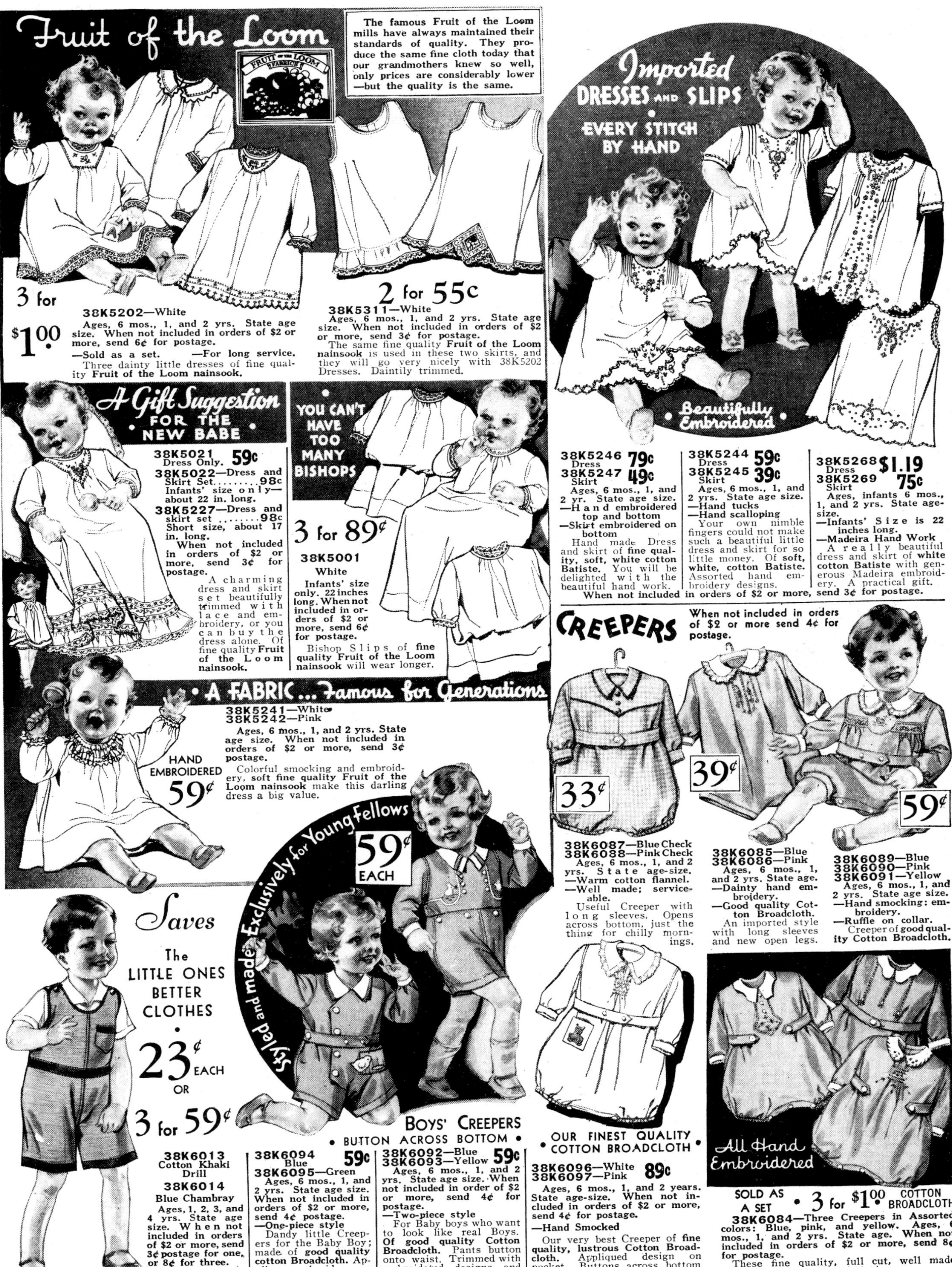
Fruit of the Loom
The famous Fruit of the Loom mills have always maintained their standards of quality. They produce the same fine cloth today that our grandmothers knew so well, only prices are considerably lower—but the quality is the same.
3 for $1.00
38K5202—White
Ages, 6 mos., 1, and 2 yrs. State age size. When not included in orders of $2 or more, send 6¢ for postage.
—Sold as a set. —For long service.
Three dainty little dresses of fine quality Fruit of the Loom nainsook.
2 for 55c
38K5311—White
Ages, 6 mos., 1, and 2 yrs. State age size. When not included in orders of $2 or more, send 3¢ for postage.
The same fine quality Fruit of the Loom nainsook is used in these two skirts, and they will go very nicely with 38K5202 Dresses. Daintily trimmed.
Imported DRESSES AND SLIPS
EVERY STITCH BY HAND
Beautifully Embroidered
38K5246 Dress 79c
38K5247 Skirt 49c
Ages, 6 mos., 1, and 2 yr. State age size.
—Hand embroidered top and bottom
—Skirt embroidered on bottom
Hand made Dress and skirt of fine quality, soft, white cotton Batiste. You will be delighted with the beautiful hand work.
38K5244 Dress 59c
38K5245 Skirt 39c
Ages, 6 mos., 1, and 2 yrs. State age size.
—Hand tucks
—Hand scalloping
Your own nimble fingers could not make such a beautiful little dress and skirt for so little money. Of soft, white, cotton Batiste. Assorted hand embroidery designs.
38K5268 Dress $1.19
38K5269 Skirt 75c
Ages, infants 6 mos., 1, and 2 yrs. State age-size.
—Infants' Size is 22 inches long.
—Madeira Hand Work
A really beautiful dress and skirt of white cotton Batiste with generous Madeira embroidery. A practical gift.
When not included in orders of $2 or more, send 3¢ for postage.
A Gift Suggestion FOR THE NEW BABE
38K5021 Dress Only. 59c
38K5022—Dress and Skirt Set.........98c
Infants' size only—about 22 in. long.
38K5227—Dress and skirt set 98c
Short size, about 17 in. long.
When not included in orders of $2 or more, send 3¢ for postage.
A charming dress and skirt set beautifully trimmed with lace and embroidery, or you can buy the dress alone. Of fine quality Fruit of the Loom nainsook.
YOU CAN'T HAVE TOO MANY BISHOPS
3 for 89¢
38K5001
White
Infants' size only. 22 inches long. When not included in orders of $2 or more, send 6¢ for postage.
Bishop Slips of fine quality Fruit of the Loom nainsook will wear longer.
A FABRIC... Famous for Generations
38K5241—White
38K5242—Pink
Ages, 6 mos., 1, and 2 yrs. State age size. When not included in orders of $2 or more, send 3¢ postage.
HAND EMBROIDERED 59¢
Colorful smocking and embroidery, soft fine quality Fruit of the Loom nainsook make this darling dress a big value.
CREEPERS
When not included in orders of $2 or more send 4¢ for postage.
33¢
39¢
59¢
38K6087—Blue Check
38K6088—Pink Check
Ages, 6 mos., 1, and 2 yrs. State age-size.
—Warm cotton flannel.
—Well made; serviceable.
Useful Creeper with long sleeves. Opens across bottom, just the thing for chilly mornings.
38K6085—Blue
38K6086—Pink
Ages, 6 mos., 1, and 2 yrs. State age.
—Dainty hand embroidery.
—Good quality Cotton Broadcloth.
An imported style with long sleeves and new open legs.
38K6089—Blue
38K6090—Pink
38K6091—Yellow
Ages, 6 mos., 1, and 2 yrs. State age size.
—Hand smocking: embroidery.
—Ruffle on collar.
Creeper of good quality Cotton Broadcloth.
Styled and made Exclusively for Young Fellows
59¢ EACH
Saves The LITTLE ONES BETTER CLOTHES
23¢ EACH OR 3 for 59¢
38K6013
Cotton Khaki Drill
38K6014
Blue Chambray
Ages, 1, 2, 3, and 4 yrs. State age size. When not included in orders of $2 or more, send 3¢ postage for one, or 8¢ for three.
Serviceable little overalls.
BOYS' CREEPERS
BUTTON ACROSS BOTTOM
38K6094 Blue 59c
38K6095—Green
Ages, 6 mos., 1, and 2 yrs. State age size. When not included in orders of $2 or more, send 4¢ postage.
—One-piece style
Dandy little Creepers for the Baby Boy; made of good quality cotton Broadcloth. Applique embroidery on pocket.
38K6092—Blue
38K6093—Yellow 59c
Ages, 6 mos., 1, and 2 yrs. State age size. When not included in order of $2 or more, send 4¢ for postage.
—Two-piece style
For Baby boys who want to look like real Boys. Of good quality Cotton Broadcloth. Pants button onto waist. Trimmed with embroidered designs and neatly piped.
OUR FINEST QUALITY COTTON BROADCLOTH
38K6096—White
38K6097—Pink 89c
Ages, 6 mos., 1, and 2 years. State age-size. When not included in orders of $2 or more, send 4¢ for postage.
—Hand Smocked
Our very best Creeper of fine quality, lustrous Cotton Broadcloth. Appliqued design on pocket. Buttons across bottom with envelope flap. Long sleeves.
All Hand Embroidered
SOLD AS A SET • 3 for $1.00 COTTON BROADCLOTH
38K6084—Three Creepers in Assorted colors: Blue, pink, and yellow. Ages, 6 mos., 1, and 2 yrs. State age. When not included in orders of $2 or more, send 8¢ for postage.
These fine quality, full cut, well made creepers are a distinct bargain.
Do Your Christmas Shopping From This Catalog
C101 P-B 149

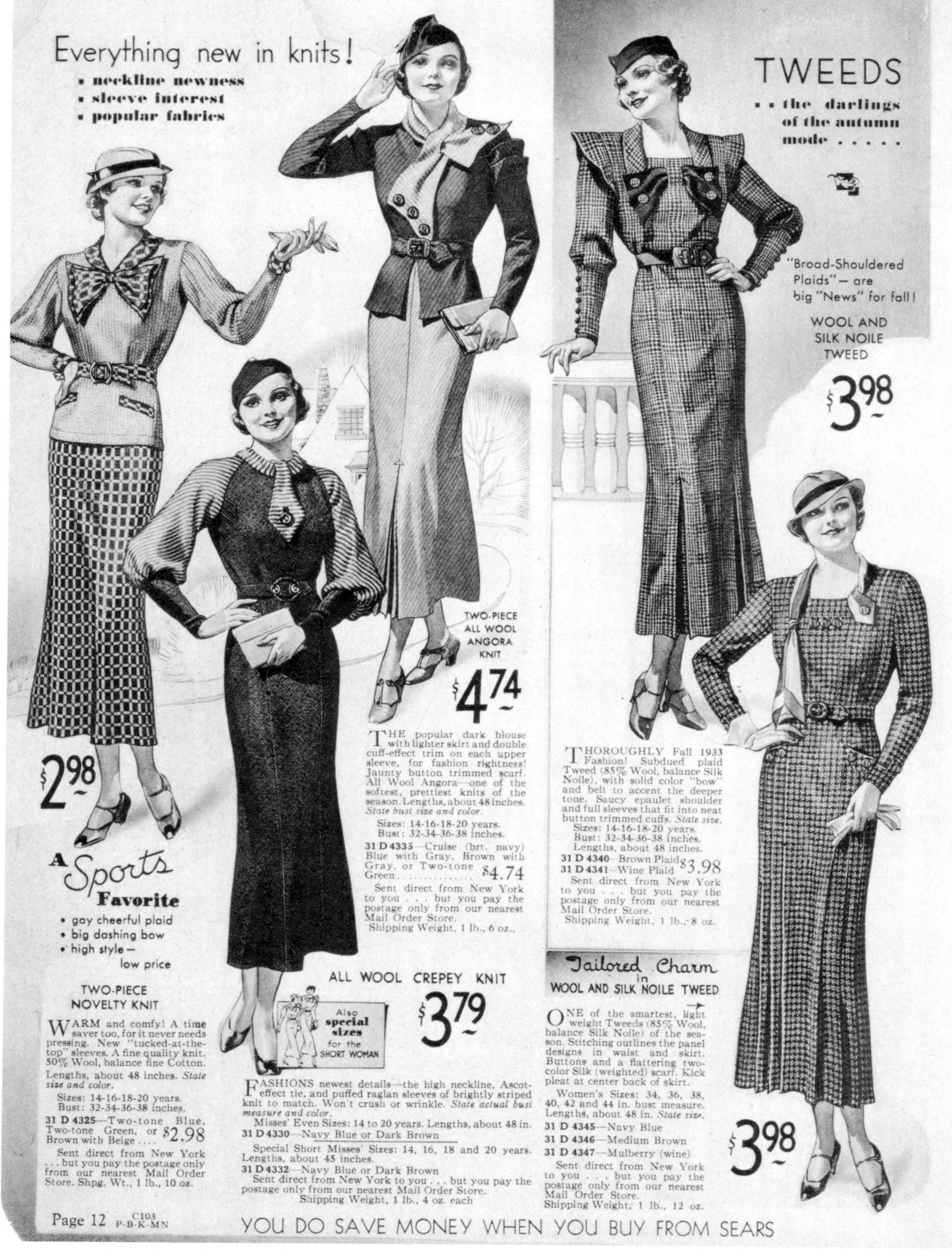
Everything new in knits!
• neckline newness
• sleeve interest
• popular fabrics
TWEEDS
• • the darlings of the autumn mode . . . . .
"Broad-Shouldered Plaids"— are big "News" for fall!
WOOL AND SILK NOILE TWEED
$3.98
TWO-PIECE ALL WOOL ANGORA KNIT
$4.74
THE popular dark blouse with lighter skirt and double cuff-effect trim on each upper sleeve, for fashion rightness! Jaunty button trimmed scarf. All Wool Angora—one of the softest, prettiest knits of the season. Lengths, about 48 inches. State bust size and color.
Sizes: 14-16-18-20 years.
Bust: 32-34-36-38 inches.
31 D 4335—Cruise (brt. navy) Blue with Gray, Brown with Gray, or Two-tone Green $4.74
Sent direct from New York to you . . . but you pay the postage only from our nearest Mail Order Store.
Shipping Weight, 1 lb., 6 oz.
THOROUGHLY Fall 1933 Fashion! Subdued plaid Tweed (85% Wool, balance Silk Noile), with solid color "bow" and belt to accent the deeper tone. Saucy epaulet shoulder and full sleeves that fit into neat button trimmed cuffs. State size.
Sizes: 14-16-18-20 years.
Bust: 32-34-36-38 inches.
Lengths, about 48 inches.
31 D 4340—Brown Plaid
31 D 4341—Wine Plaid $3.98
Sent direct from New York to you . . . but you pay the postage only from our nearest Mail Order Store.
Shipping Weight, 1 lb., 8 oz.
$2.98
A Sports Favorite
• gay cheerful plaid
• big dashing bow
• high style— low price
TWO-PIECE NOVELTY KNIT
WARM and comfy! A time saver too, for it never needs pressing. New "tucked-at-the-top" sleeves. A fine quality knit. 50% Wool, balance fine Cotton. Lengths, about 48 inches. State size and color.
Sizes: 14-16-18-20 years.
Bust: 32-34-36-38 inches.
31 D 4325—Two-tone Blue, Two-tone Green, or Brown with Beige $2.98
Sent direct from New York . . . but you pay the postage only from our nearest Mail Order Store. Shpg. Wt., 1 lb., 10 oz.
ALL WOOL CREPEY KNIT
Also special sizes for the SHORT WOMAN
$3.79
FASHIONS newest details—the high neckline, Ascot-effect tie, and puffed raglan sleeves of brightly striped knit to match. Won't crush or wrinkle. State actual bust measure and color.
Misses' Even Sizes: 14 to 20 years. Lengths, about 48 in.
31 D 4330—Navy Blue or Dark Brown
Special Short Misses' Sizes: 14, 16, 18 and 20 years. Lengths, about 45 inches.
31 D 4332—Navy Blue or Dark Brown
Sent direct from New York to you . . . but you pay the postage only from our nearest Mail Order Store.
Shipping Weight, 1 lb., 4 oz. each
Tailored Charm in WOOL AND SILK NOILE TWEED
ONE of the smartest, light weight Tweeds (85% Wool, balance Silk Noile) of the season. Stitching outlines the panel designs in waist and skirt. Buttons and a flattering two-color Silk (weighted) scarf. Kick pleat at center back of skirt.
Women's Sizes: 34, 36, 38, 40, 42 and 44 in. bust measure. Lengths, about 48 in. State size.
31 D 4345—Navy Blue
31 D 4346—Medium Brown
31 D 4347—Mulberry (wine)
Sent direct from New York to you . . . but you pay the postage only from our nearest Mail Order Store.
Shipping Weight, 1 lb., 12 oz.
$3.98
Page 12 C103 P-B-K-MN
YOU DO SAVE MONEY WHEN YOU BUY FROM SEARS

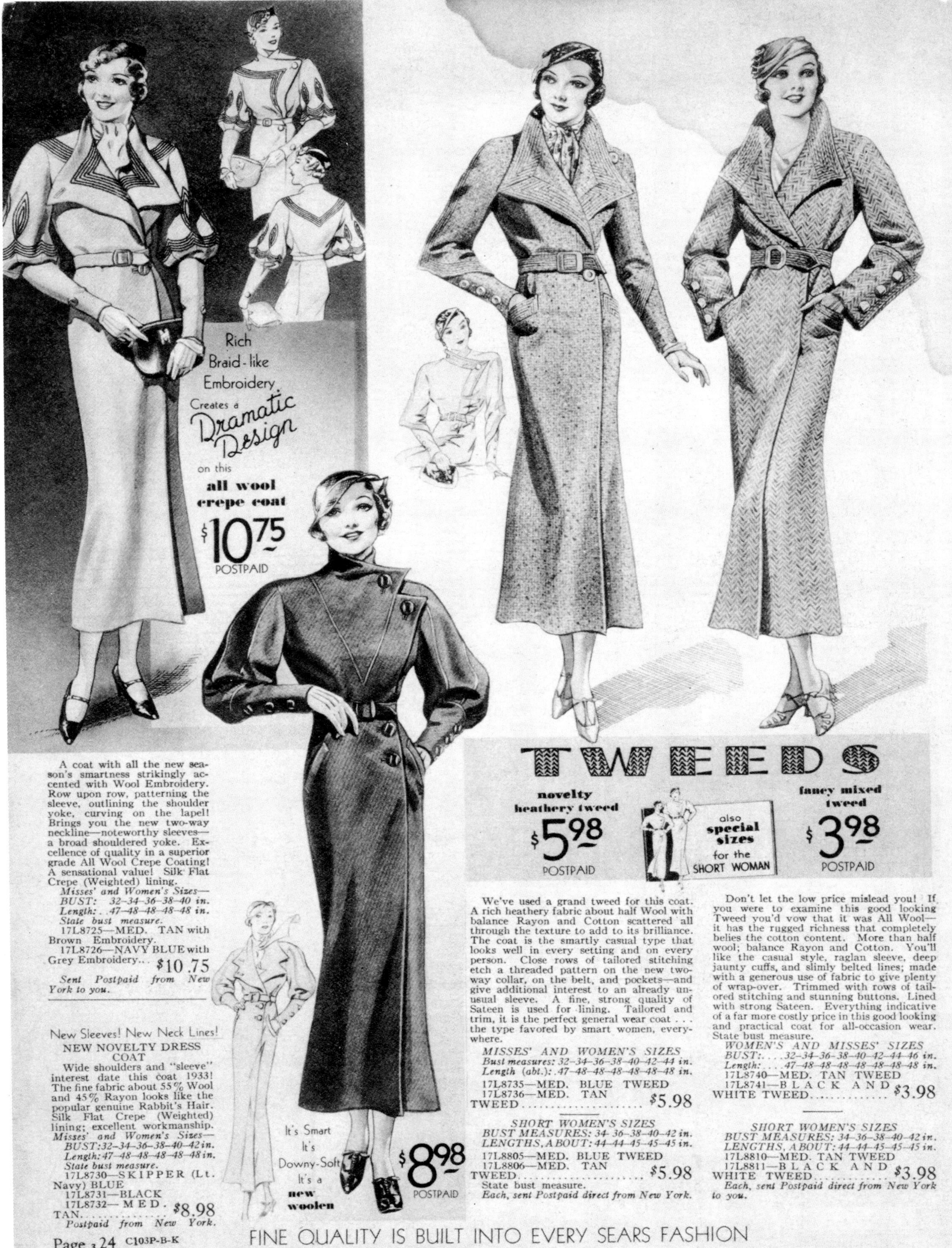
Rich
Braid-like
Embroidery
Creates a
Dramatic
Design
on this
all wool
crepe coat
$10.75
POSTPAID
A coat with all the new season's smartness strikingly accented with Wool Embroidery. Row upon row, patterning the sleeve, outlining the shoulder yoke, curving on the lapel! Brings you the new two-way neckline—noteworthy sleeves—a broad shouldered yoke. Excellence of quality in a superior grade All Wool Crepe Coating! A sensational value! Silk Flat Crepe (Weighted) lining.
Misses' and Women's Sizes—
BUST: 32–34–36–38–40 in.
Length: . .47–48–48–48–48 in.
State bust measure.
17L8725—MED. TAN with Brown Embroidery.
17L8726—NAVY BLUE with Grey Embroidery... $10.75
Sent Postpaid from New York to you.
New Sleeves! New Neck Lines!
NEW NOVELTY DRESS COAT
Wide shoulders and "sleeve" interest date this coat 1933! The fine fabric about 55% Wool and 45% Rayon looks like the popular genuine Rabbit's Hair. Silk Flat Crepe (Weighted) lining; excellent workmanship.
Misses' and Women's Sizes—
BUST:32–34–36–38–40–42 in.
Length:47–48–48–48–48–48 in.
State bust measure.
17L8730—SKIPPER (Lt. Navy) BLUE
17L8731—BLACK
17L8732—MED. TAN.............. $8.98
Postpaid from New York.
It's Smart
It's
Downy-Soft
It's a
new
woolen
$8.98
POSTPAID
TWEEDS
novelty
heathery tweed
$5.98
POSTPAID
also
special
sizes
for the
SHORT WOMAN
fancy mixed
tweed
$3.98
POSTPAID
We've used a grand tweed for this coat. A rich heathery fabric about half Wool with balance Rayon and Cotton scattered all through the texture to add to its brilliance. The coat is the smartly casual type that looks well in every setting and on every person. Close rows of tailored stitching etch a threaded pattern on the new two-way collar, on the belt, and pockets—and give additional interest to an already unusual sleeve. A fine, strong quality of Sateen is used for lining. Tailored and trim, it is the perfect general wear coat . . . the type favored by smart women, everywhere.
MISSES' AND WOMEN'S SIZES
Bust measures: 32–34–36–38–40–42–44 in.
Length (abt.): .47–48–48–48–48–48–48 in.
17L8735—MED. BLUE TWEED
17L8736—MED. TAN TWEED.................... $5.98
SHORT WOMEN'S SIZES
BUST MEASURES: 34–36–38–40–42 in.
LENGTHS, ABOUT: 44–44–45–45–45 in.
17L8805—MED. BLUE TWEED
17L8806—MED. TAN TWEED.................... $5.98
State bust measure.
Each, sent Postpaid direct from New York.
Don't let the low price mislead you! If you were to examine this good looking Tweed you'd vow that it was All Wool—it has the rugged richness that completely belies the cotton content. More than half wool; balance Rayon and Cotton. You'll like the casual style, raglan sleeve, deep jaunty cuffs, and slimly belted lines; made with a generous use of fabric to give plenty of wrap-over. Trimmed with rows of tailored stitching and stunning buttons. Lined with strong Sateen. Everything indicative of a far more costly price in this good looking and practical coat for all-occasion wear. State bust measure.
WOMEN'S AND MISSES' SIZES
BUST: . . . 32–34–36–38–40–42–44–46 in.
Length: . . . 47–48–48–48–48–48–48–48 in.
17L8740—MED. TAN TWEED
17L8741—BLACK AND WHITE TWEED............ $3.98
SHORT WOMEN'S SIZES
BUST MEASURES: 34–36–38–40–42 in.
LENGTHS, ABOUT: 44–44–45–45–45 in.
17L8810—MED. TAN TWEED
17L8811—BLACK AND WHITE TWEED............ $3.98
Each, sent Postpaid direct from New York to you.
Page 3 24 C103P-B-K
FINE QUALITY IS BUILT INTO EVERY SEARS FASHION

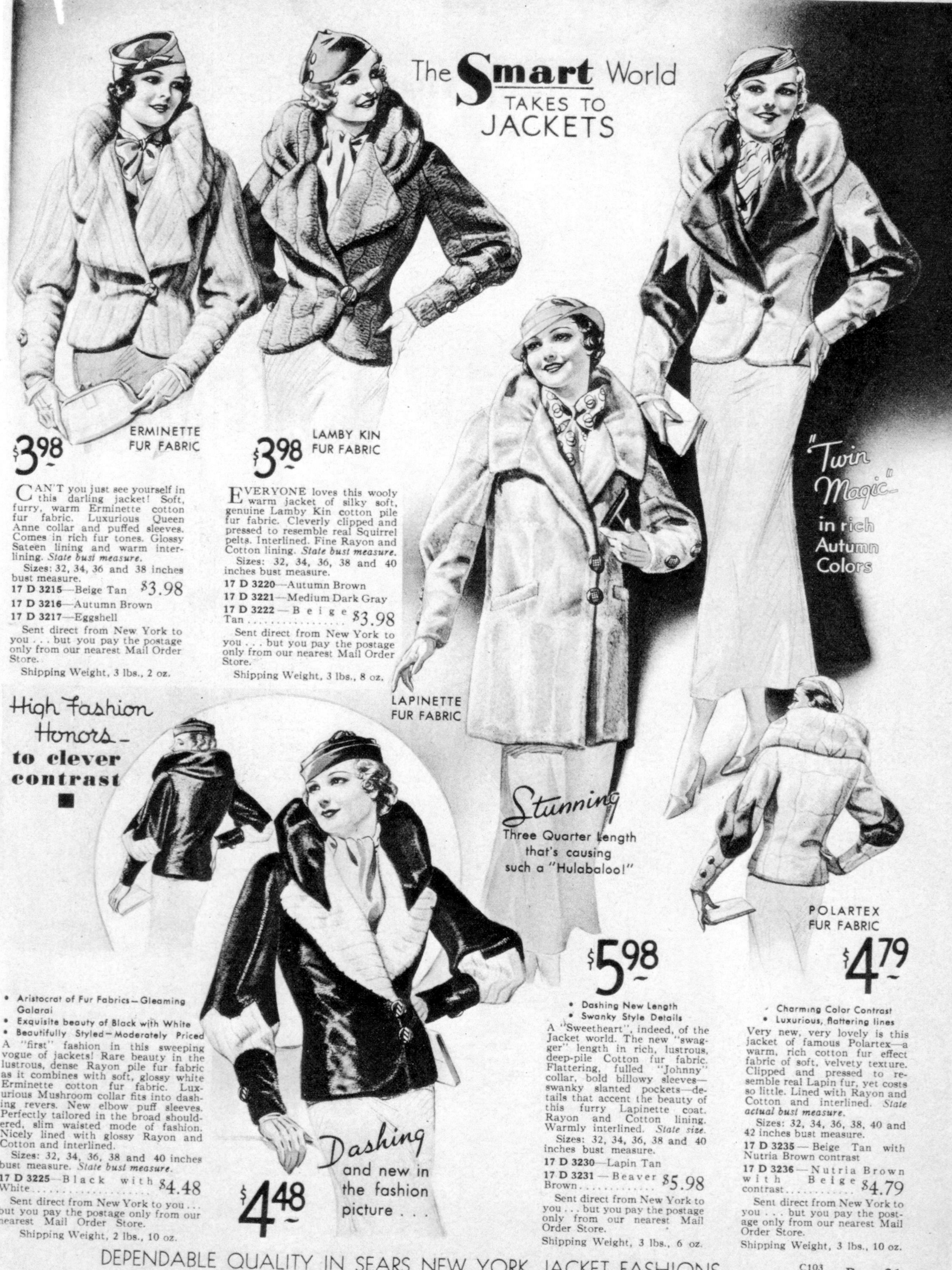

The Smart World TAKES TO JACKETS
ERMINETTE FUR FABRIC
$3.98
CAN'T you just see yourself in this darling jacket! Soft, furry, warm Erminette cotton fur fabric. Luxurious Queen Anne collar and puffed sleeves. Comes in rich fur tones. Glossy Sateen lining and warm interlining. State bust measure.
Sizes: 32, 34, 36 and 38 inches bust measure.
17 D 3215—Beige Tan $3.98
17 D 3216—Autumn Brown
17 D 3217—Eggshell
Sent direct from New York to you . . . but you pay the postage only from our nearest Mail Order Store.
Shipping Weight, 3 lbs., 2 oz.
LAMBY KIN FUR FABRIC
$3.98
EVERYONE loves this wooly warm jacket of silky soft, genuine Lamby Kin cotton pile fur fabric. Cleverly clipped and pressed to resemble real Squirrel pelts. Interlined. Fine Rayon and Cotton lining. State bust measure.
Sizes: 32, 34, 36, 38 and 40 inches bust measure.
17 D 3220—Autumn Brown
17 D 3221—Medium Dark Gray
17 D 3222—Beige Tan $3.98
Sent direct from New York to you . . . but you pay the postage only from our nearest Mail Order Store.
Shipping Weight, 3 lbs., 8 oz.
"Twin Magic" in rich Autumn Colors
LAPINETTE FUR FABRIC
High Fashion Honors— to clever contrast
Stunning
Three Quarter Length that's causing such a "Hulabaloo!"
POLARTEX FUR FABRIC
$5.98
$4.79
• Aristocrat of Fur Fabrics—Gleaming Galarai
• Exquisite beauty of Black with White
• Beautifully Styled—Moderately Priced
A "first" fashion in this sweeping vogue of jackets! Rare beauty in the lustrous, dense Rayon pile fur fabric as it combines with soft, glossy white Erminette cotton fur fabric. Luxurious Mushroom collar fits into dashing revers. New elbow puff sleeves. Perfectly tailored in the broad shouldered, slim waisted mode of fashion. Nicely lined with glossy Rayon and Cotton and interlined.
Sizes: 32, 34, 36, 38 and 40 inches bust measure. State bust measure.
17 D 3225—Black with White $4.48
Sent direct from New York to you . . . but you pay the postage only from our nearest Mail Order Store.
Shipping Weight, 2 lbs., 10 oz.
Dashing and new in the fashion picture . . .
$4.48
• Dashing New Length
• Swanky Style Details
A "Sweetheart", indeed, of the Jacket world. The new "swagger" length in rich, lustrous, deep-pile Cotton fur fabric. Flattering, fulled "Johnny" collar, bold billowy sleeves—swanky slanted pockets—details that accent the beauty of this furry Lapinette coat. Rayon and Cotton lining. Warmly interlined. State size.
Sizes: 32, 34, 36, 38 and 40 inches bust measure.
17 D 3230—Lapin Tan
17 D 3231—Beaver Brown. $5.98
Sent direct from New York to you . . . but you pay the postage only from our nearest Mail Order Store.
Shipping Weight, 3 lbs., 6 oz.
• Charming Color Contrast
• Luxurious, flattering lines
Very new, very lovely is this jacket of famous Polartex—a warm, rich cotton fur effect fabric of soft, velvety texture. Clipped and pressed to resemble real Lapin fur, yet costs so little. Lined with Rayon and Cotton and interlined. State actual bust measure.
Sizes: 32, 34, 36, 38, 40 and 42 inches bust measure.
17 D 3235—Beige Tan with Nutria Brown contrast
17 D 3236—Nutria Brown with Beige contrast $4.79
Sent direct from New York to you . . . but you pay the postage only from our nearest Mail Order Store.
Shipping Weight, 3 lbs., 10 oz.
DEPENDABLE QUALITY IN SEARS NEW YORK JACKET FASHIONS
C103 P-B-K-MN Page 21

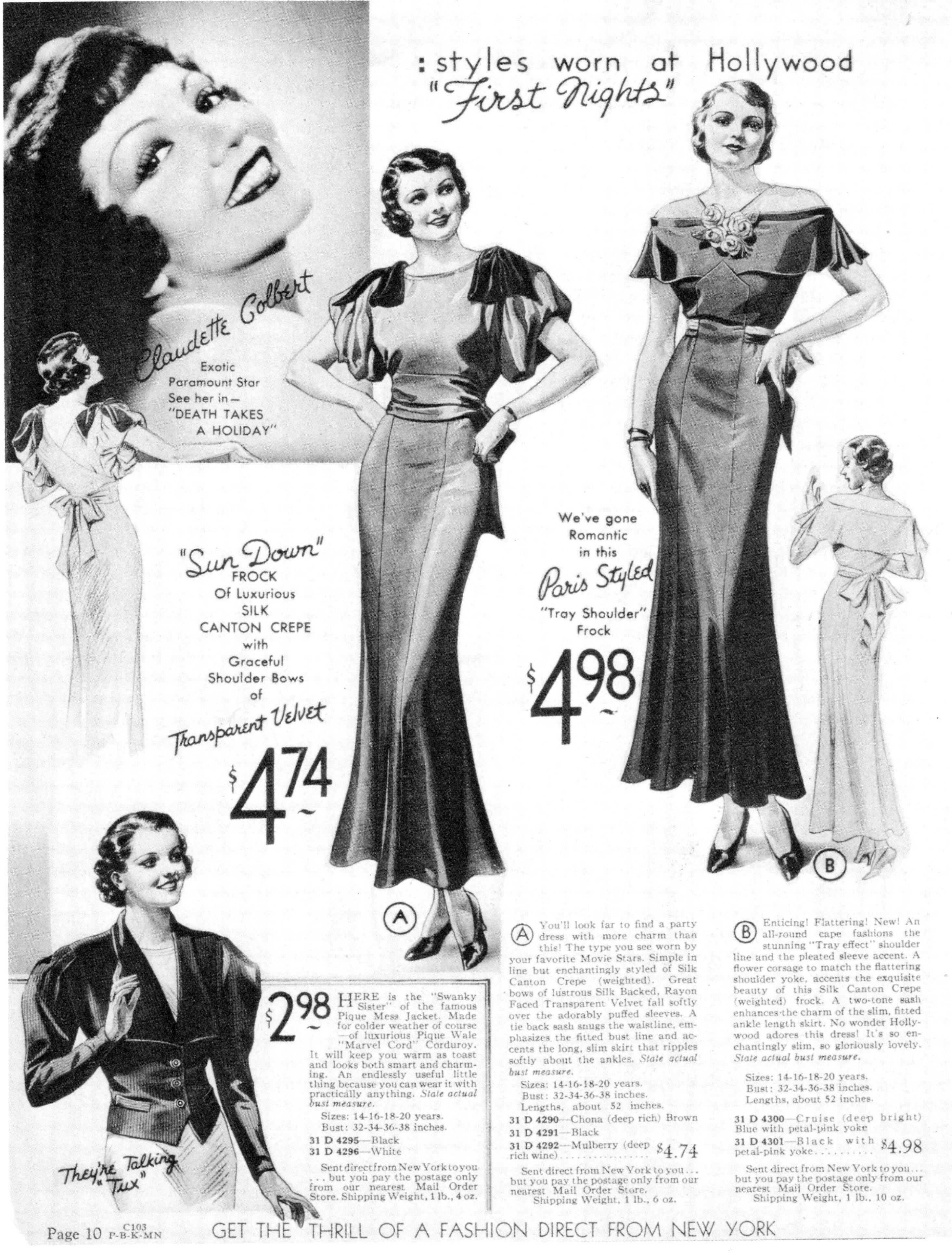

: styles worn at Hollywood
"First Nights"
Claudette Colbert
Exotic
Paramount Star
See her in—
"DEATH TAKES
A HOLIDAY"
"Sun Down"
FROCK
Of Luxurious
SILK
CANTON CREPE
with
Graceful
Shoulder Bows
of
Transparent Velvet
$4.74
We've gone
Romantic
in this
Paris Styled
"Tray Shoulder"
Frock
$4.98
A
B
They're Talking "Tux"
$2.98 HERE is the "Swanky Sister" of the famous Pique Mess Jacket. Made for colder weather of course—of luxurious Pique Wale "Marvel Cord" Corduroy. It will keep you warm as toast and looks both smart and charming. An endlessly useful little thing because you can wear it with practically anything. State actual bust measure.
Sizes: 14-16-18-20 years.
Bust: 32-34-36-38 inches.
31 D 4295—Black
31 D 4296—White
Sent direct from New York to you . . . but you pay the postage only from our nearest Mail Order Store. Shipping Weight, 1 lb., 4 oz.
(A) You'll look far to find a party dress with more charm than this! The type you see worn by your favorite Movie Stars. Simple in line but enchantingly styled of Silk Canton Crepe (weighted). Great bows of lustrous Silk Backed, Rayon Faced Transparent Velvet fall softly over the adorably puffed sleeves. A tie back sash snugs the waistline, emphasizes the fitted bust line and accents the long, slim skirt that ripples softly about the ankles. State actual bust measure.
Sizes: 14-16-18-20 years.
Bust: 32-34-36-38 inches.
Lengths, about 52 inches.
31 D 4290—Chona (deep rich) Brown
31 D 4291—Black
31 D 4292—Mulberry (deep rich wine) $4.74
Sent direct from New York to you . . . but you pay the postage only from our nearest Mail Order Store.
Shipping Weight, 1 lb., 6 oz.
(B) Enticing! Flattering! New! An all-round cape fashions the stunning "Tray effect" shoulder line and the pleated sleeve accent. A flower corsage to match the flattering shoulder yoke, accents the exquisite beauty of this Silk Canton Crepe (weighted) frock. A two-tone sash enhances the charm of the slim, fitted ankle length skirt. No wonder Hollywood adores this dress! It's so enchantingly slim, so gloriously lovely. State actual bust measure.
Sizes: 14-16-18-20 years.
Bust: 32-34-36-38 inches.
Lengths, about 52 inches.
31 D 4300—Cruise (deep bright) Blue with petal-pink yoke
31 D 4301—Black with petal-pink yoke $4.98
Sent direct from New York to you . . . but you pay the postage only from our nearest Mail Order Store.
Shipping Weight, 1 lb., 10 oz.
Page 10 C103 P-B-K-MN
GET THE THRILL OF A FASHION DIRECT FROM NEW YORK

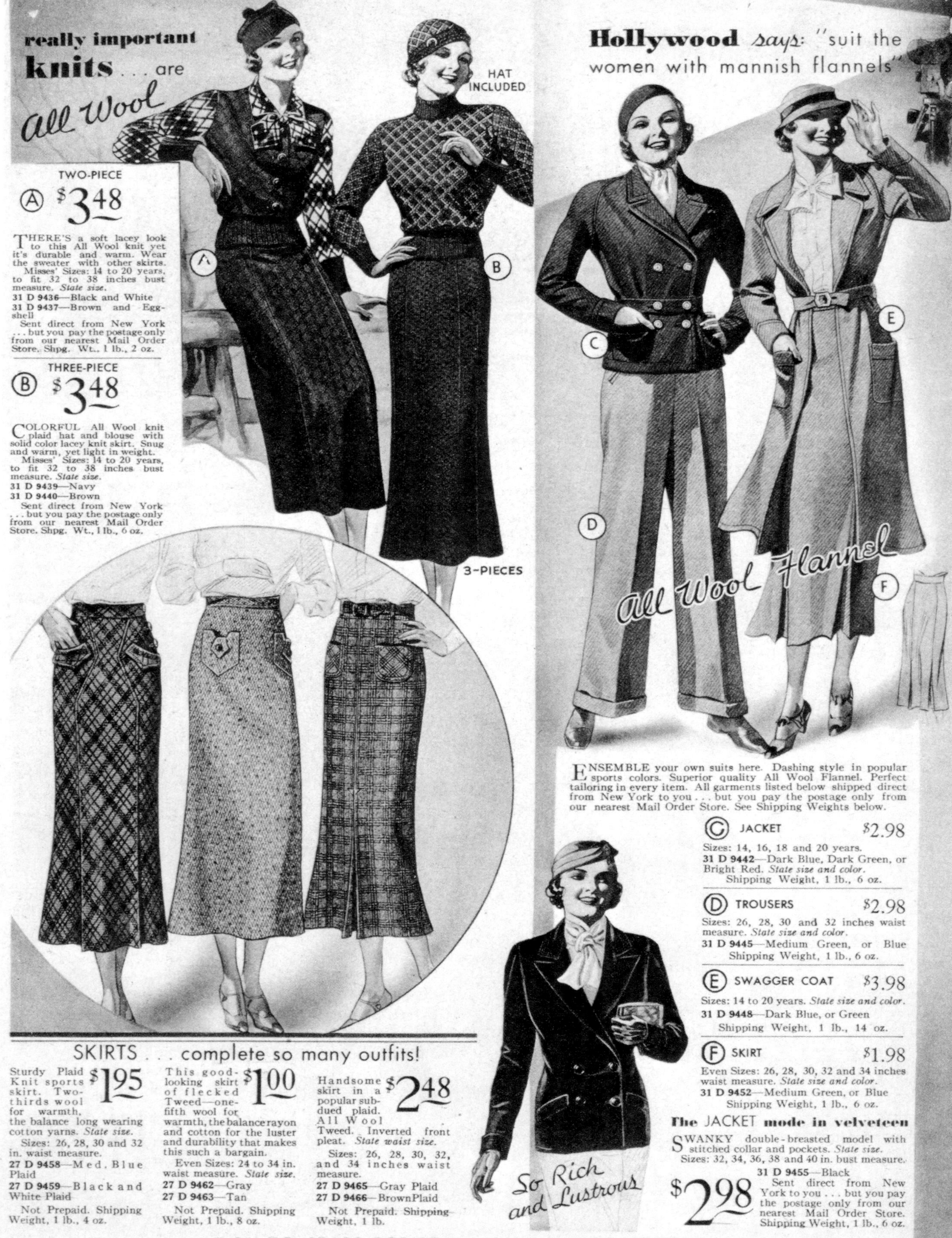

really important knits . . . are *All Wool*

HAT INCLUDED

TWO-PIECE

Ⓐ $3.48

THERE'S a soft lacey look to this All Wool knit yet it's durable and warm. Wear the sweater with other skirts.

Misses' Sizes: 14 to 20 years, to fit 32 to 38 inches bust measure. *State size.*

31 D 9436—Black and White

31 D 9437—Brown and Eggshell

Sent direct from New York . . . but you pay the postage only from our nearest Mail Order Store. Shpg. Wt., 1 lb., 2 oz.

THREE-PIECE

Ⓑ $3.48

COLORFUL All Wool knit plaid hat and blouse with solid color lacey knit skirt. Snug and warm, yet light in weight.

Misses' Sizes: 14 to 20 years, to fit 32 to 38 inches bust measure. *State size.*

31 D 9439—Navy

31 D 9440—Brown

Sent direct from New York . . . but you pay the postage only from our nearest Mail Order Store. Shpg. Wt., 1 lb., 6 oz.

3-PIECES

SKIRTS . . . complete so many outfits!

Sturdy Plaid Knit sports skirt. Two-thirds wool for warmth, the balance long wearing cotton yarns. *State size.* $1.95

Sizes: 26, 28, 30 and 32 in. waist measure.

27 D 9458—Med. Blue Plaid

27 D 9459—Black and White Plaid

Not Prepaid. Shipping Weight, 1 lb., 4 oz.

This good-looking skirt of flecked Tweed—one-fifth wool for warmth, the balance rayon and cotton for the luster and durability that makes this such a bargain. $1.00

Even Sizes: 24 to 34 in. waist measure. *State size.*

27 D 9462—Gray

27 D 9463—Tan

Not Prepaid. Shipping Weight, 1 lb., 8 oz.

Handsome skirt in a popular subdued plaid. All Wool Tweed. Inverted front pleat. *State waist size.* $2.48

Sizes: 26, 28, 30, 32, and 34 inches waist measure.

27 D 9465—Gray Plaid

27 D 9466—Brown Plaid

Not Prepaid. Shipping Weight, 1 lb.

Hollywood *says*: "suit the women with mannish flannels"

All Wool Flannel

ENSEMBLE your own suits here. Dashing style in popular sports colors. Superior quality All Wool Flannel. Perfect tailoring in every item. All garments listed below shipped direct from New York to you . . . but you pay the postage only from our nearest Mail Order Store. See Shipping Weights below.

Ⓒ JACKET $2.98

Sizes: 14, 16, 18 and 20 years.

31 D 9442—Dark Blue, Dark Green, or Bright Red. *State size and color.*

Shipping Weight, 1 lb., 6 oz.

Ⓓ TROUSERS $2.98

Sizes: 26, 28, 30 and 32 inches waist measure. *State size and color.*

31 D 9445—Medium Green, or Blue

Shipping Weight, 1 lb., 6 oz.

Ⓔ SWAGGER COAT $3.98

Sizes: 14 to 20 years. *State size and color.*

31 D 9448—Dark Blue, or Green

Shipping Weight, 1 lb., 14 oz.

Ⓕ SKIRT $1.98

Even Sizes: 26, 28, 30, 32 and 34 inches waist measure. *State size and color.*

31 D 9452—Medium Green, or Blue

Shipping Weight, 1 lb., 6 oz.

The JACKET **mode in velveteen**

SWANKY double-breasted model with stitched collar and pockets. *State size.*

Sizes: 32, 34, 36, 38 and 40 in. bust measure.

So Rich and Lustrous

$2.98

31 D 9455—Black

Sent direct from New York to you . . . but you pay the postage only from our nearest Mail Order Store. Shipping Weight, 1 lb., 6 oz.

LOOK TO SEARS FOR REAL VALUE IN SPORTSWEAR

C104 P-B-K-MN Page 45

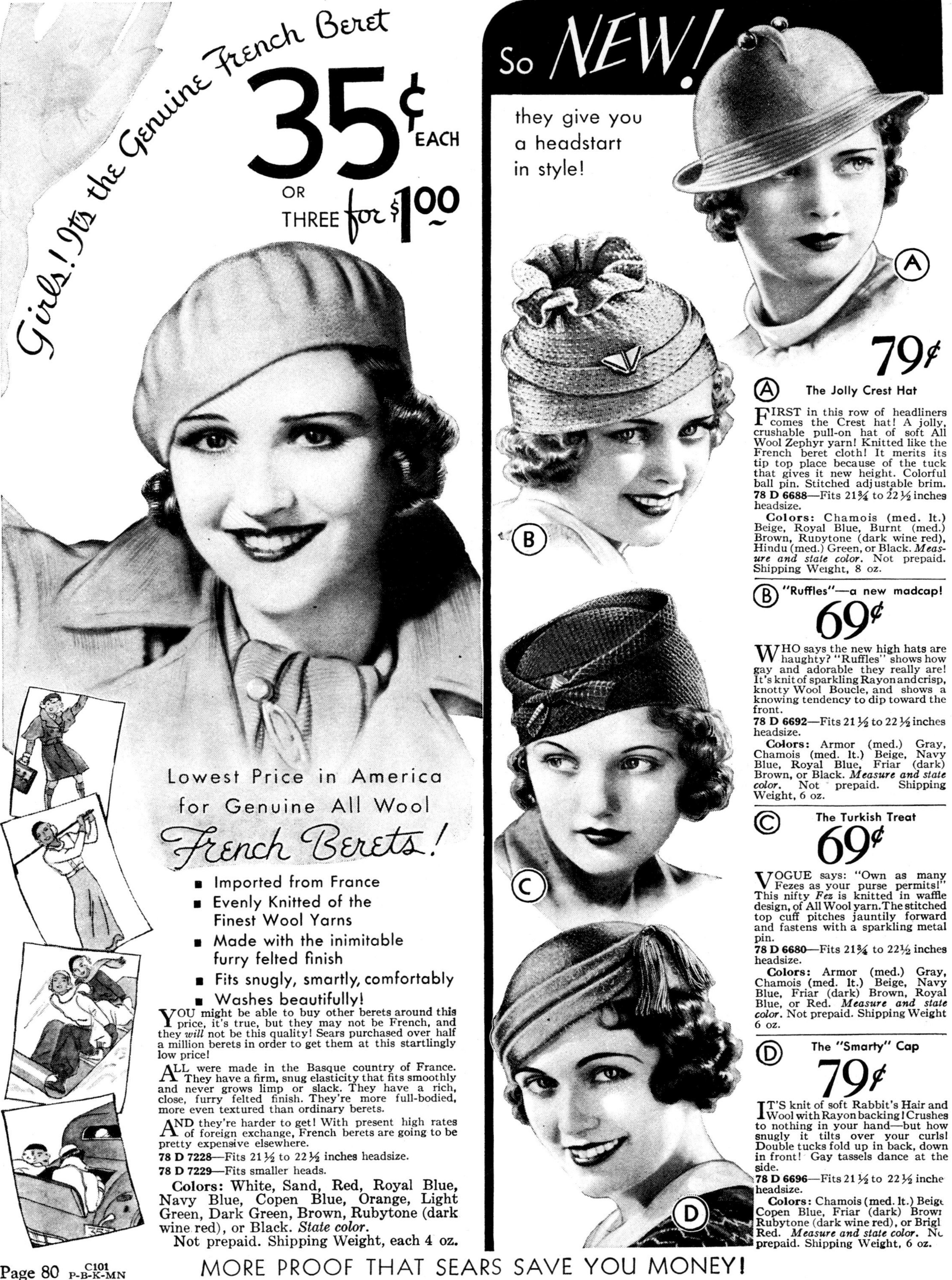

Girls! It's the Genuine French Beret
35¢ EACH
OR
THREE for $1.00
Lowest Price in America
for Genuine All Wool
French Berets!
■ Imported from France
■ Evenly Knitted of the Finest Wool Yarns
■ Made with the inimitable furry felted finish
■ Fits snugly, smartly, comfortably
■ Washes beautifully!
YOU might be able to buy other berets around this price, it's true, but they may not be French, and they will not be this quality! Sears purchased over half a million berets in order to get them at this startlingly low price!
ALL were made in the Basque country of France. They have a firm, snug elasticity that fits smoothly and never grows limp or slack. They have a rich, close, furry felted finish. They're more full-bodied, more even textured than ordinary berets.
AND they're harder to get! With present high rates of foreign exchange, French berets are going to be pretty expensive elsewhere.
78 D 7228—Fits 21½ to 22½ inches headsize.
78 D 7229—Fits smaller heads.
Colors: White, Sand, Red, Royal Blue, Navy Blue, Copen Blue, Orange, Light Green, Dark Green, Brown, Rubytone (dark wine red), or Black. State color.
Not prepaid. Shipping Weight, each 4 oz.
So NEW!
they give you a headstart in style!
A
B
C
D
79¢
(A) The Jolly Crest Hat
FIRST in this row of headliners comes the Crest hat! A jolly, crushable pull-on hat of soft All Wool Zephyr yarn! Knitted like the French beret cloth! It merits its tip top place because of the tuck that gives it new height. Colorful ball pin. Stitched adjustable brim.
78 D 6688—Fits 21¾ to 22½ inches headsize.
Colors: Chamois (med. lt.) Beige, Royal Blue, Burnt (med.) Brown, Rubytone (dark wine red), Hindu (med.) Green, or Black. Measure and state color. Not prepaid. Shipping Weight, 8 oz.
(B) "Ruffles"—a new madcap!
69¢
WHO says the new high hats are haughty? "Ruffles" shows how gay and adorable they really are! It's knit of sparkling Rayon and crisp, knotty Wool Boucle, and shows a knowing tendency to dip toward the front.
78 D 6692—Fits 21½ to 22½ inches headsize.
Colors: Armor (med.) Gray, Chamois (med. lt.) Beige, Navy Blue, Royal Blue, Friar (dark) Brown, or Black. Measure and state color. Not prepaid. Shipping Weight, 6 oz.
(C) The Turkish Treat
69¢
VOGUE says: "Own as many Fezes as your purse permits!" This nifty Fez is knitted in waffle design, of All Wool yarn. The stitched top cuff pitches jauntily forward and fastens with a sparkling metal pin.
78 D 6680—Fits 21¾ to 22½ inches headsize.
Colors: Armor (med.) Gray, Chamois (med. lt.) Beige, Navy Blue, Friar (dark) Brown, Royal Blue, or Red. Measure and state color. Not prepaid. Shipping Weight 6 oz.
(D) The "Smarty" Cap
79¢
IT'S knit of soft Rabbit's Hair and Wool with Rayon backing! Crushes to nothing in your hand—but how snugly it tilts over your curls! Double tucks fold up in back, down in front! Gay tassels dance at the side.
78 D 6696—Fits 21½ to 22½ inche headsize.
Colors: Chamois (med. lt.) Beige Copen Blue, Friar (dark) Brown Rubytone (dark wine red), or Brigl Red. Measure and state color. Nc prepaid. Shipping Weight, 6 oz.
Page 80 C101 P-B-K-MN
MORE PROOF THAT SEARS SAVE YOU MONEY!

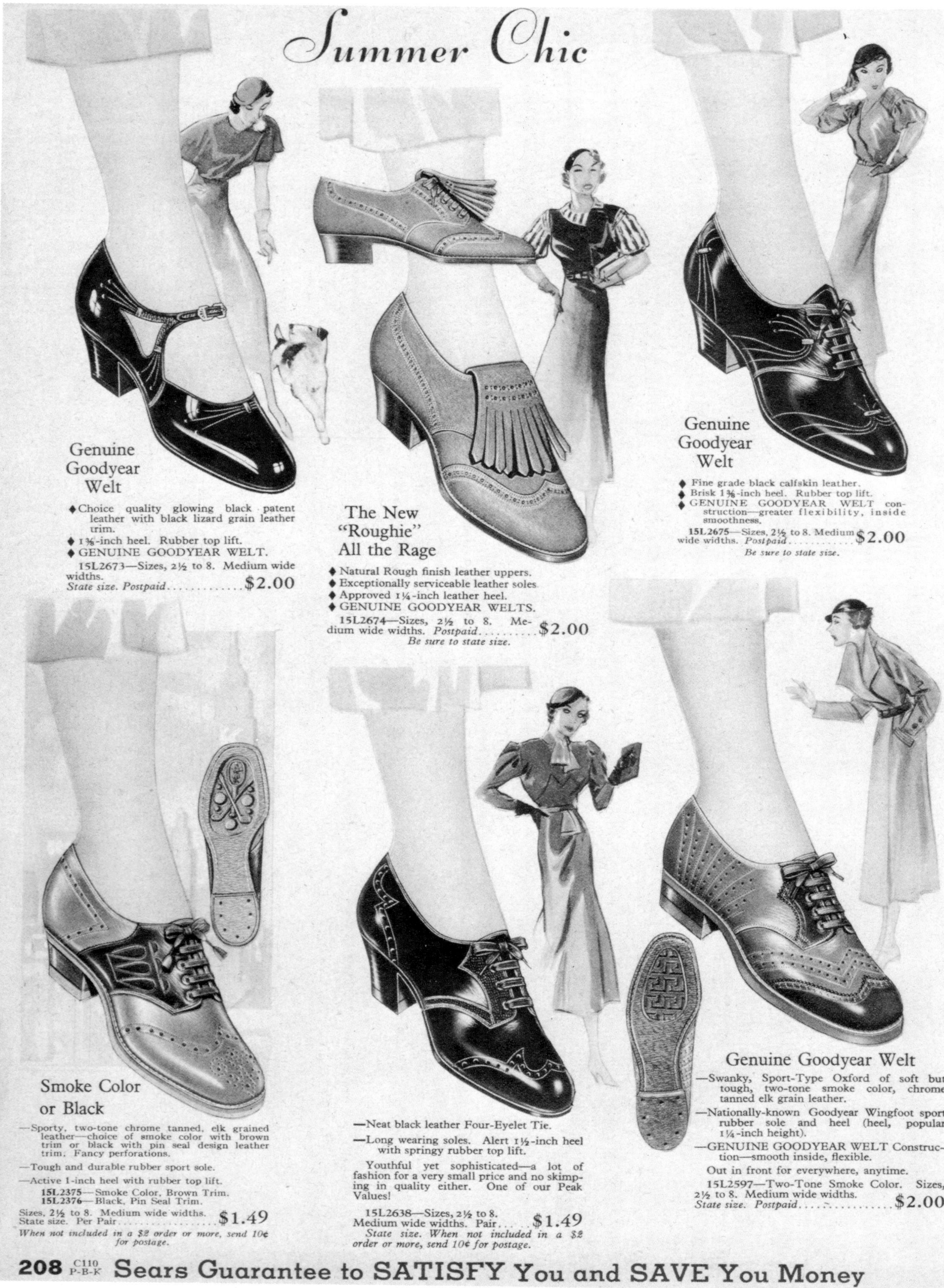
Summer Chic
Genuine Goodyear Welt
♦ Choice quality glowing black patent leather with black lizard grain leather trim.
♦ 1⅜-inch heel. Rubber top lift.
♦ GENUINE GOODYEAR WELT.
15L2673—Sizes, 2½ to 8. Medium wide widths.
State size. Postpaid............. $2.00
The New "Roughie" All the Rage
♦ Natural Rough finish leather uppers.
♦ Exceptionally serviceable leather soles
♦ Approved 1¼-inch leather heel.
♦ GENUINE GOODYEAR WELTS.
15L2674—Sizes, 2½ to 8. Medium wide widths. Postpaid.......... $2.00
Be sure to state size.
Genuine Goodyear Welt
♦ Fine grade black calfskin leather.
♦ Brisk 1⅜-inch heel. Rubber top lift.
♦ GENUINE GOODYEAR WELT construction—greater flexibility, inside smoothness.
15L2675—Sizes, 2½ to 8. Medium wide widths. Postpaid............ $2.00
Be sure to state size.
Smoke Color or Black
—Sporty, two-tone chrome tanned, elk grained leather—choice of smoke color with brown trim or black with pin seal design leather trim. Fancy perforations.
—Tough and durable rubber sport sole.
—Active 1-inch heel with rubber top lift.
15L2375—Smoke Color, Brown Trim.
15L2376—Black, Pin Seal Trim.
Sizes, 2½ to 8. Medium wide widths. State size. Per Pair.................. $1.49
When not included in a $2 order or more, send 10¢ for postage.
—Neat black leather Four-Eyelet Tie.
—Long wearing soles. Alert 1½-inch heel with springy rubber top lift.
Youthful yet sophisticated—a lot of fashion for a very small price and no skimping in quality either. One of our Peak Values!
15L2638—Sizes, 2½ to 8. Medium wide widths. Pair..... $1.49
State size. When not included in a $2 order or more, send 10¢ for postage.
Genuine Goodyear Welt
—Swanky, Sport-Type Oxford of soft but tough, two-tone smoke color, chrome tanned elk grain leather.
—Nationally-known Goodyear Wingfoot sport rubber sole and heel (heel, popular 1¼-inch height).
—GENUINE GOODYEAR WELT Construction—smooth inside, flexible.
Out in front for everywhere, anytime.
15L2597—Two-Tone Smoke Color. Sizes, 2½ to 8. Medium wide widths.
State size. Postpaid................ $2.00
208 C110 P-B-K Sears Guarantee to SATISFY You and SAVE You Money

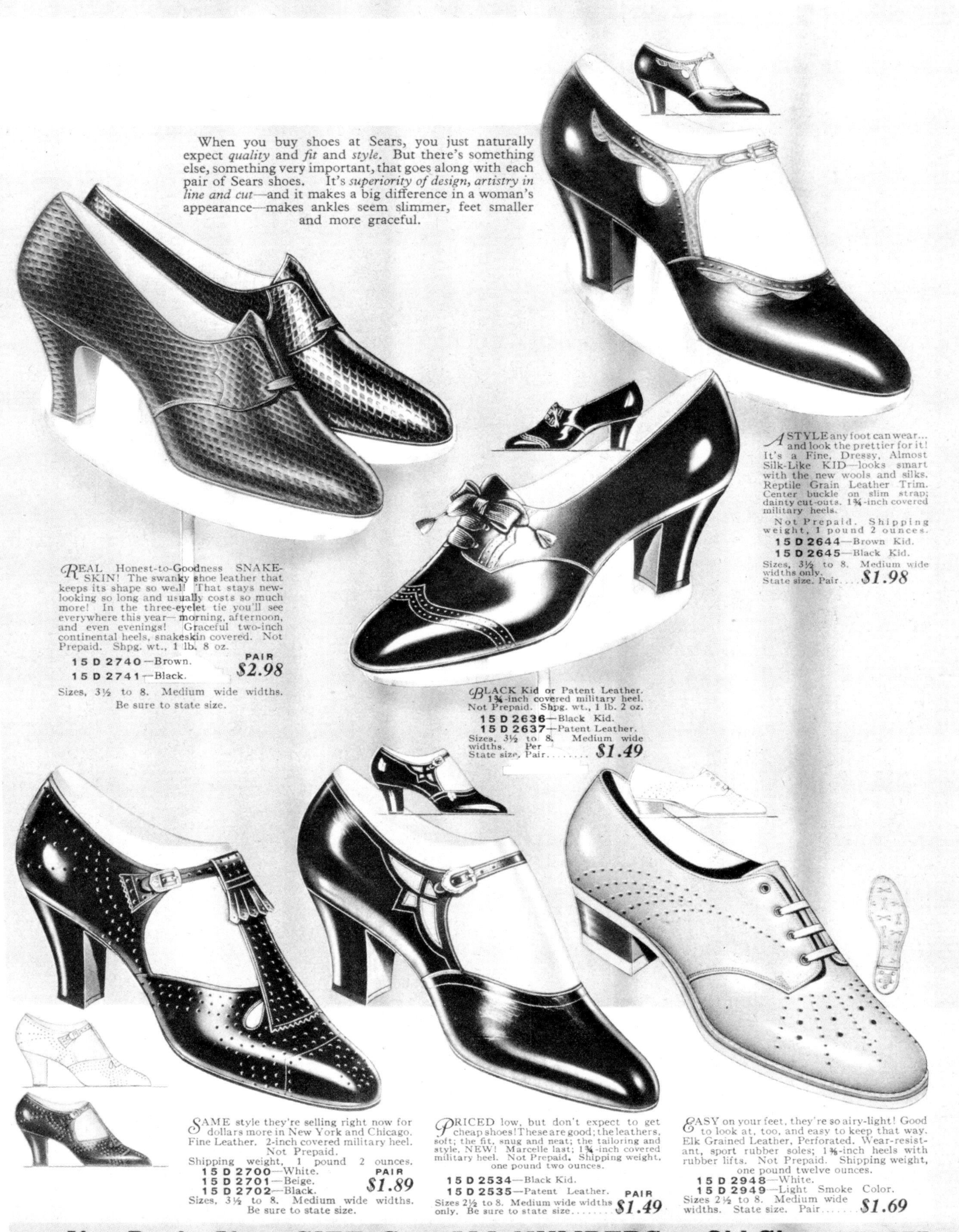
When you buy shoes at Sears, you just naturally expect *quality* and *fit* and *style*. But there's something else, something very important, that goes along with each pair of Sears shoes. It's *superiority of design, artistry in line and cut*—and it makes a big difference in a woman's appearance—makes ankles seem slimmer, feet smaller and more graceful.
REAL Honest-to-Goodness SNAKE-SKIN! The swanky shoe leather that keeps its shape so well! That stays new-looking so long and usually costs so much more! In the three-eyelet tie you'll see everywhere this year—morning, afternoon, and even evenings! Graceful two-inch continental heels, snakeskin covered. Not Prepaid. Shpg. wt., 1 lb. 8 oz.
15 D 2740—Brown.
15 D 2741—Black.
PAIR $2.98
Sizes, 3½ to 8. Medium wide widths. Be sure to state size.
BLACK Kid or Patent Leather. 1¾-inch covered military heel. Not Prepaid. Shpg. wt., 1 lb. 2 oz.
15 D 2636—Black Kid.
15 D 2637—Patent Leather.
Sizes, 3½ to 8. Medium wide widths. Per State size. Pair........ $1.49
A STYLE any foot can wear... and look the prettier for it! It's a Fine, Dressy, Almost Silk-Like KID—looks smart with the new wools and silks. Reptile Grain Leather Trim. Center buckle on slim strap; dainty cut-outs. 1¾-inch covered military heels.
Not Prepaid. Shipping weight, 1 pound 2 ounces.
15 D 2644—Brown Kid.
15 D 2645—Black Kid.
Sizes, 3½ to 8. Medium wide widths only. State size. Pair.... $1.98
SAME style they're selling right now for dollars more in New York and Chicago. Fine Leather. 2-inch covered military heel. Not Prepaid.
Shipping weight, 1 pound 2 ounces.
15 D 2700—White.
15 D 2701—Beige.
15 D 2702—Black.
PAIR $1.89
Sizes, 3½ to 8. Medium wide widths. Be sure to state size.
PRICED low, but don't expect to get cheap shoes! These are good; the leathers, soft; the fit, snug and neat; the tailoring and style, NEW! Marcelle last; 1¾-inch covered military heel. Not Prepaid. Shipping weight, one pound two ounces.
15 D 2534—Black Kid.
15 D 2535—Patent Leather.
PAIR
Sizes 2½ to 8. Medium wide widths only. Be sure to state size........ $1.49
EASY on your feet, they're so airy-light! Good to look at, too, and easy to keep that way. Elk Grained Leather, Perforated. Wear-resistant, sport rubber soles; 1⅜-inch heels with rubber lifts. Not Prepaid. Shipping weight, one pound twelve ounces.
15 D 2948—White.
15 D 2949—Light Smoke Color.
Sizes 2½ to 8. Medium wide widths. State size. Pair....... $1.69
If in Doubt About SIZE, Give ALL NUMBERS in Old Shoe
C117P-B K-MN 2 255

A Colorful Scarf is the Spice of the Outfit!

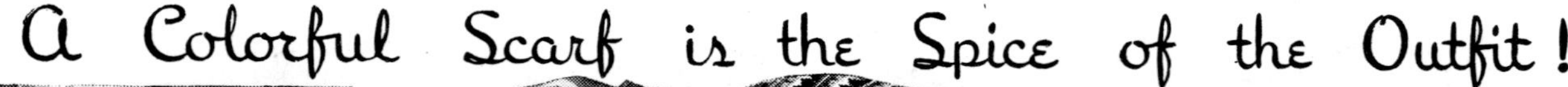

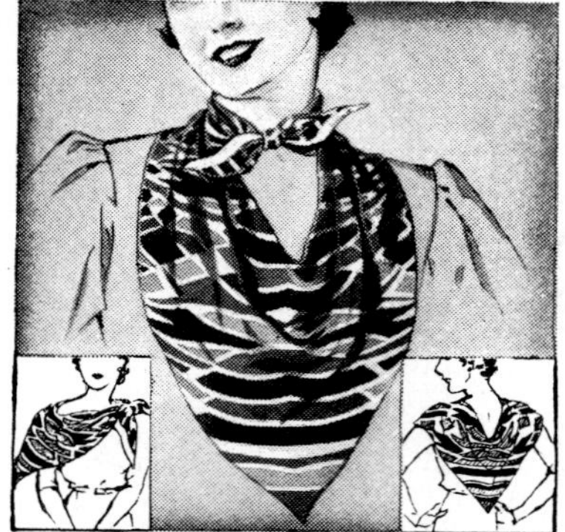

49c So Many Ways You Can Wear It!

18 D 4547—Fling this smart colorful V-shaped scarf over your shoulders and see how it glorifies your frock! Ends can be crossed in front and tucked under a belt, too! Good heavy Printed (weighted), Silk Crepe de Chine. Length, about 37 in. Predominating colors: **Tan and Brown, Navy and Copenhagen or Red and Black. State color.** Not Prepaid. Shpg. wt., 4 oz.

De Luxe Gift
Sylvia Sidney
Beloved PARAMOUNT Star inspires this style!

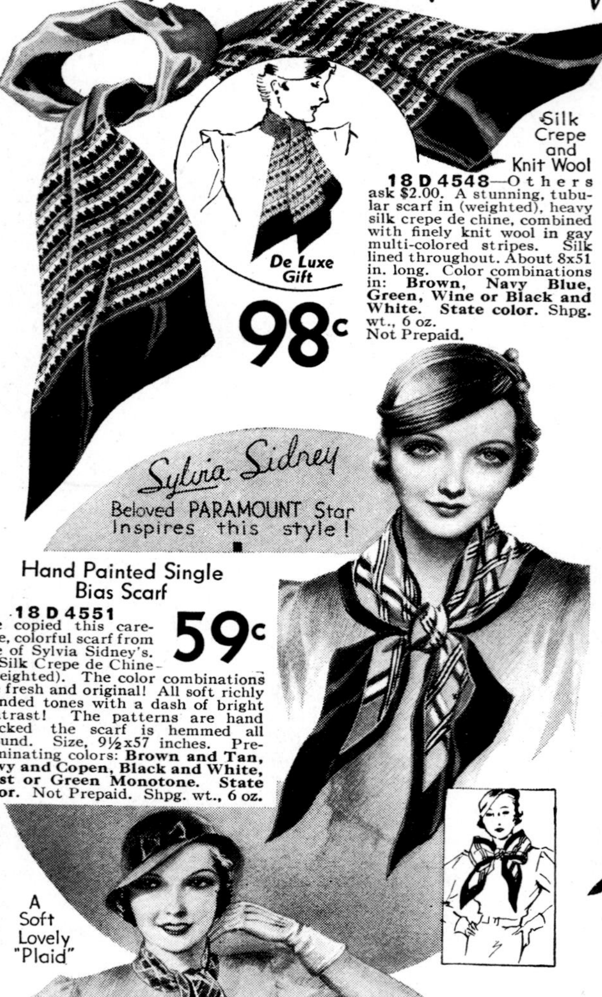

Silk Crepe and Knit Wool

98c

18 D 4548—Others ask $2.00. A stunning, tubular scarf in (weighted), heavy silk crepe de chine, combined with finely knit wool in gay multi-colored stripes. Silk lined throughout. About 8x51 in. long. Color combinations in: **Brown, Navy Blue, Green, Wine or Black and White. State color.** Shpg. wt., 6 oz. Not Prepaid.

Hand Painted on Both Sides **98c**

18 D 4549—It's that swanky, **shorter style! It's tubular**—keeps its shape better because of the double texture. And it flaunts a gay block pattern in the most fashionable new color combination! All done by hand! Neat, fringed ends. Fine, smooth, French Silk (Weighted) Crepe. Size, 9x44 in. Main Colors: **Brown and Tan; Navy and Copenhagen; Black and White or Wine Monotone. State color.** Not Prepaid. Shpg. wt., 6 oz.

Hand Painted Single Bias Scarf

18 D 4551 **59c**

We copied this carefree, colorful scarf from one of Sylvia Sidney's. Silk Crepe de Chine (Weighted). The color combinations are fresh and original! All soft richly blended tones with a dash of bright contrast! The patterns are hand blocked the scarf is hemmed all around. Size, 9½x57 inches. Predominating colors: **Brown and Tan, Navy and Copen, Black and White, Rust or Green Monotone. State color.** Not Prepaid. Shpg. wt., 6 oz.

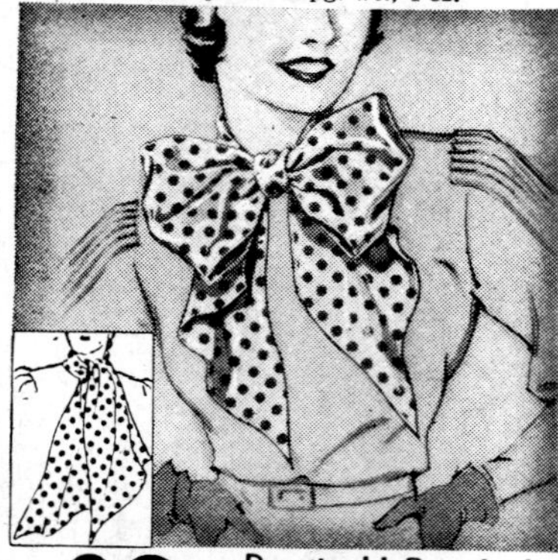

39c Practical! Popular! Polka Dots!

18 D 4550—The great Garbo wore a polka dot scarf when she returned to Hollywood! Wear yours in a fluffy bow—a middy knot or an ascot fling! The scarf's Printed, Silk Crepe de Chine (Weighted), about 8¼x54 inches. Main colors: **White with Black dots, Navy with White dots, Tan with Brown dots or Red with White dots. State color.** Not Prepaid. Shpg. wt., 6 oz.

A Soft Lovely "Plaid"

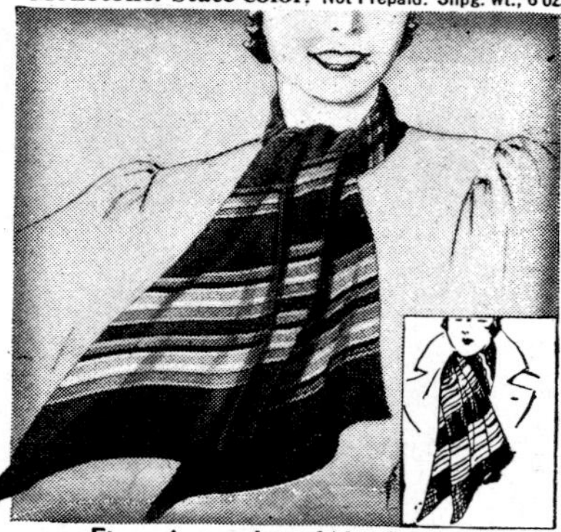

Fine Australian Wool Scarf!

18 D 4552—Light and fine and soft as silk! Slips through a finger ring as easily as ribbon! **59c**

Yet what bland, caressing warmth it holds! What brave, bright color stripes it flaunts! What a grand, comfy neckpiece it is for suit, coat or leather jacket! All fine wool, in sheer lattice weave. Size, about 9½x53 inches. Background colors: **Brown, Dark Blue, Red or Sand. State color.** Not Prepaid. Shpg. wt., 6 oz.

a bright thought for *Gifts*... they'll be more than welcome!

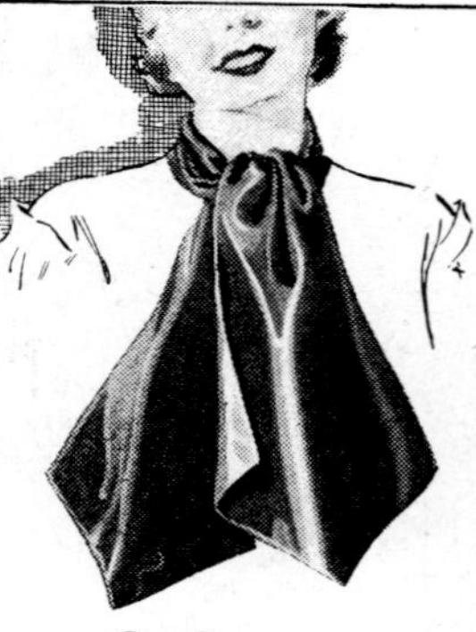

39c 2-Way Reversible Tubular Ascot

18 D 4553—Two-textured, All Rayon fabric—and beautifully tailored! Wear it Taffeta side out—and it looks like a dark, monotone scarf! Wear it Satin side out—and it's a stunning, 2-tone neckpiece: one end in dark color, one end in flashing light-toned contrast! Tapered-in at the center, widened smartly and wedge-shaped at the ends. Length, about 41 inches. Colors: **Navy and Copenhagen, Black and White, Red and White or Solid White. State color.** Not Prepaid. Shpg. wt., 4 oz.

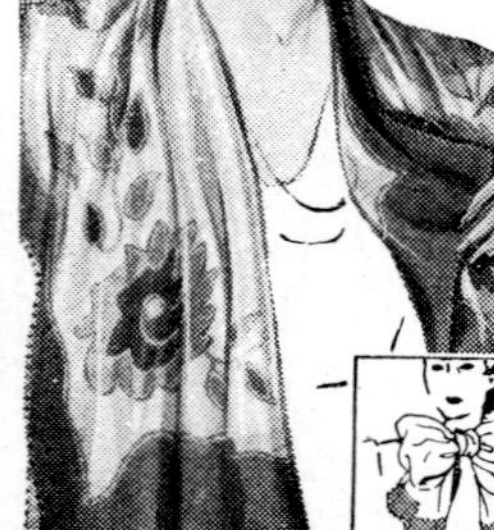

Smart Bow Effect

Hand Painted Silk Chiffon **69c**

18 D 4554

The airy folds of this sheer filmy (weighted silk) scarf fluff up around the shoulders and make a lovely soft frame for your face. Its delicate pastel colors are applied by hand and beautifully blended! Picot edged all around. Its full gauzy length measures 33x48 in. Background colors: **Pink, Orchid, Tan, Powder Blue or White and Black Combinations. State color.** Not Prepaid. Shpg. wt., 4 oz.

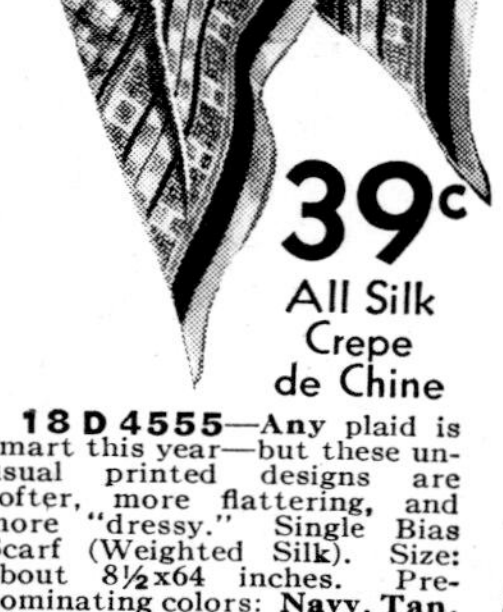

39c All Silk Crepe de Chine

18 D 4555—Any plaid is smart this year—but these unusual printed designs are softer, more flattering, and more "dressy." Single Bias Scarf (Weighted Silk). Size: about 8½x64 inches. Predominating colors: **Navy, Tan, Wine, Green or Black and White. State color.** Not Prepaid. Shpg. wt., 6 oz.

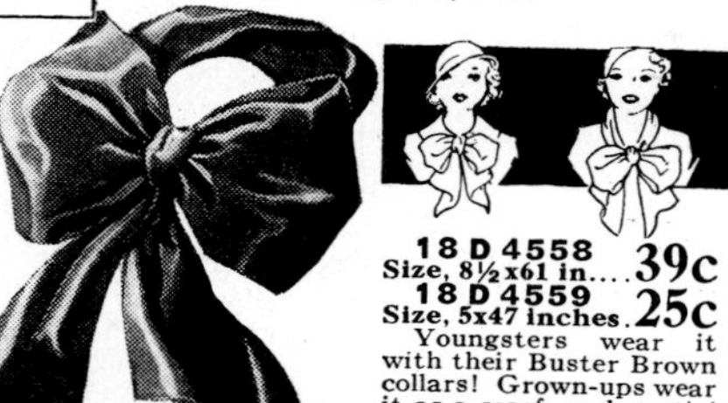

The "Scarf-Tie"

18 D 4558 Size, 8½x61 in.... **39c**
18 D 4559 Size, 5x47 inches.. **25c**

Youngsters wear it with their Buster Brown collars! Grown-ups wear it as a scarf, sash or tie! Gleaming Celanese satin. Colors: **White, Black, Red or Navy Blue. State color.** Not Prepaid. Shpg. wt., 4 oz.

Chic Tubular Scarf

69c Hand Painted Silk Crepe

18 D 4556

Here's a slim French **Silk** (weighted) crepe ascot that just fills in the neck of your coat! It's **lined** to hold its shape—**hand blocked** to give you original color patterns and jauntily finished with diagonally cut ends. So nicely made that it's a decidedly smart gift. Lgth. about 52 in. Predominating colors: **Brown, Navy Blue, Red or Green. State color.** Not Prepaid. Shpg. wt., 4 oz.

79c Hand Painted Tubular Scarf

18 D 4557 — A handsome Scarf that you **may** buy for a gift, but you'll long to keep for yourself! And why shouldn't you! It's of heavy French silk (weighted) crepe—and the gay carefree colors are blocked in by hand! The scarf is **lined** with solid colored silk to hold its shape, to drape gracefully and to wear well! Length, about 50 inches. Main Colors: **Brown, Navy Blue, Red or Green. State color.** Not Prepaid. Shpg. wt., 6 oz.

 Do Your CHRISTMAS SHOPPING From SEARS Catalogs

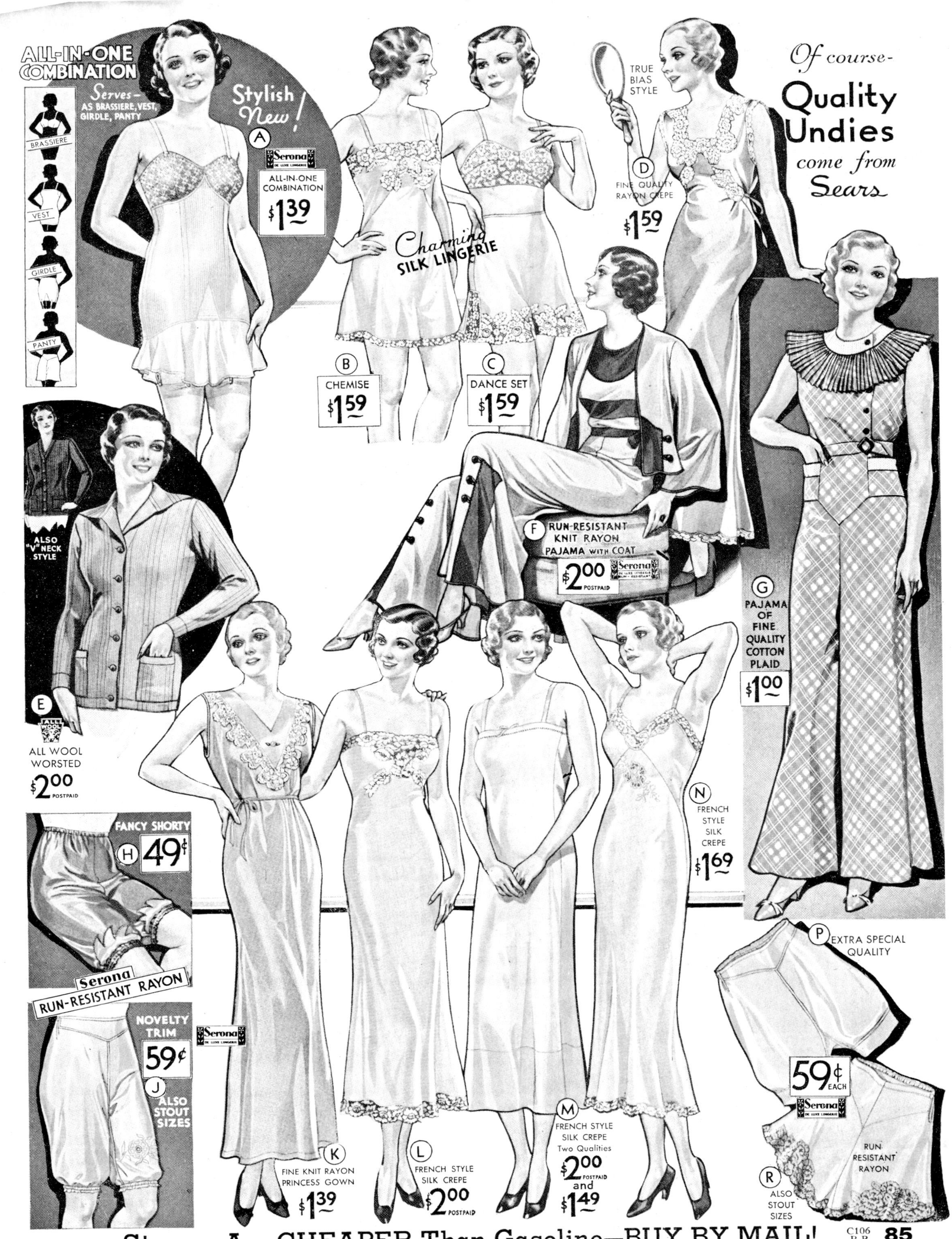
ALL-IN-ONE COMBINATION
Serves– AS BRASSIERE, VEST, GIRDLE, PANTY
BRASSIERE
VEST
GIRDLE
PANTY
Stylish New!
A
Serona DE LUXE LINGERIE
ALL-IN-ONE COMBINATION
$1.39
Charming SILK LINGERIE
B
CHEMISE
$1.59
C
DANCE SET
$1.59
TRUE BIAS STYLE
D
FINE QUALITY RAYON CREPE
$1.59
Of course- Quality Undies come from Sears
ALSO "V" NECK STYLE
E
ALL WOOL
ALL WOOL WORSTED
$2.00 POSTPAID
F
RUN-RESISTANT KNIT RAYON PAJAMA WITH COAT
$2.00 POSTPAID
Serona
G
PAJAMA OF FINE QUALITY COTTON PLAID
$1.00
FANCY SHORTY
H
49¢
Serona
RUN-RESISTANT RAYON
NOVELTY TRIM
59¢
J
ALSO STOUT SIZES
Serona
N
FRENCH STYLE SILK CREPE
$1.69
P
EXTRA SPECIAL QUALITY
59¢ EACH
Serona
RUN-RESISTANT RAYON
R
ALSO STOUT SIZES
K
FINE KNIT RAYON PRINCESS GOWN
$1.39
L
FRENCH STYLE SILK CREPE
$2.00 POSTPAID
M
FRENCH STYLE SILK CREPE
Two Qualities
$2.00 POSTPAID and $1.49

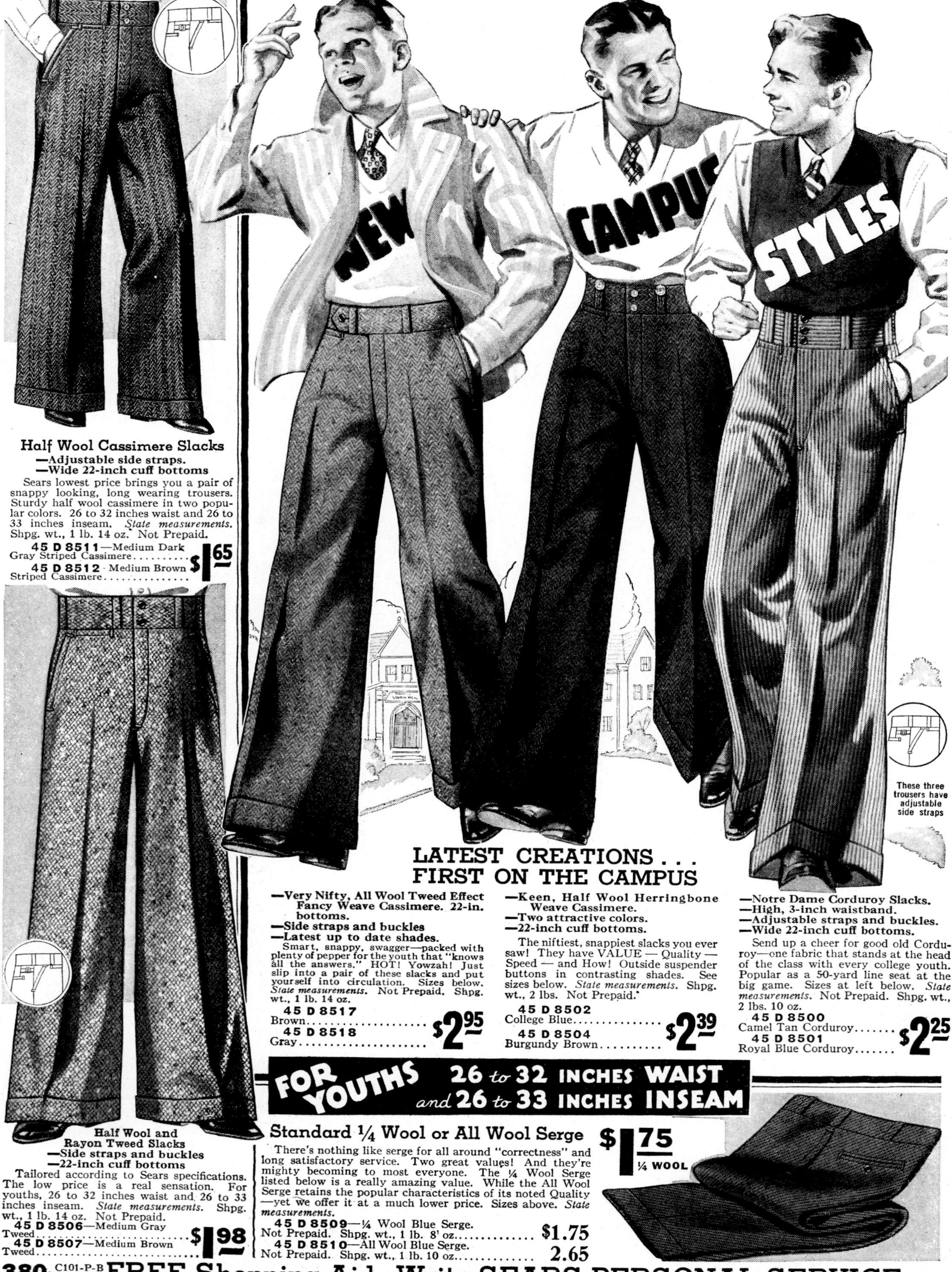
NEW
CAMPUS
STYLES
Half Wool Cassimere Slacks
—Adjustable side straps.
—Wide 22-inch cuff bottoms
Sears lowest price brings you a pair of snappy looking, long wearing trousers. Sturdy half wool cassimere in two popular colors. 26 to 32 inches waist and 26 to 33 inches inseam. State measurements. Shpg. wt., 1 lb. 14 oz. Not Prepaid.
45 D 8511—Medium Dark Gray Striped Cassimere..........
45 D 8512 Medium Brown Striped Cassimere..............
$1.65
These three trousers have adjustable side straps
LATEST CREATIONS...
FIRST ON THE CAMPUS
—Very Nifty, All Wool Tweed Effect Fancy Weave Cassimere. 22-in. bottoms.
—Side straps and buckles
—Latest up to date shades.
Smart, snappy, swagger—packed with plenty of pepper for the youth that "knows all the answers." HOT! Yowzah! Just slip into a pair of these slacks and put yourself into circulation. Sizes below. State measurements. Not Prepaid. Shpg. wt., 1 lb. 14 oz.
45 D 8517 Brown....................
45 D 8518 Gray....................
$2.95
—Keen, Half Wool Herringbone Weave Cassimere.
—Two attractive colors.
—22-inch cuff bottoms.
The niftiest, snappiest slacks you ever saw! They have VALUE — Quality — Speed — and How! Outside suspender buttons in contrasting shades. See sizes below. State measurements. Shpg. wt., 2 lbs. Not Prepaid.
45 D 8502 College Blue..............
45 D 8504 Burgundy Brown..........
$2.39
—Notre Dame Corduroy Slacks.
—High, 3-inch waistband.
—Adjustable straps and buckles.
—Wide 22-inch cuff bottoms.
Send up a cheer for good old Corduroy—one fabric that stands at the head of the class with every college youth. Popular as a 50-yard line seat at the big game. Sizes at left below. State measurements. Not Prepaid. Shpg. wt., 2 lbs. 10 oz.
45 D 8500 Camel Tan Corduroy.......
45 D 8501 Royal Blue Corduroy.......
$2.25
FOR YOUTHS 26 to 32 INCHES WAIST and 26 to 33 INCHES INSEAM
Half Wool and Rayon Tweed Slacks
—Side straps and buckles
—22-inch cuff bottoms
Tailored according to Sears specifications. The low price is a real sensation. For youths, 26 to 32 inches waist and 26 to 33 inches inseam. State measurements. Shpg. wt., 1 lb. 14 oz. Not Prepaid.
45 D 8506—Medium Gray Tweed..............................
45 D 8507—Medium Brown Tweed..............................
$1.98
Standard 1/4 Wool or All Wool Serge
$1.75 1/4 WOOL
There's nothing like serge for all around "correctness" and long satisfactory service. Two great values! And they're mighty becoming to most everyone. The 1/4 Wool Serge listed below is a really amazing value. While the All Wool Serge retains the popular characteristics of its noted Quality—yet we offer it at a much lower price. Sizes above. State measurements.
45 D 8509—1/4 Wool Blue Serge. Not Prepaid. Shpg. wt., 1 lb. 8 oz.............. $1.75
45 D 8510—All Wool Blue Serge. Not Prepaid. Shpg. wt., 1 lb. 10 oz.............. 2.65

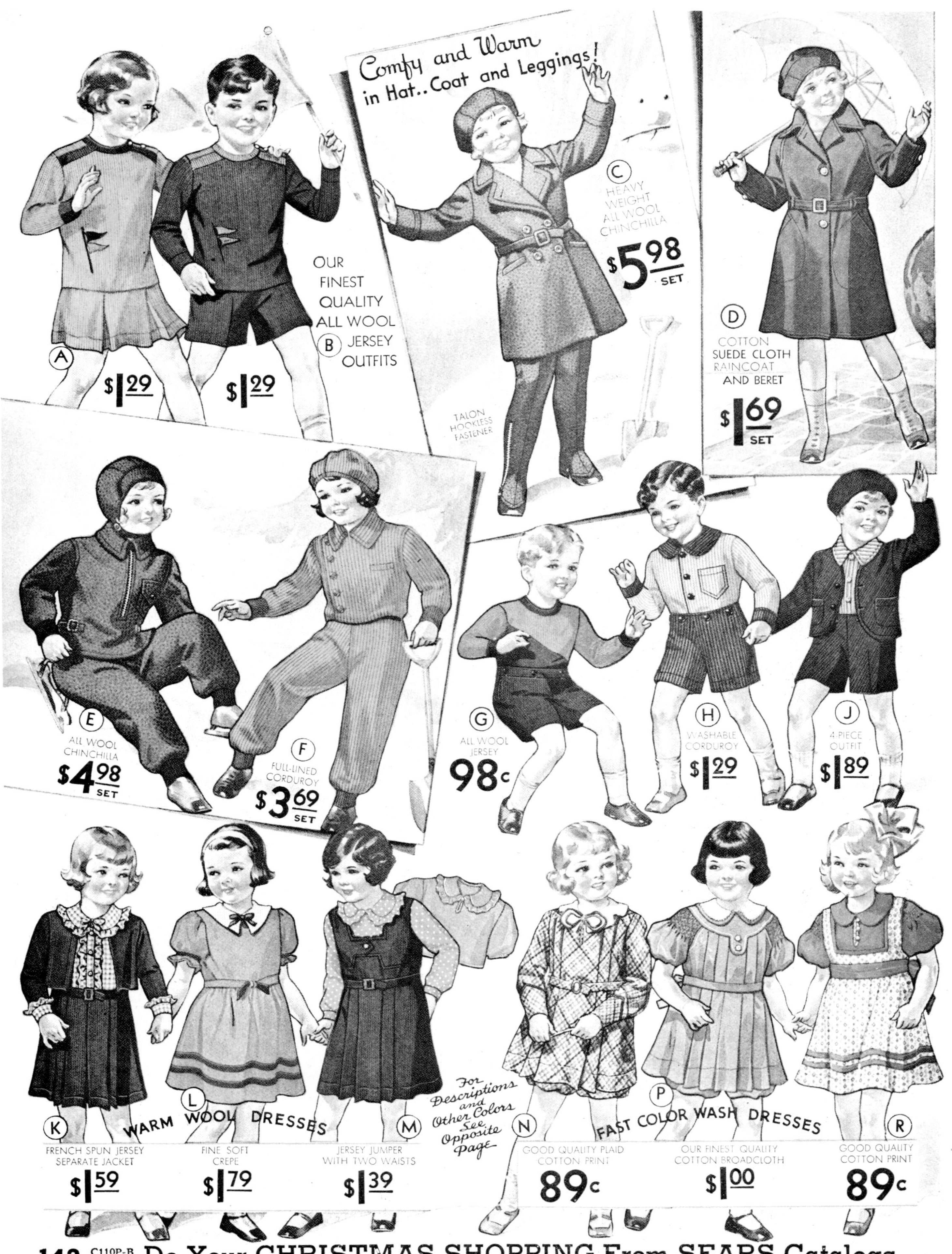

OUR FINEST QUALITY ALL WOOL JERSEY OUTFITS
A $1.29
B $1.29
Comfy and Warm in Hat.. Coat and Leggings!
C HEAVY WEIGHT ALL WOOL CHINCHILLA
$5.98 SET
TALON HOOKLESS FASTENER
D COTTON SUEDE CLOTH RAINCOAT AND BERET
$1.69 SET
E ALL WOOL CHINCHILLA
$4.98 SET
F FULL-LINED CORDUROY
$3.69 SET
G ALL WOOL JERSEY
98c
H WASHABLE CORDUROY
$1.29
J 4-PIECE OUTFIT
$1.89
WARM WOOL DRESSES
K FRENCH SPUN JERSEY SEPARATE JACKET
$1.59
L FINE SOFT CREPE
$1.79
M JERSEY JUMPER WITH TWO WAISTS
$1.39
For Descriptions and Other Colors See Opposite Page
FAST COLOR WASH DRESSES
N GOOD QUALITY PLAID COTTON PRINT
89c
P OUR FINEST QUALITY COTTON BROADCLOTH
$1.00
R GOOD QUALITY COTTON PRINT
89c

Suits STEP BRISKLY INTO SPRING FASHION

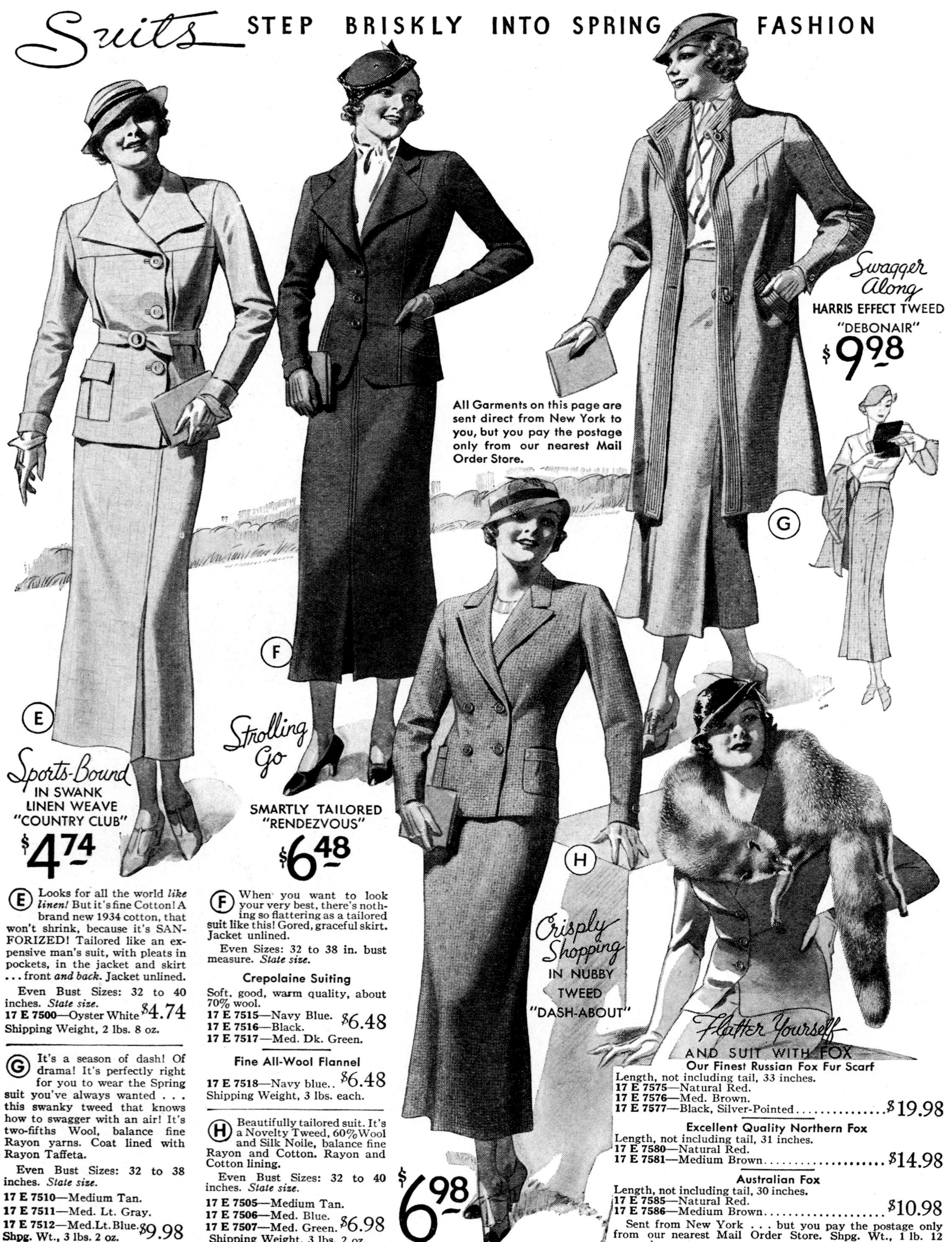

(E) Looks for all the world *like linen!* But it's fine Cotton! A brand new 1934 cotton, that won't shrink, because it's SANFORIZED! Tailored like an expensive man's suit, with pleats in pockets, in the jacket and skirt . . . front *and back*. Jacket unlined.

Even Bust Sizes: 32 to 40 inches. *State size.*
17 E 7500—Oyster White $4.74
Shipping Weight, 2 lbs. 8 oz.

(G) It's a season of dash! Of drama! It's perfectly right for you to wear the Spring suit you've always wanted . . . this swanky tweed that knows how to swagger with an air! It's two-fifths Wool, balance fine Rayon yarns. Coat lined with Rayon Taffeta.

Even Bust Sizes: 32 to 38 inches. *State size.*
17 E 7510—Medium Tan.
17 E 7511—Med. Lt. Gray.
17 E 7512—Med.Lt.Blue. $9.98
Shpg. Wt., 3 lbs. 2 oz.

(F) When you want to look your very best, there's nothing so flattering as a tailored suit like this! Gored, graceful skirt. Jacket unlined.

Even Sizes: 32 to 38 in. bust measure. *State size.*

Crepolaine Suiting

Soft, good, warm quality, about 70% wool.
17 E 7515—Navy Blue.
17 E 7516—Black. $6.48
17 E 7517—Med. Dk. Green.

Fine All-Wool Flannel

17 E 7518—Navy blue.. $6.48
Shipping Weight, 3 lbs. each.

(H) Beautifully tailored suit. It's a Novelty Tweed, 60% Wool and Silk Noile, balance fine Rayon and Cotton. Rayon and Cotton lining.

Even Bust Sizes: 32 to 40 inches. *State size.*
17 E 7505—Medium Tan.
17 E 7506—Med. Blue.
17 E 7507—Med. Green. $6.98
Shipping Weight, 3 lbs. 2 oz.

Our Finest Russian Fox Fur Scarf

Length, not including tail, 33 inches.
17 E 7575—Natural Red.
17 E 7576—Med. Brown.
17 E 7577—Black, Silver-Pointed.............. $19.98

Excellent Quality Northern Fox

Length, not including tail, 31 inches.
17 E 7580—Natural Red.
17 E 7581—Medium Brown.................. $14.98

Australian Fox

Length, not including tail, 30 inches.
17 E 7585—Natural Red.
17 E 7586—Medium Brown.................. $10.98

Sent from New York . . . but you pay the postage only from our nearest Mail Order Store. Shpg. Wt., 1 lb. 12 oz. each.

do your friends know about Sears New York-to-you fashion service?

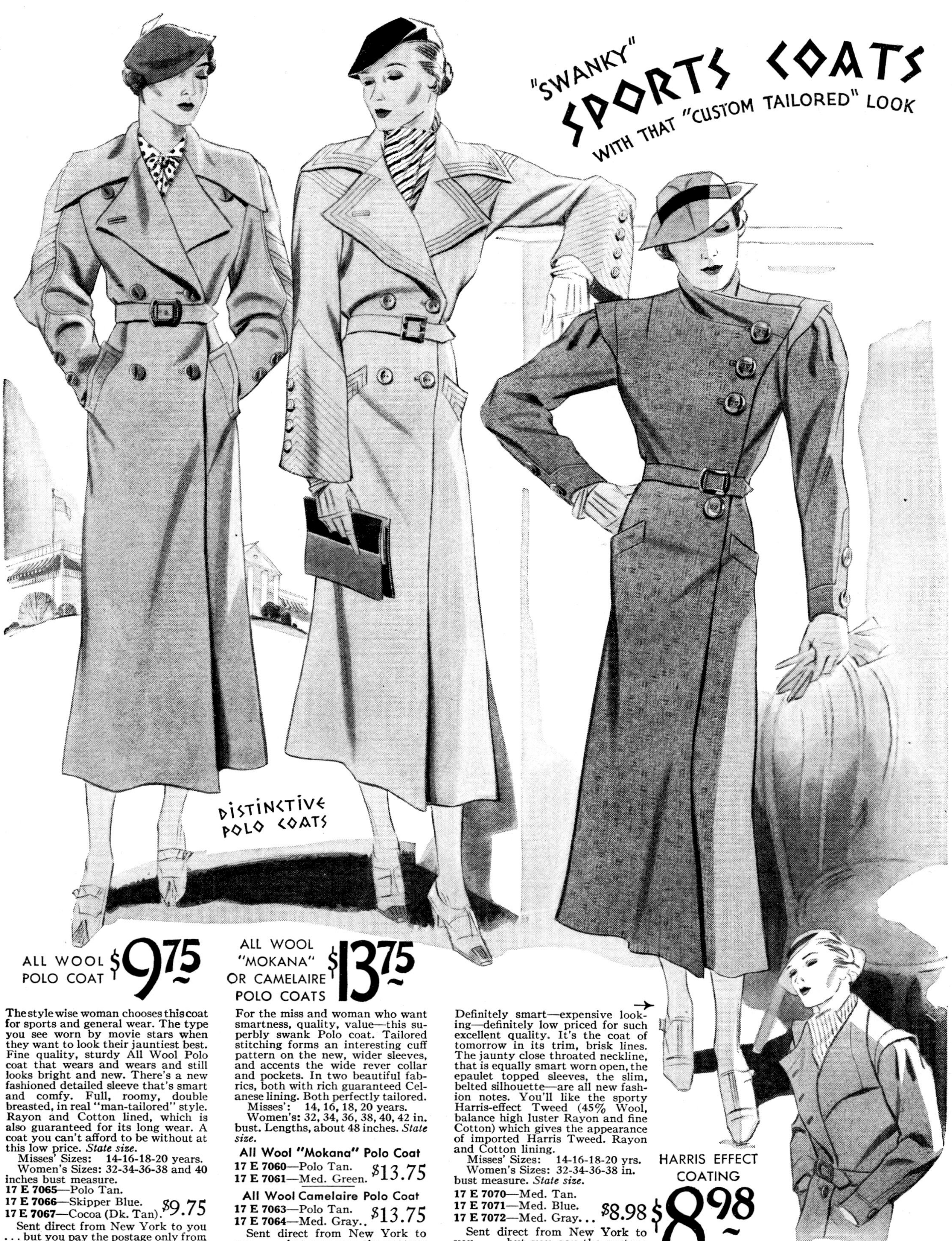

ALL WOOL POLO COAT $9.75

The style wise woman chooses this coat for sports and general wear. The type you see worn by movie stars when they want to look their jauntiest best. Fine quality, sturdy All Wool Polo coat that wears and wears and still looks bright and new. There's a new fashioned detailed sleeve that's smart and comfy. Full, roomy, double breasted, in real "man-tailored" style. Rayon and Cotton lined, which is also guaranteed for its long wear. A coat you can't afford to be without at this low price. *State size.*

Misses' Sizes: 14-16-18-20 years.
Women's Sizes: 32-34-36-38 and 40 inches bust measure.
17 E 7065—Polo Tan.
17 E 7066—Skipper Blue.
17 E 7067—Cocoa (Dk. Tan). $9.75

Sent direct from New York to you . . . but you pay the postage only from our nearest Mail Order Store. Shipping Weight, 3 lbs. 8 oz.

ALL WOOL "MOKANA" OR CAMELAIRE POLO COATS $13.75

For the miss and woman who want smartness, quality, value—this superbly swank Polo coat. Tailored stitching forms an interesting cuff pattern on the new, wider sleeves, and accents the wide rever collar and pockets. In two beautiful fabrics, both with rich guaranteed Celanese lining. Both perfectly tailored.

Misses': 14, 16, 18, 20 years.
Women's: 32, 34, 36, 38, 40, 42 in. bust. Lengths, about 48 inches. *State size.*

All Wool "Mokana" Polo Coat
17 E 7060—Polo Tan.
17 E 7061—Med. Green. $13.75

All Wool Camelaire Polo Coat
17 E 7063—Polo Tan.
17 E 7064—Med. Gray.. $13.75

Sent direct from New York to you . . . but you pay the postage only from our nearest Mail Order Store. Shipping Weight, 4 lbs.

HARRIS EFFECT COATING $8.98

Definitely smart—expensive looking—definitely low priced for such excellent quality. It's the coat of tomorrow in its trim, brisk lines. The jaunty close throated neckline, that is equally smart worn open, the epaulet topped sleeves, the slim, belted silhouette—are all new fashion notes. You'll like the sporty Harris-effect Tweed (45% Wool, balance high luster Rayon and fine Cotton) which gives the appearance of imported Harris Tweed. Rayon and Cotton lining.

Misses' Sizes: 14-16-18-20 yrs.
Women's Sizes: 32-34-36-38 in. bust measure. *State size.*
17 E 7070—Med. Tan.
17 E 7071—Med. Blue.
17 E 7072—Med. Gray... $8.98

Sent direct from New York to you . . . but you pay the postage only from our nearest Mail Order Store. Shipping Weight, 3 lbs. 8 oz.

extra style...quality...value...it's safe to save at Sears

insure
your
figure lines
Wear this new "Softie"
THE SUCCESS OF YOUR
DRESS DEPENDS ON
YOUR FOUNDATION
$5.98
$4.98
the newest "party-times" are subtly "curve" revealing

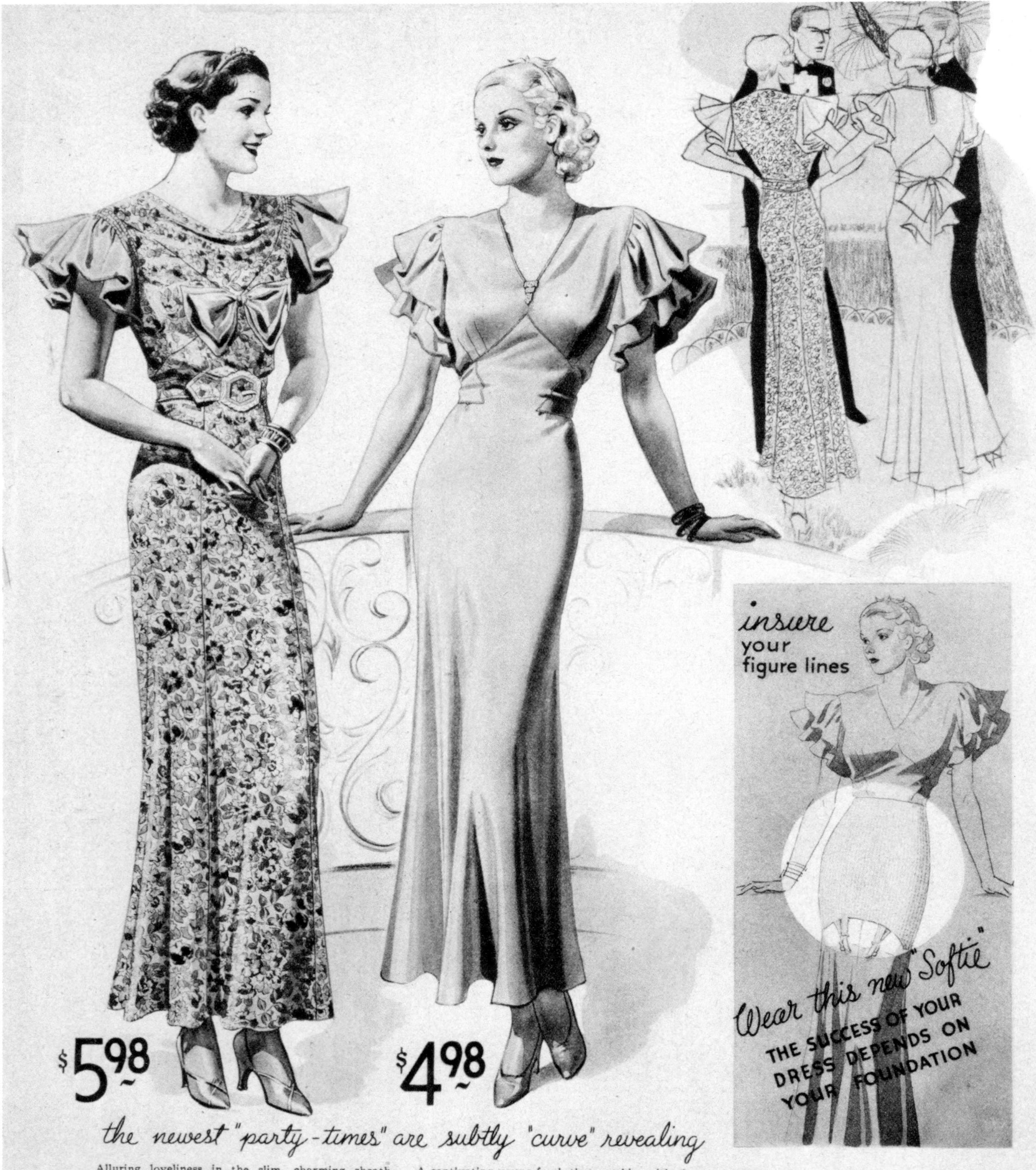

Alluring loveliness in the slim, charming sheath silhouette. The All Rayon Print is the new service weight sheer—drapes like softest Chiffon, yet has the close weave of fine silk. Crisp, rustling Celanese Taffeta fashions the "swish" fly-away shirred sleeves and gay bow. The long slender skirt falls in soft, full folds about the ankles. It's inexpensive, too. *State size.*

Misses' Sizes: 14-16-18-20 years.

Bust Measures: 32-34-36-38 inches.

31 E 6032 — Summery Print on Light Ground........................ $5.98

Sent direct from New York to you . . . but you pay the postage only from our nearest Mail Order Store. Shipping Weight, 1 lb. 6 oz.

A captivating young frock that sparkles with charm from its tiered puff sleeves to the ankle swirling, slim fitting, bias cut skirt. A tie back sash gives the new "nipped" waistline. A new dull finish, fine quality All Rayon Canton Crepe is used. The gleaming neck clip is of rhinestones. *State size.*

Misses' Sizes: 14-16-18-20 years.
Bust Measures: 32-34-36-38 inches.

31 E 6028—Blue Lilac (Blue with Lavender cast).

31 E 6029—Applemint (Lt. Brt. Green).

31 E 6030—Ash Rose.

31 E 6031—National (Deep Brt.) Blue.... $4.98

Sent direct from New York to you . . . but you pay the postage only from our nearest Mail Order Store. Shipping Weight, 1 lb. 6 oz.

Watch out for dangerous curves—even you slim young things! Nothing spoils the beauty of a smart dress like uncurbed curves! This two-way-stretch step-in does a grand job at smoothing you out, and giving you the molded lines you should have! It's soft, firm knit elastic . . . stretches with you when you bend; never "rides" out of place. No need, ever, to yank it down! Length, about 14½ in. This is a nationally known quality that sells under another name at $5.00! Not Prepaid. Shipping Weight, 14 oz.

18 E 492—Tearose color. Sizes to fit Waists 24, 25, 26, 27, 28, 29, 30, 31 and 32 inches. *Give waist and hip measurements taken over dress.* $2.98

your friends will want to know of Sears New York fashion service

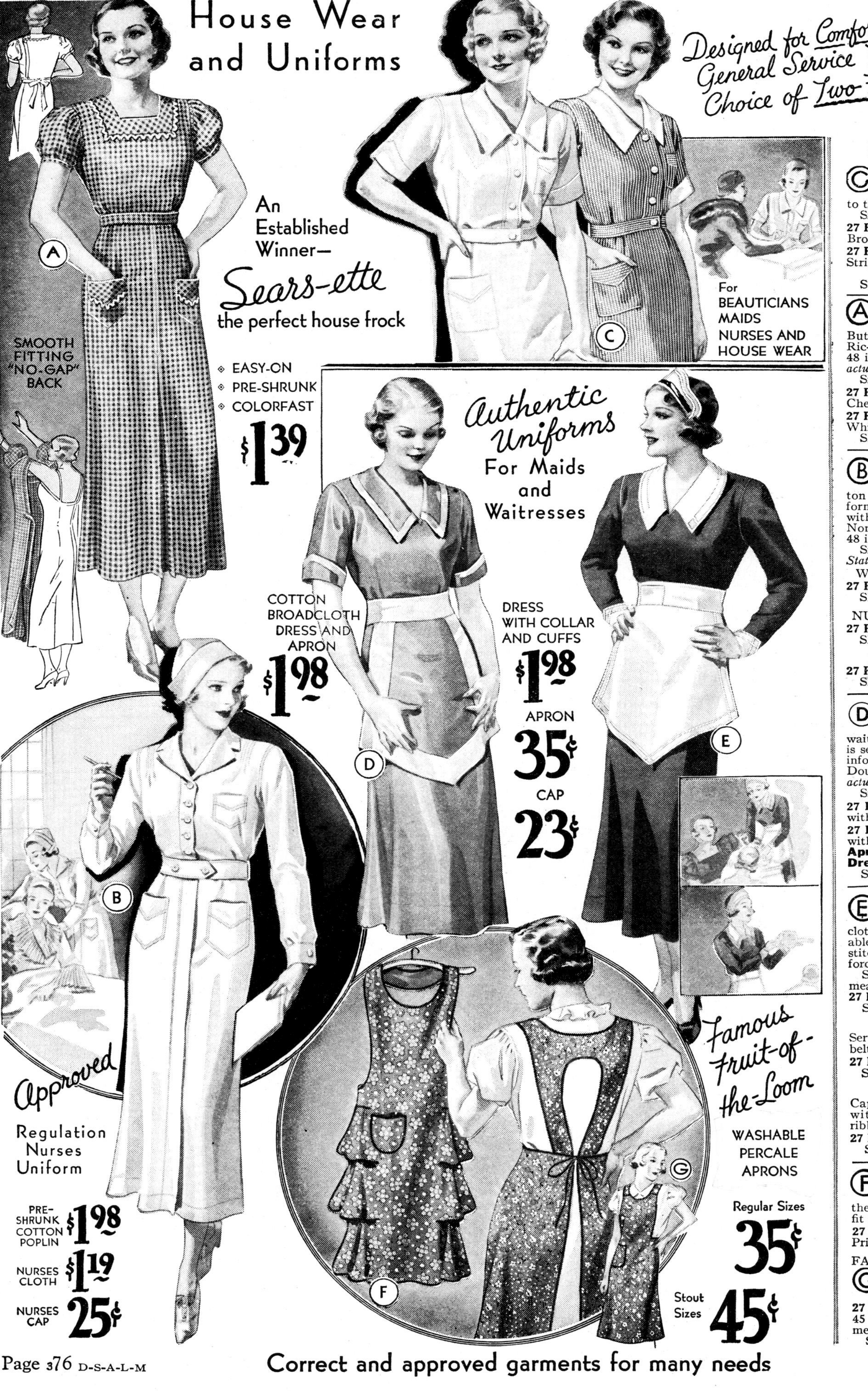

EACH **94¢**

(C) Expertly tailored uniforms, made in two fine qualities of cotton. Open to the waist. *State size.*
Sizes: 32 to 44 in. bust.
27 F 9539—White Broadcloth........ 94¢
27 F 9540—Navy and White Striped Percale.... 94¢
Shipping wgt., 12 oz. each

(A) Sears-ette, the perfect fitting house dress. Made of a famous cotton print. Button fastening at shoulder. Ric-Rac trim. Length, about 48 inches. Easy to iron. *State actual bust measure.*
Sizes: 32 to 42 in. bust.
27 F 4789—Copen and White Check.
27 F 4790—Red and White Check...... $1.39
Shipping weight, 12 oz.

(B) Furnished in choice of two fabrics, fine quality, pre-shrunk two-ply cotton poplin, and nurses' uniform cloth. Opens to the waist with ocean pearl buttons. Non-rip cuffs. Lengths, about 48 inches.
Sizes: 32 to 44 in. bust. *State bust measure.*
WHITE POPLIN
27 F 9535......... $1.98
Shipping weight, 1 lb. 8 oz.
NURSES' CLOTH
27 F 9537—White.. $1.19
Shipping weight, 1 lb. 6 oz.
NURSES' CAP
27 F 9538—White..... 25¢
Shipping weight, 6 oz.

(D) Our finest quality Cotton Broadcloth makes this two-piece, two-tone waitress' uniform. The apron is separate. The dress has reinforced pockets in the skirt. Double stitched seams. *State actual bust measure.*
Sizes: 32 to 44 in. bust.
27 F 3065 — Medium Green with Tan trimming.
27 F 3066 — Medium Tan with Brown trimming.
Apron and Dress............. $1.98
Shipping weight, 1 lb. 6 oz.

(E) Neat, sturdy, and excellently made dress of finest Cotton Broadcloth. Service cloth, detachable cuffs and collar. Double stitched seams. Two reinforced patch pockets.
Sizes: 34 to 44 in. bust measure. *State size.*
27 F 9500—Black.. $1.98
Shipping weight, 1 lb. 6 oz.

WHITE APRON
Service Cloth. All around belt.
27 F 9503........... 35¢
Shipping weight, 6 oz.

WHITE CAP
Cap of good quality organdy with black all silk satin ribbon.
27 F 9504........... 23¢
Shipping weight, 3 oz.

(F) Made of nationally known, durable and long-wearing Fruit-of-the-Loom Percale. Sizes to fit 32 to 44 in. bust measure.
27 F 9565 — Fancy Print Slip-over Apron. 35¢

FANCY PRINT COVERALL
(G) **27 F 9567**—To fit Regular Sizes: 38 to 44 in. bust....... 35¢
27 F 9569—To fit Stout Sizes 45 to 53 in. bust measure............ 45¢
Shipping weight, each 6 oz

Correct and approved garments for many needs

Setting the pace FOR STYLE AND VALUE in Sports Apparel
Ahoy There!
See my 3-PIECE MARINE OUTFIT
BLOUSE SLACKS HAT
$1.49
New SWEAT SHIRT
85¢
SLACKS
$1.19
A
B
Good looking togs, Mary! wish I could afford them!
Oh, yes you can, Helen just order from Sears!
Save at Sears ON STYLISH RIDING TOGS
WHIPCORD JODPHURS
$3.48
RIDING BREECHES
Whipcord - Gabardine
$2.98 $2.69
JACKET - SHIRT
$1.98 98¢
C
D
POLO SHIRT
85¢
E
IT'S SHORTS for Sports
98¢
TWIN SWEATERS With Matching SKIRT—
Summer's Indispensable
$2.98
F

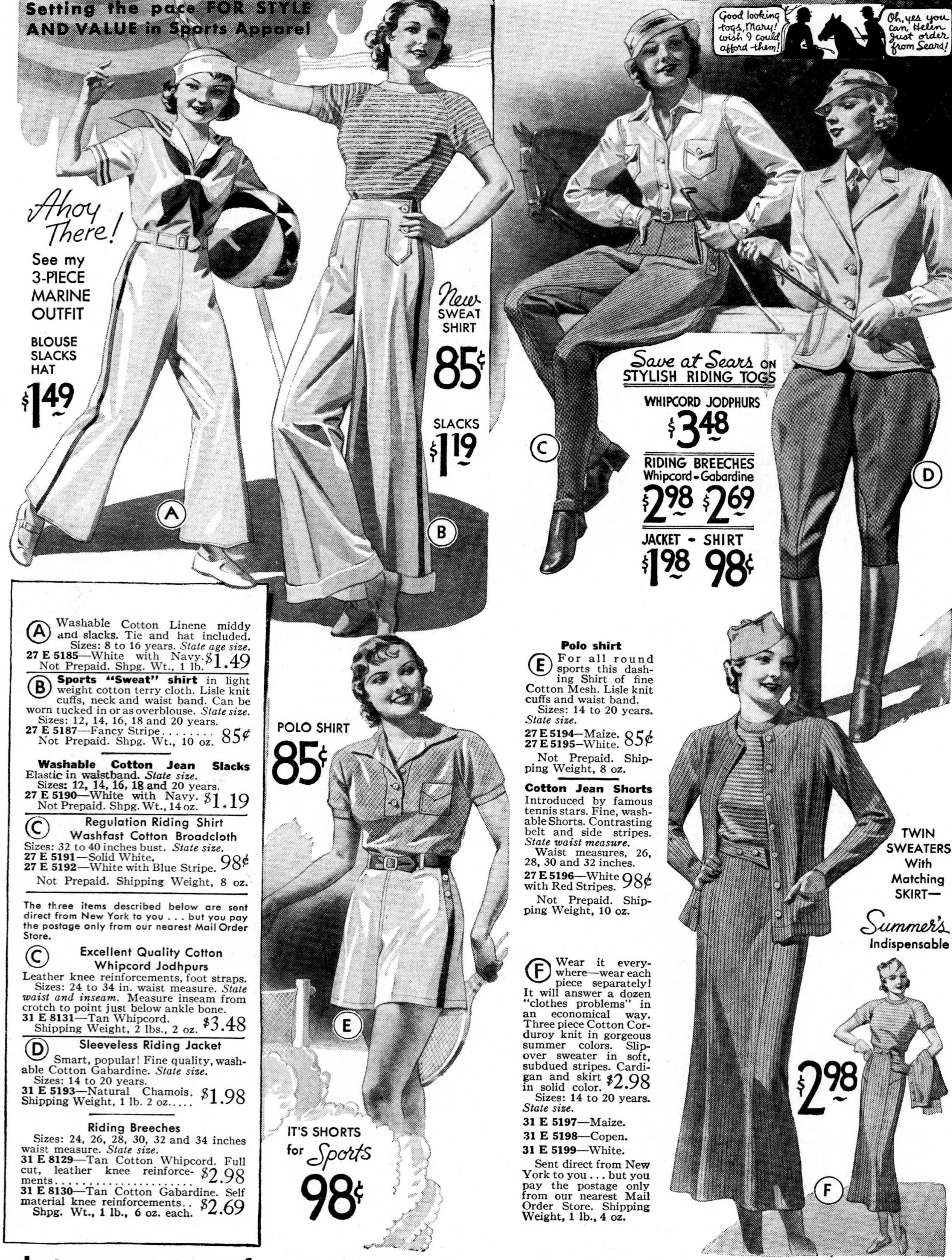

(A) Washable Cotton Linene middy and slacks. Tie and hat included. Sizes: 8 to 16 years. *State age size.*
27 E 5185—White with Navy. $1.49
Not Prepaid. Shpg. Wt., 1 lb.

(B) Sports "Sweat" shirt in light weight cotton terry cloth. Lisle knit cuffs, neck and waist band. Can be worn tucked in or as overblouse. *State size.*
Sizes: 12, 14, 16, 18 and 20 years.
27 E 5187—Fancy Stripe........ 85¢
Not Prepaid. Shpg. Wt., 10 oz.

Washable Cotton Jean Slacks
Elastic in waistband. *State size.*
Sizes: 12, 14, 16, 18 and 20 years.
27 E 5190—White with Navy. $1.19
Not Prepaid. Shpg. Wt., 14 oz.

(C) Regulation Riding Shirt
Washfast Cotton Broadcloth
Sizes: 32 to 40 inches bust. *State size.*
27 E 5191—Solid White.
27 E 5192—White with Blue Stripe. 98¢
Not Prepaid. Shipping Weight, 8 oz.

The three items described below are sent direct from New York to you . . . but you pay the postage only from our nearest Mail Order Store.

(C) Excellent Quality Cotton Whipcord Jodhpurs
Leather knee reinforcements, foot straps. Sizes: 24 to 34 in. waist measure. *State waist and inseam.* Measure inseam from crotch to point just below ankle bone.
31 E 8131—Tan Whipcord. $3.48
Shipping Weight, 2 lbs., 2 oz.

(D) Sleeveless Riding Jacket
Smart, popular! Fine quality, washable Cotton Gabardine. *State size.*
Sizes: 14 to 20 years.
31 E 5193—Natural Chamois. $1.98
Shipping Weight, 1 lb. 2 oz.....

Riding Breeches
Sizes: 24, 26, 28, 30, 32 and 34 inches waist measure. *State size.*
31 E 8129—Tan Cotton Whipcord. Full cut, leather knee reinforcements.................... $2.98
31 E 8130—Tan Cotton Gabardine. Self material knee reinforcements.. $2.69
Shpg. Wt., 1 lb., 6 oz. each.

Polo shirt
(E) For all round sports this dashing Shirt of fine Cotton Mesh. Lisle knit cuffs and waist band.
Sizes: 14 to 20 years. *State size.*
27 E 5194—Maize.
27 E 5195—White. 85¢
Not Prepaid. Shipping Weight, 8 oz.

Cotton Jean Shorts
Introduced by famous tennis stars. Fine, washable Shorts. Contrasting belt and side stripes. *State waist measure.*
Waist measures, 26, 28, 30 and 32 inches.
27 E 5196—White with Red Stripes. 98¢
Not Prepaid. Shipping Weight, 10 oz.

(F) Wear it everywhere—wear each piece separately! It will answer a dozen "clothes problems" in an economical way. Three piece Cotton Corduroy knit in gorgeous summer colors. Slipover sweater in soft, subdued stripes. Cardigan and skirt in solid color. $2.98
Sizes: 14 to 20 years. *State size.*
31 E 5197—Maize.
31 E 5198—Copen.
31 E 5199—White.
Sent direct from New York to you . . . but you pay the postage only from our nearest Mail Order Store. Shipping Weight, 1 lb., 4 oz.

whatever sport you favor get your togs at Sears and save

Our finest
soft velvety
Genuine
SUEDE LEATHER
fully lined with
rich Rayon
and Cotton
$7.89
C
For those who
want . . .
Finer
Jackets
these
GENUINE
LEATHERS
A
button-up
Cossack
Style
fine quality
SUEDE LEATHER
$5.98
Genuine
GLOVE LEATHER
$4.98
D
Genuine
SUEDE LEATHER
with Easy-on-Talon
Fastener
Only $5.48
"Talon Fastener"
Ultra
Smart
collarless jacket
FINE
SUEDE LEATHER
$6.48
B
WITH
BUTTON
FRONT
$5.74
selected quality
Genuine
GLOVE LEATHER
warm wool
flannel lining
$6.89

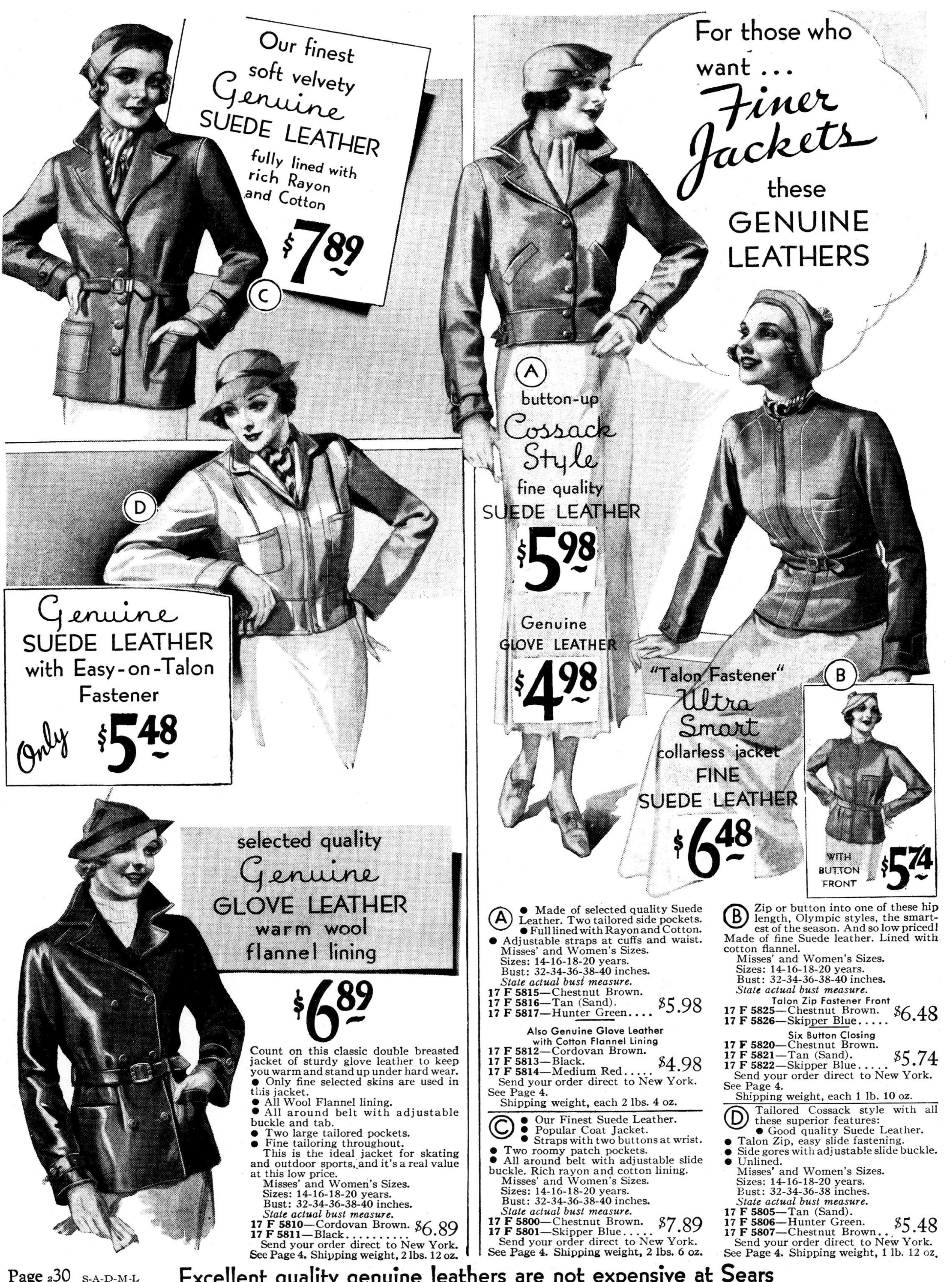

Count on this classic double breasted jacket of sturdy glove leather to keep you warm and stand up under hard wear.
● Only fine selected skins are used in this jacket.
● All Wool Flannel lining.
● All around belt with adjustable buckle and tab.
● Two large tailored pockets.
● Fine tailoring throughout.

This is the ideal jacket for skating and outdoor sports, and it's a real value at this low price.

Misses' and Women's Sizes.
Sizes: 14-16-18-20 years.
Bust: 32-34-36-38-40 inches.
State actual bust measure.

17 F 5810—Cordovan Brown.
17 F 5811—Black.......... $6.89

Send your order direct to New York. See Page 4. Shipping weight, 2 lbs. 12 oz.

(A) ● Made of selected quality Suede Leather. Two tailored side pockets.
● Full lined with Rayon and Cotton.
● Adjustable straps at cuffs and waist.

Misses' and Women's Sizes.
Sizes: 14-16-18-20 years.
Bust: 32-34-36-38-40 inches.
State actual bust measure.

17 F 5815—Chestnut Brown.
17 F 5816—Tan (Sand).
17 F 5817—Hunter Green.... $5.98

Also Genuine Glove Leather with Cotton Flannel Lining

17 F 5812—Cordovan Brown.
17 F 5813—Black.
17 F 5814—Medium Red..... $4.98

Send your order direct to New York. See Page 4.
Shipping weight, each 2 lbs. 4 oz.

(C) ● Our Finest Suede Leather.
● Popular Coat Jacket.
● Straps with two buttons at wrist.
● Two roomy patch pockets.
● All around belt with adjustable slide buckle. Rich rayon and cotton lining.

Misses' and Women's Sizes.
Sizes: 14-16-18-20 years.
Bust: 32-34-36-38-40 inches.
State actual bust measure.

17 F 5800—Chestnut Brown.
17 F 5801—Skipper Blue..... $7.89

Send your order direct to New York. See Page 4. Shipping weight, 2 lbs. 6 oz.

(B) Zip or button into one of these hip length, Olympic styles, the smartest of the season. And so low priced! Made of fine Suede leather. Lined with cotton flannel.

Misses' and Women's Sizes.
Sizes: 14-16-18-20 years.
Bust: 32-34-36-38-40 inches.
State actual bust measure.

Talon Zip Fastener Front

17 F 5825—Chestnut Brown.
17 F 5826—Skipper Blue..... $6.48

Six Button Closing

17 F 5820—Chestnut Brown.
17 F 5821—Tan (Sand).
17 F 5822—Skipper Blue..... $5.74

Send your order direct to New York. See Page 4.
Shipping weight, each 1 lb. 10 oz.

(D) Tailored Cossack style with all these superior features:
● Good quality Suede Leather.
● Talon Zip, easy slide fastening.
● Side gores with adjustable slide buckle.
● Unlined.

Misses' and Women's Sizes.
Sizes: 14-16-18-20 years.
Bust: 32-34-36-38 inches.
State actual bust measure.

17 F 5805—Tan (Sand).
17 F 5806—Hunter Green.
17 F 5807—Chestnut Brown.. $5.48

Send your order direct to New York. See Page 4. Shipping weight, 1 lb. 12 oz.

Excellent quality genuine leathers are not expensive at Sears

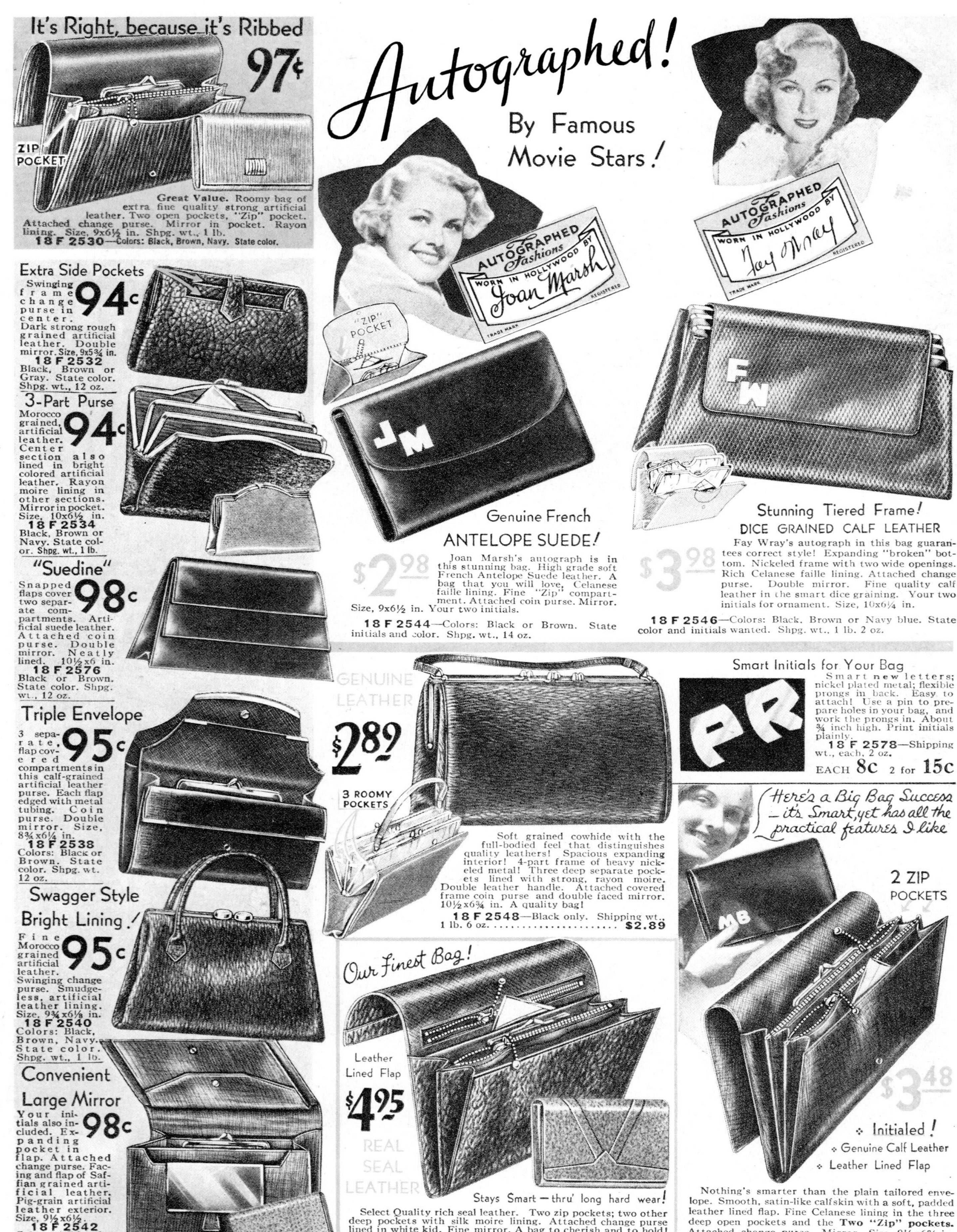
It's Right, because it's Ribbed
97¢
ZIP POCKET
Great Value. Roomy bag of extra fine quality strong artificial leather. Two open pockets, "Zip" pocket. Attached change purse. Mirror in pocket. Rayon lining. Size, 9x6½ in. Shpg. wt., 1 lb.
18 F 2530—Colors: Black, Brown, Navy. State color.
Autographed!
By Famous Movie Stars!
AUTOGRAPHED Fashions WORN IN HOLLYWOOD BY Joan Marsh TRADE MARK REGISTERED
AUTOGRAPHED Fashions WORN IN HOLLYWOOD BY Fay Wray TRADE MARK REGISTERED
Extra Side Pockets
94c
Swinging frame change purse in center. Dark strong rough grained artificial leather. Double mirror. Size, 9x5¾ in.
18 F 2532
Black, Brown or Gray. State color. Shpg. wt., 12 oz.
3-Part Purse
94c
Morocco grained, artificial leather. Center section also lined in bright colored artificial leather. Rayon moire lining in other sections. Mirror in pocket. Size, 10x6½ in.
18 F 2534
Black, Brown or Navy. State color. Shpg. wt., 1 lb.
"Suedine"
98c
Snapped flaps cover two separate compartments. Artificial suede leather. Attached coin purse. Double mirror. Neatly lined. 10½x6 in.
18 F 2576
Black or Brown. State color. Shpg. wt., 12 oz.
Triple Envelope
95c
3 separate, flap covered compartments in this calf-grained artificial leather purse. Each flap edged with metal tubing. Coin purse. Double mirror. Size, 8¾x6¼ in.
18 F 2538
Colors: Black or Brown. State color. Shpg. wt. 12 oz.
Swagger Style
Bright Lining!
95c
Fine Morocco grained artificial leather. Swinging change purse. Smudgeless, artificial leather lining. Size, 9¾x6⅛ in.
18 F 2540
Colors: Black, Brown, Navy. State color. Shpg. wt., 1 lb.
Convenient
Large Mirror
98c
Your initials also included. Expanding pocket in flap. Attached change purse. Facing and flap of Saffian grained artificial leather. Pig-grain artificial leather exterior. Size, 9½x6½.
18 F 2542
Colors: Black, Brown or Red. State color and initials. Shpg. wt., 1 lb. 2 oz.
FD
"ZIP" POCKET
JM
Genuine French
ANTELOPE SUEDE!
$2.98
Joan Marsh's autograph is in this stunning bag. High grade soft French Antelope Suede leather. A bag that you will love. Celanese faille lining. Fine "Zip" compartment. Attached coin purse. Mirror. Size, 9x6½ in. Your two initials.
18 F 2544—Colors: Black or Brown. State initials and color. Shpg. wt., 14 oz.
FW
Stunning Tiered Frame!
DICE GRAINED CALF LEATHER
$3.98
Fay Wray's autograph in this bag guarantees correct style! Expanding "broken" bottom. Nickeled frame with two wide openings. Rich Celanese faille lining. Attached change purse. Double mirror. Fine quality calf leather in the smart dice graining. Your two initials for ornament. Size, 10x6¼ in.
18 F 2546—Colors: Black, Brown or Navy blue. State color and initials wanted. Shpg. wt., 1 lb. 2 oz.
GENUINE LEATHER
$2.89
3 ROOMY POCKETS
Soft grained cowhide with the full-bodied feel that distinguishes quality leathers! Spacious expanding interior! 4-part frame of heavy nickeled metal! Three deep separate pockets lined with strong, rayon moire. Double leather handle. Attached covered frame coin purse and double faced mirror. 10½x6¾ in. A quality bag!
18 F 2548—Black only. Shipping wt., 1 lb. 6 oz. $2.89
Smart Initials for Your Bag
PR
Smart new letters; nickel plated metal; flexible prongs in back. Easy to attach! Use a pin to prepare holes in your bag, and work the prongs in. About ¾ inch high. Print initials plainly.
18 F 2578—Shipping wt., each, 2 oz.
EACH 8c 2 for 15c
Here's a Big Bag Success – it's Smart, yet has all the practical features I like
MB
2 ZIP POCKETS
Our Finest Bag!
Leather Lined Flap
$4.95
REAL SEAL LEATHER
Stays Smart—thru' long hard wear!
Select Quality rich seal leather. Two zip pockets; two other deep pockets with silk moire lining. Attached change purse lined in white kid. Fine mirror. A bag to cherish and to hold! Size, 9½x6¾ in.
18 F 2550—Colors: Black or Dark Brown. State color. Shpg. wt., 1 lb. 6 oz. $4.95
$3.48
Initialed!
Genuine Calf Leather
Leather Lined Flap
Nothing's smarter than the plain tailored envelope. Smooth, satin-like calfskin with a soft, padded leather lined flap. Fine Celanese lining in the three deep open pockets and the Two "Zip" pockets. Attached change purse. Mirror. Size, 9½x6¾ in. And your two initials are included.
18 F 2552—Colors: Black or Brown. State color and print initials. Shpg. wt., 1 lb. 2 oz.
You'll Find the Smartest Bags at Sears
3 AMLDS 91

It's new! and dramatic! the hollywood halo hat!
$1.98
Autographed
WORN IN HOLLYWOOD BY Loretta Young REGISTERED TRADE MARK
an authentic "movie" style marked with this label!

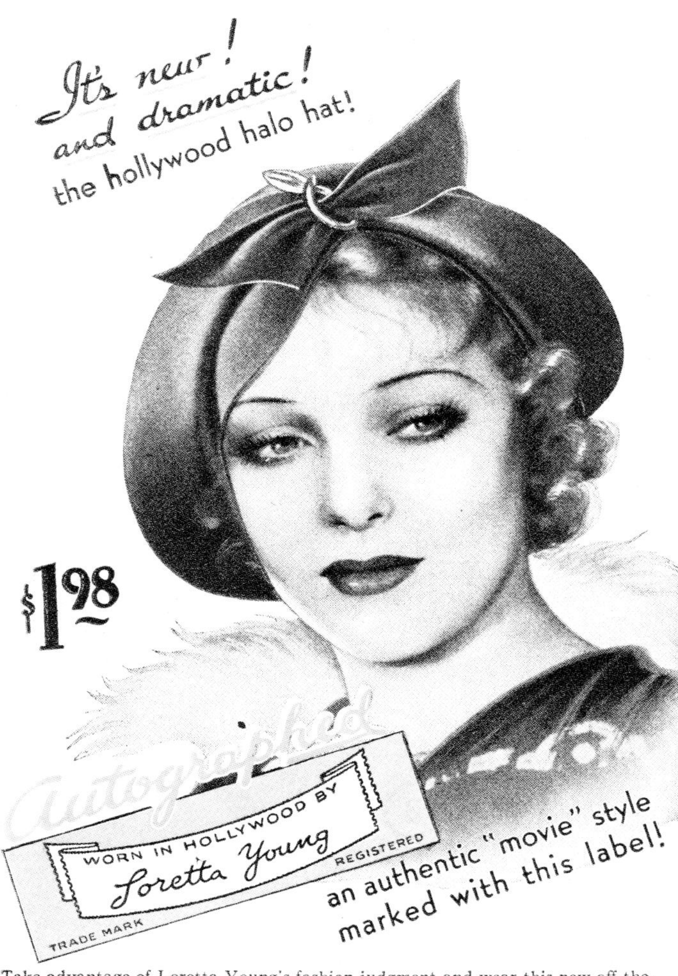

Take advantage of Loretta Young's fashion judgment and wear this new off-the-face hat! It's *different*, it's young looking, it's striking! There's something of the angel's halo and something of the buccaneer's bravado in its dramatic, folded-back brim, its snug eye-line bandeau, its gay folded felt bow. Made of fine quality all wool body felt, with a colorful composition loop over the bow. Loretta Young has this hat in her personal wardrobe for Fall wear.

78 F 7305—Fits 22 to 22½ inches headsize. **Colors:** Black or Jaffa (Dark) Brown. *Measure and state color.* Shpg. Wt., 1 lb. $1.98

$1.29

youthful! in a dignified way!

Ⓐ We know! You want to look young, but you'd hate to go to extremes about it! We have just the hat for you! With a comfortable, good sized crown, a pleasant dipping brim and a flattering veil that's kind to tired eyes! The hat is fine quality all wool body felt with a cockade of two-tone ribbons in front.

78 F 7520—Fits 22¼ to 22¾ inches headsize.

78 F 7521—Fits 23 to 23½ inches headsize.

Colors: Black, Jaffa (Dark) Brown or Cruise (Navy) Blue. *State color.* Shpg. Wt., 1 lb........ $1.29

79¢

bright colored corduroy

Ⓑ We nominate this bright corduroy hat for every smart woman's wardrobe, no matter how many other hats she has! Because it does wonders at "lighting up" Fall costumes! It's rich and lovely. It's made in a style that is becoming to every one! And it's a colorful fashion that all can afford at this low price.

78 F 7620—Fits 22 to 22½ inches headsize.

Colors: Royal Blue, Brt. Red, Med. Green or Rust Brown. *State color.* Shpg. Wt., 1 lb......... 79¢

Ⓒ Satin comes in as regularly as Autumn—and here's a stunning rayon satin hat that you can wear with late summer prints as well as with your winter coat! Made in the typical 1934 Fashion, with the brim turned snugly up against the crown in back; turned flatteringly down in front. Stitched all-over to give the smart, semi-quilted effect. A stitched rayon satin strip divides the crown. Two-tone ribbon band.

78 F 7405—Fits 22 to 22½ inches headsize.

Colors: Black only. Shipping Weight, 1 lb.......... $1.39

$1.39

stitched satin!

Wool Felt

$1.39

a good large headsize with smart "patent" flowers

If it's hard to find hats that fit, here's the choice for you! It's grand and comfortable, and it adds smartness to your outfit! For this hat is trimmed with artificial patent leather—the newest accent for Fall hats! The all wool body felt is a fine, pliable quality brushed to a soft gloss and stitched with rich guimp braid. Truly, an unusual value.

78 F 7525—Fits 22½ to 23 inches.

78 F 7526—Fits 23¼ to 23¾ inches.

Colors: Black or Cruise (Navy) Blue. *Measure and state color.* Shipping Weight, 1 lb. $1.39

$1.19

there's news in the droop of this flattering brim!

We call it the "mushroom" brim—and you'll recognize it as one of the smartest styles in your fashion magazines! Flattering, too, because it shadows your eyes glamorously. Made of all wool body felt, brushed to a rich, furry finish; banded with shiny patent leather cloth brightened with a metal pin.

78 F 7495—Fits 22 to 22½ inches.

78 F 7496—Fits 22¾ to 23¼ inches.

Colors: Black, Jaffa (Dark) Brown or Cruise (Navy) Blue. *State color.* Shpg. Wt., 1 lb........ $1.19

MEASURE THIS WAY

88¢

Value! in the spotlight!

We want to call your attention to the *low* price of this smart hat! Because it leaves no excuse for wearing last year's style! This is a good pliable all wool body felt blocked with the new shallower crown and the slightly wider brim that you find even in the most expensive models. Metal ornament. One of those classic styles that *everyone* can wear. We've tried it on many different types of women and we know.

78 F 7410—Fits 22 to 22½ inches headsize.

Colors: Black, Jaffa (Dark) Brown or Cruise (Navy) Blue. *Measure and state color.* Shipping Weight, 1 lb........... 88¢

Every new dress deserves a new hat!

You're "IN THE SWIM"—with a suit that FITS!
HOW TO ORDER
Measure your chest or bust and state size desired. If size is uneven, order the next larger even size. If you are taller or stouter than average, order one size larger. Do not guess your size. Use a tape measure.
ALL WOOL $1.98 MEN'S
ADJUSTABLE BACK
WOMEN'S $2.79
WOMEN'S AND MISSES' SIZES
FINE ZEPHYR WOOL
WOMEN'S AND MISSES' SIZES
Fit-Rite SWIM SUITS
ALL WOOL $1.98 WOMEN'S
SPECIAL $1.79
FOR GIRLS ALL WOOL WITH GAY APPLIQUE
2 to 6 Yrs. 85¢
ALL WOOL
$1.19
FOR BOYS OR GIRLS ALL WOOL
Men! The SEARS QUALITY That Fits, and Lasts!
Men's 2-Ply All Wool Worsted
Close, heavy knit elastic rib stitch, so that it fits snugly, comfortably, the way only fine suits can! One piece speed style; attached trunks; reinforced crotch. Not Prepaid. Shipping Weight, 14 oz.
18 E 800—Even Sizes: 34 to 46 in. chest. Colors: Black or Royal Blue. State size and color $2.98
Men's 100% All Wool Worsted
Same style suit as above. A good quality. Not Prepaid. Shipping Weight, 14 oz.
18 E 802—Even Sizes: 34 to 46 in. chest. Colors: Royal Blue, Black, Navy Blue, Maroon. State size and color $1.98
Boys' 100% All Wool Worsted
Medium weight speed style suit as above. Not Prepaid. Shpg. Wt., 8 oz.
18 E 600—Sizes: 8, 10, 12 and 14 years. Colors: Navy Blue, Royal Blue or Maroon. State size and color $1.69
Men's Cotton Speed Suit
Good quality. Not Prepaid. Shipping Weight, 10 oz.
18 E 830—Navy Blue. Sizes: 36, 38, 40, 42 and 44 inches chest. State size .... 79¢
Boys' Cotton Speed Style Suit
Not Prepaid. Shipping Weight, 8 oz.
18 E 630—Navy Blue. Sizes: 8, 10, 12 and 14 years. State size .... 65¢
(A) Adjust the back straps to suit yourself! 100% All Wool Zephyr yarn in elastic rib stitch knit. Not Prepaid.
18 E 932—Women's. Even Sizes: 34 to 44 in. bust. Colors: Belgium (med) Blue, Poppy Glo (Orange), Jade Green, Black. State size and color. Shipping Weight, 12 oz. $2.79
18 E 732—Misses'. Sizes: 28, 30, 32 and 34 in. bust. Colors: Belgium (med) Blue, Poppy Glo (Orange), Jade Green, Jockey Red. State size and color. Shipping Weight, 8 oz $2.48
(B) All wool worsted; rib stitch knit. Crossed straps. Assorted appliques. Not Prepaid. Shipping Weight, 6 oz.
18 E 530—Sizes: 2, 4 and 6 years. Colors: Red, (med) Blue or Green. State size and color .... 85¢
(C) Low back underarm cutouts. All wool worsted; rib stitch knit. White belt. Shpg. Wt., 5 oz.
18 E 532 — Sizes: 2, 4, 6 and 8 years. Colors: Red, Blue or Green trunks. All white uppers. State size and color $1.19
Women's Suit All Wool Zephyr
(D) Fine knit, soft, hugs the body snugly. Low sun back. Reinforced crotch. Shpg. Wt., 14 oz.
18 E 904—Even Bust Sizes: 34 to 46 in. Colors: French (med) Blue, Jap Red, Jade Green, Royal Blue or Black. State size and color .. $2.98
Women's Suit of All Wool Worsted
Styled as above, but in elastic rib stitch. Not Prepaid. Shpg. Wt., 12 oz.
18 E 902—Even Bust Sizes: 34 to 46 in. Colors: Jade Green, Black, Royal Blue, Jockey Red. State size and color $1.98
Misses' All Wool Worsted Suit in rib stitch. Deep sun back. Shpg. Wt., 8 oz.
18 E 700—Sizes: 8, 10, 12 and 14 years. Colors: Jockey Red, French (med) Blue or Jade Green. State size and color $1.69
Misses' All Wool Worsted Suits
(E) Medium low back. Firmly knit. Neat appliques. Shipping Weight, 8 oz.
18 E 702—Sizes: 8, 10, 12 and 14 years. Colors: Jade Green, Jockey Red, Belgian (med) Blue, Poppy Glo (Orange). State size and color $1.79
Misses' Knit Cotton Suit
Well made. Medium low sun-back. Not Prepaid. Shipping Weight, 8 oz.
18 E 730—Sizes: 8, 10, 12 and 14 years. Jockey Red only. State size .... 65¢
"ZIP" The Top Comes Off
GET THAT SUMMER TAN IN TRUNKS
SPEEDSHIRTS For Wear with Trunks
25¢
DURO-TEX CAP
Brand new LATEX cap; resists strain and puncture. Shpg. Wt., 2 oz. State color.
18 E 1012—White, Green, Red or Blue.
BATHING SLIPPERS
29¢ pr.
18 E 1030 — Women's Sizes: 3 to 7. No half sizes. Colors: Red, Blue, Green or White. Shpg. Wt., 10 oz.
SWIM BELT
White web belt, 1⅜ in. wide. Metal buckle. Shpg. Wt., 4 oz.
18 E 1004—Sizes to fit up to 44 in. waist. State size. 21¢
MEN'S
KIDDIES
BOYS
WARM WOOL WORSTED
The suit for a real swimmer! No binding—leaves you freedom for long strokes! Top section slips off easily. $2.98
No belt. Not Prepaid. Shpg. Wt., 12 oz.
18 E 806—Navy Trunks: white top. White side strips. Sizes: 34, 36, 38, 40 and 42 inches chest. State size.
Gigolo trunks in all wool worsted, elastic rib stitch. Web belt. Asst. applique designs. Shpg. Wt. 4 oz. 79¢
18 E 528—Ages: 2, 4 and 6 years. Colors: Red, Royal Blue or Green. State size and color.
—All Wool Zephyr
Pocket at side; imitation fly front. White side stripes and web belt. Not Prepaid. Shipping Weight, 14 oz.
18 E 846—Even Sizes: 28 to 40 in. waist. Colors: Navy or Royal Blue. State size and color. $2.39
—All Wool Worsted
Elastic rib knit trunks styled like above. No pocket or fly front.
18 E 840—Navy Blue or Royal Blue. Even Sizes: 28 to 40 in. waist. State size. Shipping Weight, 12 oz. $1.69
—All Wool Worsted Elastic rib stitch knit. High, snug-fitting waist. White web belt and side stripes, Shpg. Wt., 10 oz. $1.49
18 E 640—Colors: Navy or Royal Blue. Even Sizes: 24 to 30 in. waist.
—Men's White All Wool Zephyr Speed Shirt
Fine, soft quality. Open bottom. Shpg. Wt., 12 oz. State size.
18 E 850—Even Sizes: 34 to 44 in. chest... $1.85
—Boys' All Wool Worsted. Same style as above in elastic rib stitch. Not Prepaid. Shpg. Wt., 12 oz. State size.
18 E 650—Sizes: 28, 30, 32 and 34 in. chest. $1.45

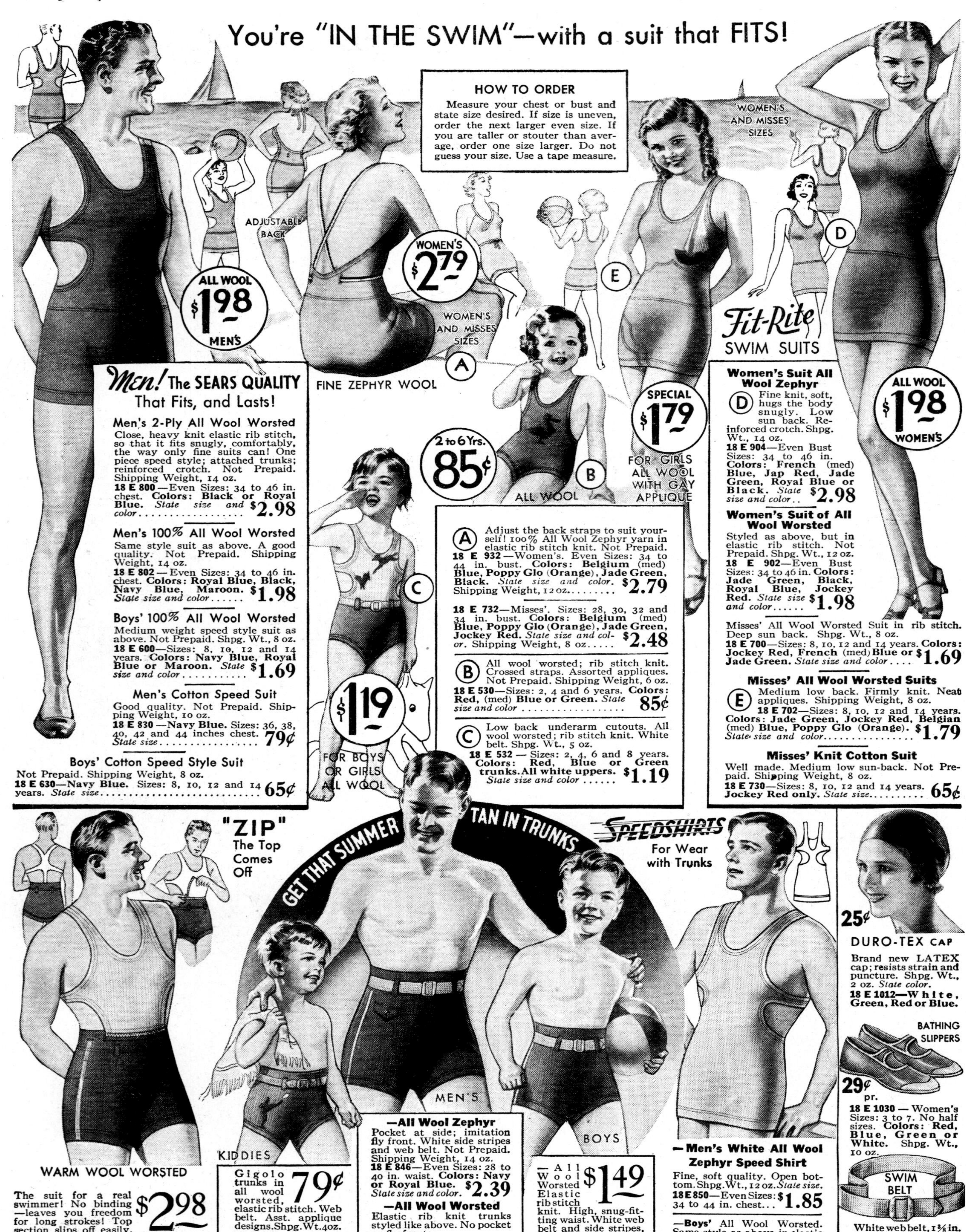

please measure carefully to determine your size

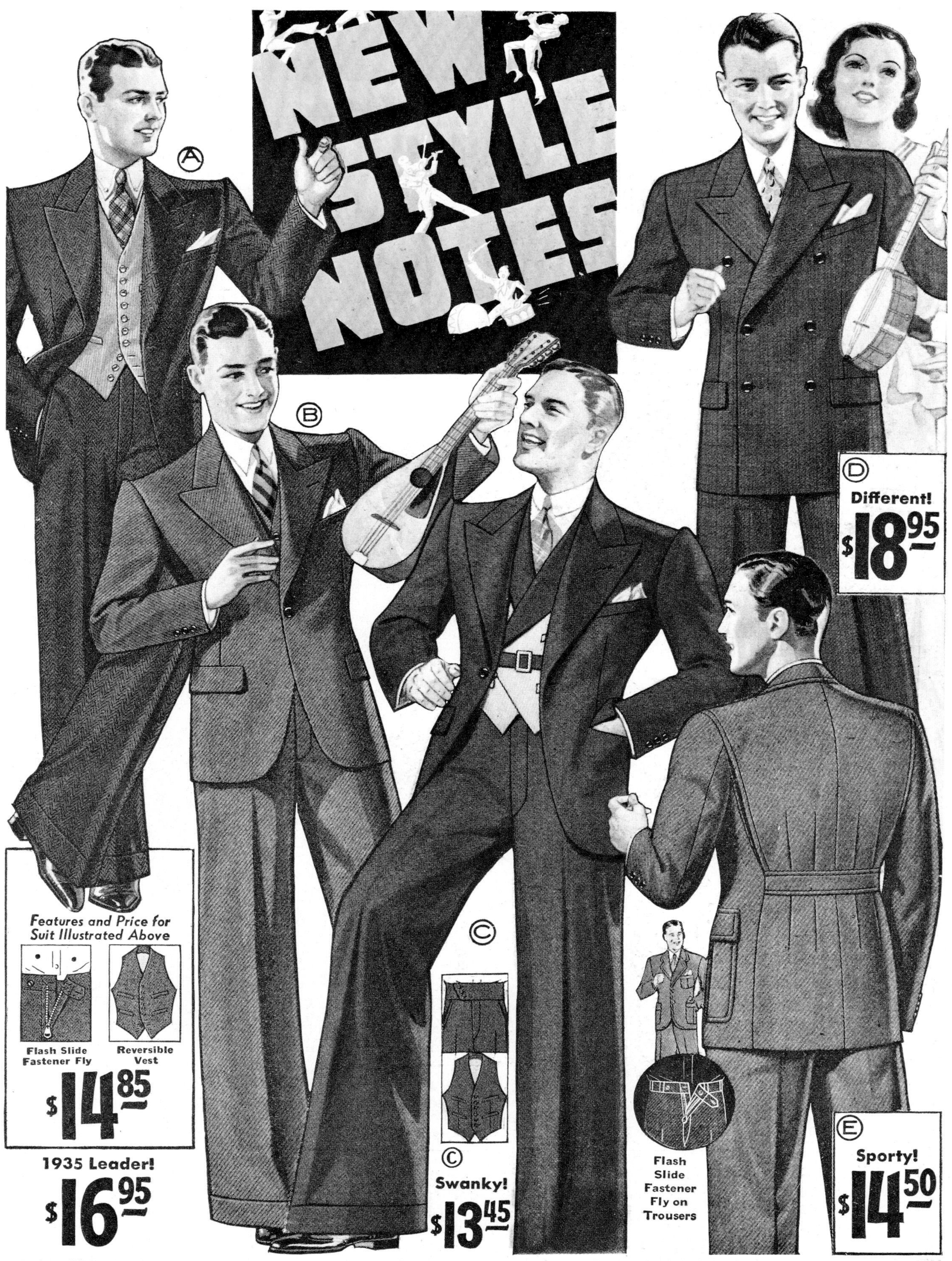

PRICES in This Book Are for MAIL ORDERS Only

Nubby Tweed $3.98 or Monotone Suiting $4.98
Smart Spring Tweed $6.98
Crepolaine with Pique' Vest $7.95
C
D
E
Rich Novelty Diagonal Weave
$8.98

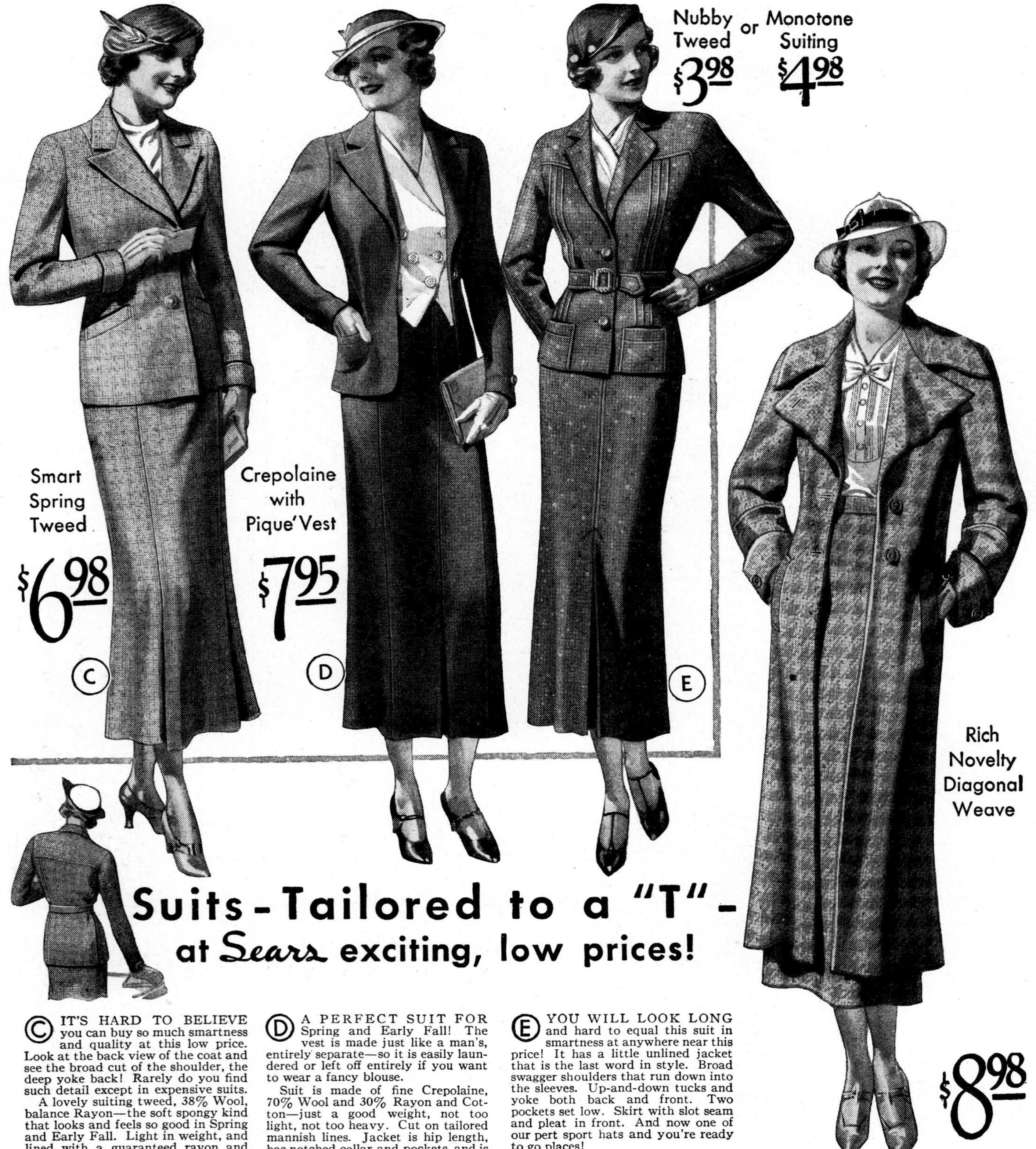

Suits-Tailored to a "T"- at Sears exciting, low prices!

Ⓒ IT'S HARD TO BELIEVE you can buy so much smartness and quality at this low price. Look at the back view of the coat and see the broad cut of the shoulder, the deep yoke back! Rarely do you find such detail except in expensive suits.

A lovely suiting tweed, 38% Wool, balance Rayon—the soft spongy kind that looks and feels so good in Spring and Early Fall. Light in weight, and lined with a guaranteed rayon and cotton. Hip length jacket. Has notched collar and two-button closing. Straight line skirt with front pleats. A suit famous for keeping its shape and staying in style—you'll feel "right" in it for seasons to come. You won't find a smarter one, and we don't believe you'll find a better value!

Misses' Sizes: 14-16-18-20 yrs.
Women's Sizes: 32-34-36-38-40-42 in. bust measure. *State bust measure.*

17 H 9720—Medium Tan
17 H 9721—Med. Light Blue
17 H 9722—Medium Light Gray.................. $6.98

Sent direct from New York to you . . . but you pay the postage only from our nearest Mail Order House. See Page 12. Shipping weight, 2 lbs. 12 oz.

Ⓓ A PERFECT SUIT FOR Spring and Early Fall! The vest is made just like a man's, entirely separate—so it is easily laundered or left off entirely if you want to wear a fancy blouse.

Suit is made of fine Crepolaine, 70% Wool and 30% Rayon and Cotton—just a good weight, not too light, not too heavy. Cut on tailored mannish lines. Jacket is hip length, has notched collar and pockets, and is lined with fine quality Rayon and Cotton. Straight line skirt with front pleats.

Remember, it's cleverly feminine to be a little mannish—Anne Williams suggests new square-toe oxfords (which you'll find on our interesting shoe pages) to wear with this trim, tailored outfit.

Misses' Sizes: 14-16-18-20 yrs.
Women's Sizes: 32-34-36-38 in. bust measure. *State actual bust measure.*

17 H 9725—Navy Blue.... $7.95

Sent direct from New York to you but you pay postage only from our nearest Mail Order House. See page 12. Shipping weight, 2 lbs. 14 oz.

Ⓔ YOU WILL LOOK LONG and hard to equal this suit in smartness at anywhere near this price! It has a little unlined jacket that is the last word in style. Broad swagger shoulders that run down into the sleeves. Up-and-down tucks and yoke both back and front. Two pockets set low. Skirt with slot seam and pleat in front. And now one of our pert sport hats and you're ready to go places!

Misses' Sizes: 14-16-18-20 yrs.
Women's Sizes: 32-34-36-38 in. bust measure. *State actual bust measure.*

Monotone Suiting
three-fifths Wool, balance Rayon

17 H 9730—Light Navy Blue
17 H 9731—Medium Tan
17 H 9732—Medium Gray. $4.98

Novelty Tweed
one-third Wool, balance Rayon

17 H 9735—Medium Green
17 H 9736—Medium Blue
17 H 9737—Med. Lt. Brown $3.98

Sent direct from New York to you but you pay postage only from our nearest Mail Order House. See page 12. Shipping weight, each, 1 lb. 14 oz.

YOU'LL BE AMAZED AT THE BEAUTY OF this fabric! Soft and smooth—but exceedingly sporty! A rich novelty diagonal weave—38% wool and 62% rayon. The rayon gives it a richer texture than if it were all wool. The coat is the new long 45 inch style, cut on the latest swagger lines. Smart worn with skirt or as separate coat. Coat lined with long wearing rayon and cotton.

Misses' Sizes: 14-16-18-20 years.
Women's Sizes: 32-34-36-38-40-42 in. bust measure. *State actual bust measure.*

17 H 9740—Copper Tan Mixture
17 H 9741—Medium Blue Mixture
17 H 9742—Golden Tan Mixture...... $8.98

Sent direct from New York to you. See Page 12. Shipping weight, 3 lbs. 10 oz.

Get Sears New York-to-you habit—and save. See page 12.

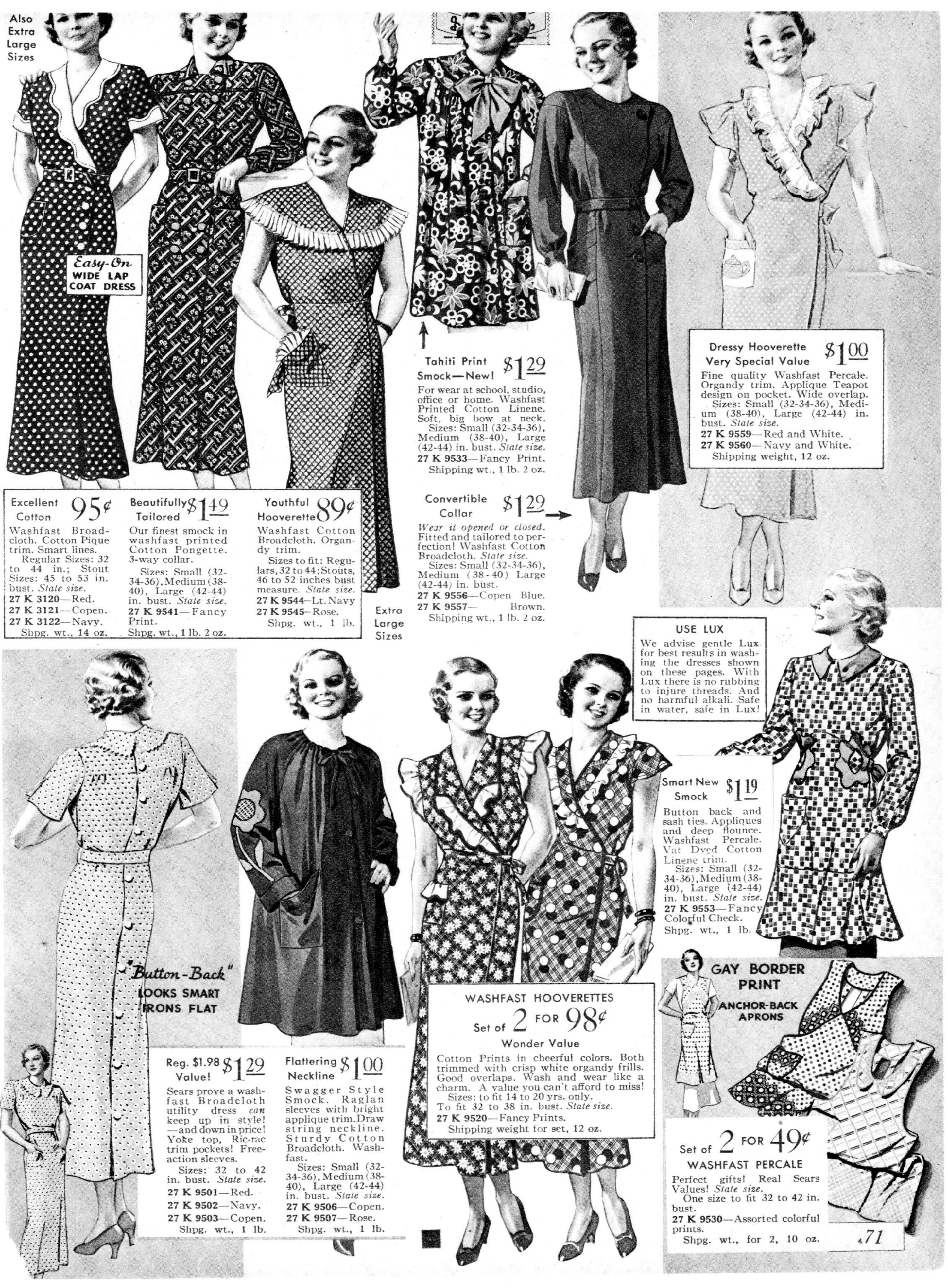

Also Extra Large Sizes
Easy-On WIDE LAP COAT DRESS
Excellent Cotton 95¢
Washfast Broadcloth. Cotton Pique trim. Smart lines.
Regular Sizes: 32 to 44 in.; Stout Sizes: 45 to 53 in. bust. State size.
27 K 3120—Red.
27 K 3121—Copen.
27 K 3122—Navy.
Shpg. wt., 14 oz.
Beautifully Tailored $1.49
Our finest smock in washfast printed Cotton Pongette. 3-way collar.
Sizes: Small (32-34-36), Medium (38-40), Large (42-44) in. bust. State size.
27 K 9541—Fancy Print.
Shpg. wt., 1 lb. 2 oz.
Youthful Hooverette 89¢
Washfast Cotton Broadcloth. Organdy trim.
Sizes to fit: Regulars, 32 to 44; Stouts, 46 to 52 inches bust measure. State size.
27 K 9544—Lt. Navy
27 K 9545—Rose.
Shpg. wt., 1 lb.
Extra Large Sizes
Tahiti Print Smock—New! $1.29
For wear at school, studio, office or home. Washfast Printed Cotton Linene. Soft, big bow at neck.
Sizes: Small (32-34-36), Medium (38-40), Large (42-44) in. bust. State size.
27 K 9533—Fancy Print.
Shipping wt., 1 lb. 2 oz.
Convertible Collar $1.29
Wear it opened or closed. Fitted and tailored to perfection! Washfast Cotton Broadcloth. State size.
Sizes: Small (32-34-36), Medium (38-40) Large (42-44) in. bust.
27 K 9556—Copen Blue.
27 K 9557—Brown.
Shipping wt., 1 lb. 2 oz.
Dressy Hooverette Very Special Value $1.00
Fine quality Washfast Percale. Organdy trim. Applique Teapot design on pocket. Wide overlap.
Sizes: Small (32-34-36), Medium (38-40), Large (42-44) in. bust. State size.
27 K 9559—Red and White.
27 K 9560—Navy and White.
Shipping weight, 12 oz.
USE LUX
We advise gentle Lux for best results in washing the dresses shown on these pages. With Lux there is no rubbing to injure threads. And no harmful alkali. Safe in water, safe in Lux!
Smart New Smock $1.19
Button back and sash ties. Appliques and deep flounce. Washfast Percale. Vat Dyed Cotton Linene trim.
Sizes: Small (32-34-36), Medium (38-40), Large (42-44) in. bust. State size.
27 K 9553—Fancy Colorful Check.
Shpg. wt., 1 lb.
"Button-Back" LOOKS SMART IRONS FLAT
Reg. $1.98 Value! $1.29
Sears prove a washfast Broadcloth utility dress can keep up in style! —and down in price! Yoke top, Ric-rac trim pockets! Free-action sleeves.
Sizes: 32 to 42 in. bust. State size.
27 K 9501—Red.
27 K 9502—Navy.
27 K 9503—Copen.
Shpg. wt., 1 lb.
Flattering Neckline $1.00
Swagger Style Smock. Raglan sleeves with bright applique trim. Draw string neckline. Sturdy Cotton Broadcloth. Washfast.
Sizes: Small (32-34-36), Medium (38-40), Large (42-44) in. bust. State size.
27 K 9506—Copen.
27 K 9507—Rose.
Shpg. wt., 1 lb.
WASHFAST HOOVERETTES
Set of 2 FOR 98¢
Wonder Value
Cotton Prints in cheerful colors. Both trimmed with crisp white organdy frills. Good overlaps. Wash and wear like a charm. A value you can't afford to miss!
Sizes: to fit 14 to 20 yrs. only.
To fit 32 to 38 in. bust. State size.
27 K 9520—Fancy Prints.
Shipping weight for set, 12 oz.
GAY BORDER PRINT
ANCHOR-BACK APRONS
Set of 2 FOR 49¢
WASHFAST PERCALE
Perfect gifts! Real Sears Values! State size.
One size to fit 32 to 42 in. bust.
27 K 9530—Assorted colorful prints.
Shpg. wt., for 2, 10 oz.
471

AUTOGRAPHED FASHIONS

At Sears Savings!

The Dress

THIS IS ONE OF MY FAVORITE Autograph Fashions and one I am delighted to tell you about because it has so many last-minute fashion features! The long tunic is very youthful and slenderizing! It's very new, too, and so is the slit skirt! (Skirts are not slit high as in the old "hobble" skirts, you know, but just through the hem at the side—a much more wearable style.) Notice the svelte fitted line of this dress about the waist. It cuts up into the important V under the bust, and has a half belt that buckles in the back. The dress is a rich quality Silk Canton Crepe (weighted) with a jabot and two buttons, and collars and cuffs of lovely lace. The lace collar is not the ordinary kind, but very crisp and chic—and so cleverly made you'd know it was an advanced 1935 style the minute you looked at it! Loretta Young Autographed Label in every dress.

ANNE WILLIAMS.

Misses' Sizes: 14-16-18-20 years.
Bust Measures: 32-34-36-38 inches.
Lengths, about 49 inches. *State size.*

31 H 8628—Romany Blue (Lt. Navy).
31 H 8629—Rich Med. Green.
31 H 8630—Peacock Blue........ $4.98

Sent direct from New York to you . . . but you pay the postage only from our nearest Mail Order House. See Page 12. Shipping weight, 1 lb. 14 oz.

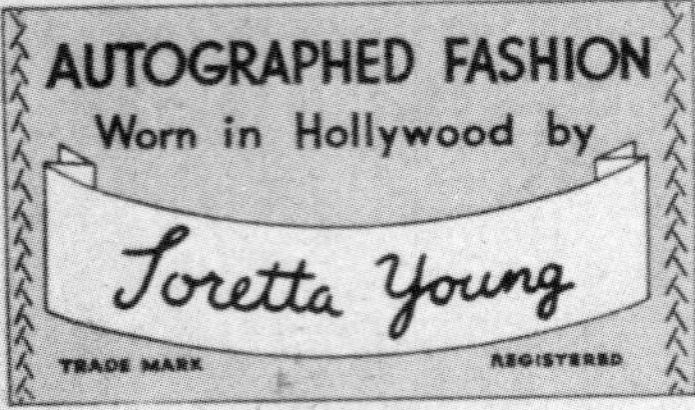

The Coat

THIS GORGEOUS COAT IS TYPICAL of the fine coats offered by Sears in this Fashion presentation! *Made in the very newest style in one of the very newest fabrics!* An ALL-WOOL BARK WEAVE CREPE with beautiful hard worsted finish . . . the kind seen in the most expensive coats. Buy Treebark Calfskin Oxfords to match. (See Shoe Pages).

Like most fashions worn by Loretta Young, it is made on simple smart lines with just enough trimming to set off the richness of the fabric. The inside of the double collar is lined with rayon faille in contrasting shade, a fresh youthful touch for Spring and Summer!

The coat is lined throughout with an extra fine quality Silk Crepe (weighted). A single flower on the left lapel gives an extra dashing air. A really stunning style you can wear everywhere—*and an exclusive Sears autographed fashion* with Loretta Young Label.

Misses' Sizes: 14-16-18-20 years.
Women's Sizes: 32-34-36-38-40-42-44-46 inches bust measure. *State actual bust measure.*
Lengths, about 49 inches.

17 H 9100—Navy Blue.
17 H 9101—Rich Black.
17 H 9102—Medium Tan......... $9.95

Sent direct from New York to you but you pay postage only from our nearest Mail Order House. See page 12.
Shipping weight, 2 lbs. 12 oz.

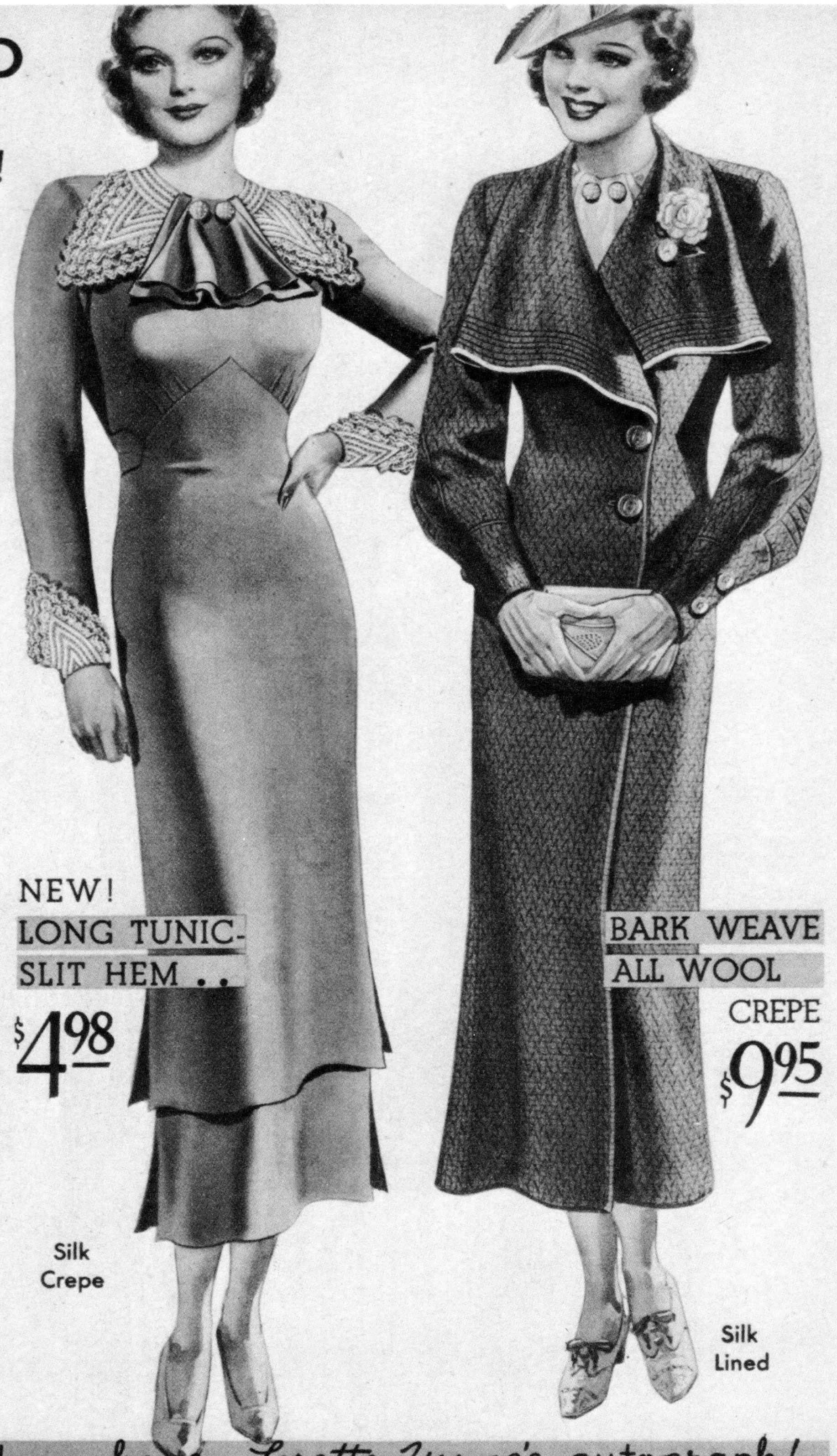

NEW!
LONG TUNIC-
SLIT HEM . .
$4.98

Silk Crepe

BARK WEAVE
ALL WOOL
CREPE
$9.95

Silk Lined

these, too—have Loretta Young's autograph!

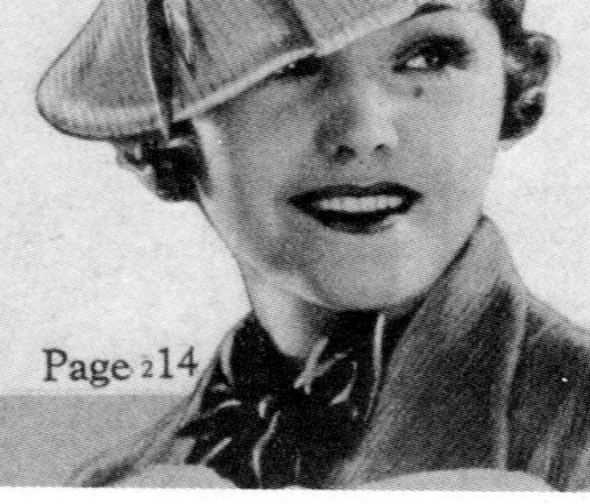

THE SMART, LARGE, SOFT BERET OF CELLOMAT Visca Cloth! Bright quills are backed with pin—can be attached at any angle. Shipping weight. 10 oz.
78 H 6770—Fits 21½ to 22½ in. headsize........ $1.59
Colors: Beige Sand, Navy, White. *Measure, state color.*

A BAG THAT MATCHES THE SHOE EXACTLY! Line for line! Color for color! Made of fine artificial leather in smooth, washable calf finish. Zip compartment, 2 other pockets, rayon lined flap. Attached frame top coin purse. Size 5¾ x 8 in. Mirror in pocket. Shipping weight, 12 oz.
18 H 2510—Colors: Beige or Navy Blue. *State color.* 95¢
Oxfords to match. See Page 268.................. **$1.98**
Order these accessories from Sears nearest Mail Order House.

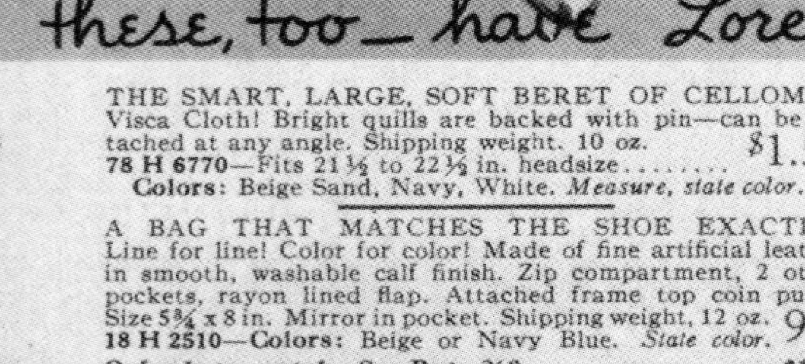

Page 214

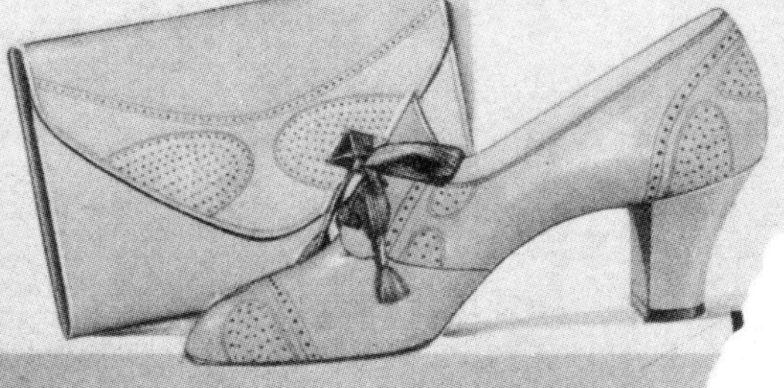

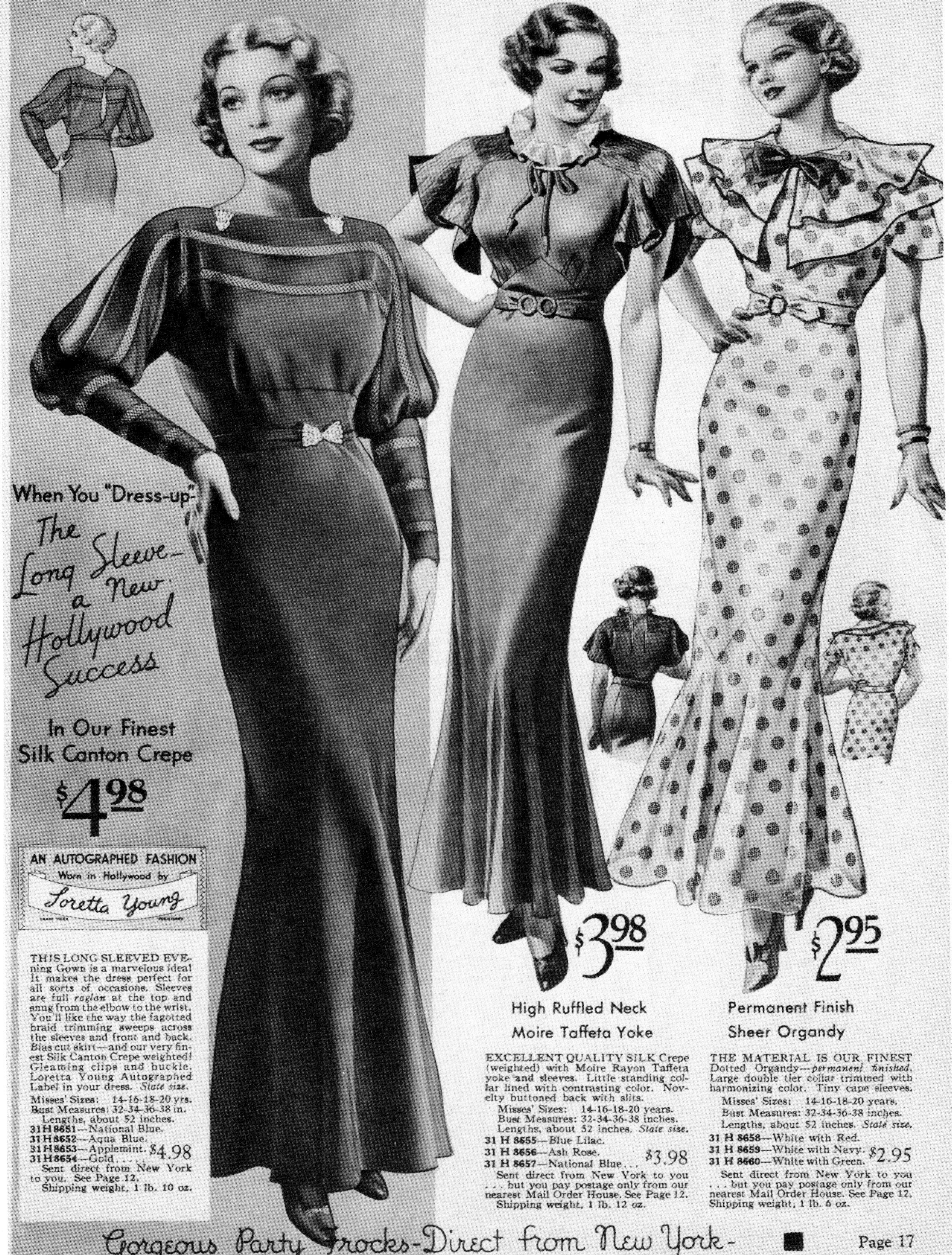
When You "Dress-up"
The Long Sleeve—a New Hollywood Success
In Our Finest Silk Canton Crepe
$4.98
AN AUTOGRAPHED FASHION
Worn in Hollywood by
Loretta Young
THIS LONG SLEEVED EVENING Gown is a marvelous idea! It makes the dress perfect for all sorts of occasions. Sleeves are full *raglan* at the top and snug from the elbow to the wrist. You'll like the way the fagotted braid trimming sweeps across the sleeves and front and back. Bias cut skirt—and our very finest Silk Canton Crepe weighted! Gleaming clips and buckle. Loretta Young Autographed Label in your dress. *State size.*
Misses' Sizes: 14-16-18-20 yrs.
Bust Measures: 32-34-36-38 in.
Lengths, about 52 inches.
31 H 8651—National Blue.
31 H 8652—Aqua Blue.
31 H 8653—Applemint.
31 H 8654—Gold $4.98
Sent direct from New York to you. See Page 12.
Shipping weight, 1 lb. 10 oz.
$3.98
High Ruffled Neck
Moire Taffeta Yoke
EXCELLENT QUALITY SILK Crepe (weighted) with Moire Rayon Taffeta yoke and sleeves. Little standing collar lined with contrasting color. Novelty buttoned back with slits.
Misses' Sizes: 14-16-18-20 years.
Bust Measures: 32-34-36-38 inches.
Lengths, about 52 inches. *State size.*
31 H 8655—Blue Lilac.
31 H 8656—Ash Rose.
31 H 8657—National Blue . . . $3.98
Sent direct from New York to you . . . but you pay postage only from our nearest Mail Order House. See Page 12.
Shipping weight, 1 lb. 12 oz.
$2.95
Permanent Finish
Sheer Organdy
THE MATERIAL IS OUR FINEST Dotted Organdy—*permanent finished.* Large double tier collar trimmed with harmonizing color. Tiny cape sleeves.
Misses' Sizes: 14-16-18-20 years.
Bust Measures: 32-34-36-38 inches.
Lengths, about 52 inches. *State size.*
31 H 8658—White with Red.
31 H 8659—White with Navy.
31 H 8660—White with Green. $2.95
Sent direct from New York to you . . . but you pay postage only from our nearest Mail Order House. See Page 12.
Shipping weight, 1 lb. 6 oz.
Gorgeous Party Frocks—Direct from New York—
Page 17

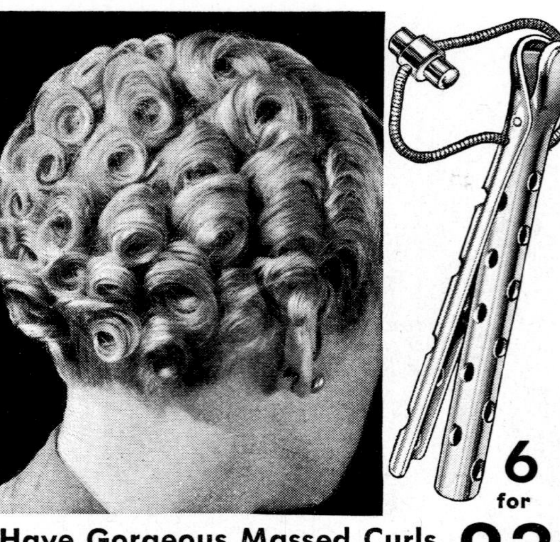

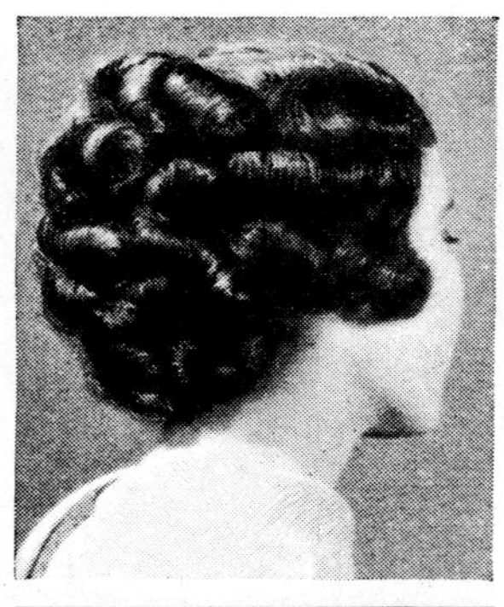

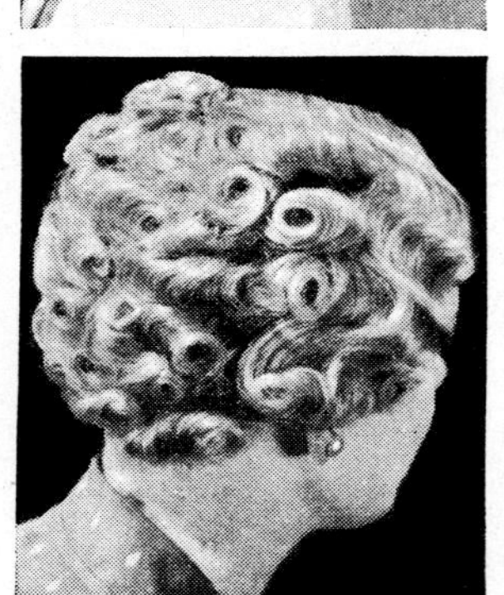

6 for 23c

Have Gorgeous Massed Curls With Kurley Kew Kurlers

—Light Weight, Perforated Aluminum—Hair dries Quickly
—Metal Cap-end locks Curler Securely
—Gives Smooth Roll Curls—No Frizzing

Lots of curls . . . "and worn high" adds Lady Fashion! With Kurley Kew Kurlers it's easy to fix your hair just like photograph. Complete instructions with each set. Lengths, 2½ or 3 in. **State length.** Shipping weight, 2 ounces.
25 K 9040—Set of six curlers. **Now**............... 23c

8 for 23c

Curly Lox Curlers

Use for cluster curls—or ringlet ends. Rayon covered wire with rubber sleeve and metal compressor. Curler slides out without unrolling curl. Directions included. Shpg. wt., 3 oz.
25 K 9005
Card of **8** Curlers...... 23c

5 for 45c

Wide Wave Curlers

A favorite curler for ringlet ends, round curls or all over waves. Flat metal—length about 3 inches. Instructions included. Shipping weight, 3 oz.
25 K 9048
Set of **5**........... 45c

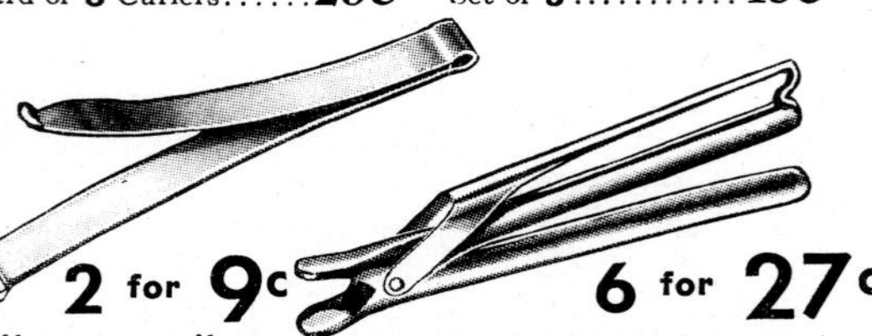

2 for 9c

"Link Lok" Curlers

Easy to open and close. Slip through the hair easily, lock in any position. Length, about 3 inches. Instructions included. Shipping weight, 2 ounces.
25 K 9044
2 for.................... 9c

6 for 27c

Metal End Curlers

Finish your coiffure with end ringlets—easy to do with a set of these curlers. Made of metal with strong spring. Length, 3⅜ inches. Curling instructions included. Shpg. wt., 3 oz.
25 K 9046
6 for............... 27c

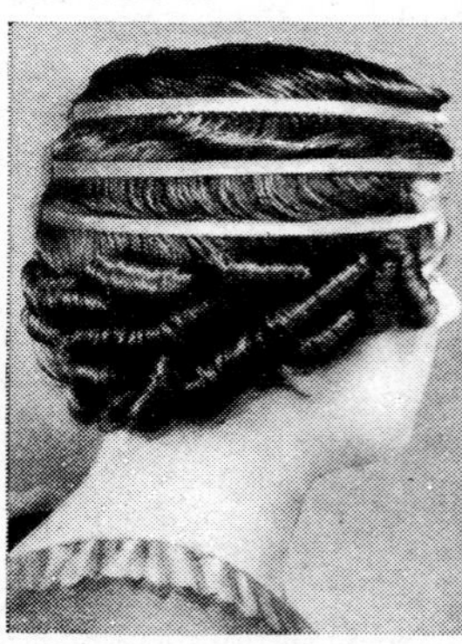

7 for 79c

Only 1 Needed! 59c Ea.

Madame "X" Aids to a Lovely Coiffure

Most wonderful waving combs ever invented! For getting the effect of an expert swirl, finger wave, or the new pompadour style. Each comb 14 inches long. Celluloid. Special large rubber band holds it in place. Full instructions for waving your own hair. Shipping weight, 3 ounces.
25 K 9032
3 in Set................. 89c

Famous Madame X water wave combs . . . for a lovely wave-set . . . amazing results obtained due to the patented construction. Rubber bands clip over knobs, holding securely. Celluloid. Instructions included. Shipping weight, 4 ounces.
25 K 9033
7 combs.............. 79c

"Roll-N-Pin" End Curler . . . the quick way to curl ends wet or dry, instantly without heat. (Curler is not left in hair.) So marvelous you'll wonder how you ever got along without it. Sliding composition bar with metal pin. Length, about 7¼ in. Can be carried in purse. Illustrated directions. Shipping weight, 4 oz.
25 K 9025—Each....... 59c

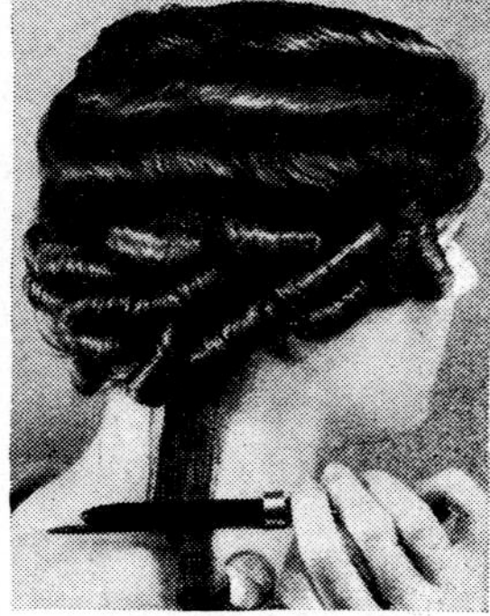

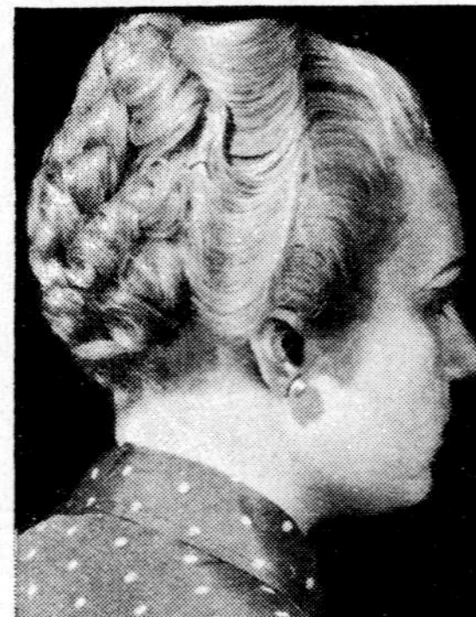

Marcels

Continuous waves all around the head easy with Baldwin marcellers. Flexible perfumed rubber curlers. Length, about 4⅜ inches. Shpg. wt., 7 oz.
Price Reduced.
25 K 9036
6 for....... 37c

Vassar Wavers

For end-curls, waves or long bob croquignole curls. Flexible rubber with center opening. Length, about 4 in. Comfortable, easy to use. Shipping weight, 2 ounces.
25 K 9021
6 for...... 15c

"Kid" Curlers

Leather covered —flexible. Old time favorites because they can be used to obtain so many different effects. Length, 5 inches. Shipping weight, 2 ounces.
25 K 9068
16 for....... 9c

Hair Roller

Keep your growing "bob" tidy. Catches up all loose ends into a neat roll at back of neck. Invisible, no pins necessary. Brown celluloid. Shipping weight, 2 ounces.
25 K 9020
Each.......... 9c

For Long "Bobs"

For the Bob-Roll or making "doughnuts" over ears or at back. Grasps ends firmly. 9-in. rayon covered wire. Black or Brown. **State color.** Shipping weight, 2 oz.
25 K 9071
2 for....... 9c

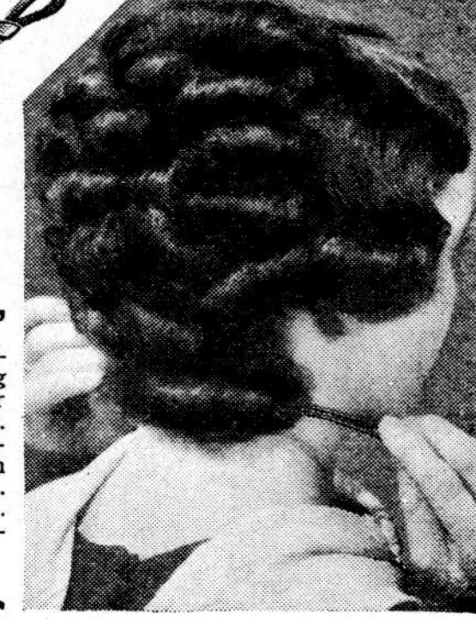

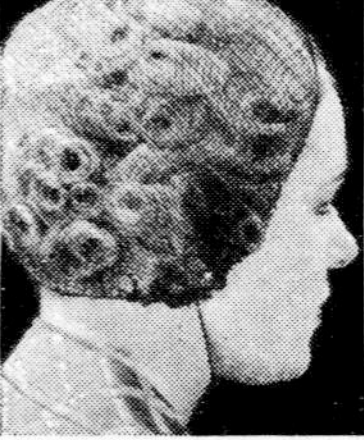

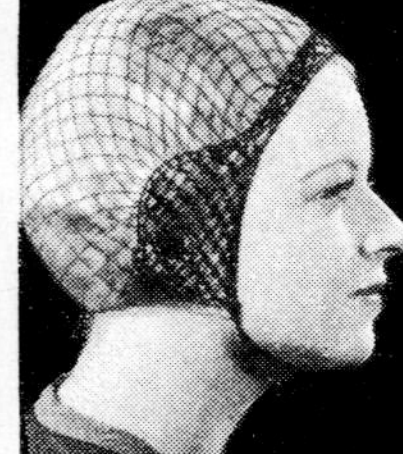

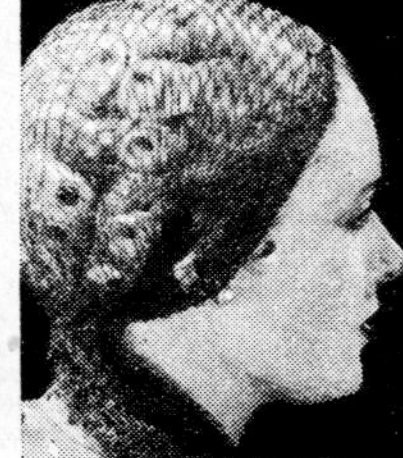

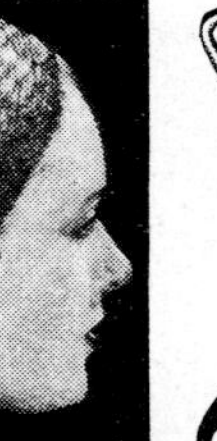

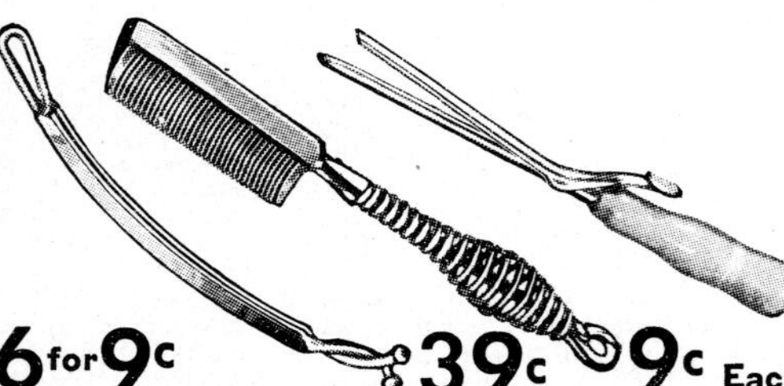

6 for 9c 39c 9c Each

Rayon Net Cap

Tailored cap style lustrous rayon net . . . with ties. Colors: **White, Orchid, Brown, or Black. State color.** Shpg. wt., ea., 1 oz.
25 K 9076
Each............... 19c

Similar style cap, of cotton net. **State color.**
25 K 9074
for................. 17c

Knotless Style

Newest of all wave nets. Rayon weave—no elastic across front to mark forehead—no knots at sides. **Brown only.** Shipping weight, 2 ounces.
25 K 9075
2 for.......... 17c

Fine Rayon

Keeps waves in place until dry. Imported wave cap. Elastic chin strap. No elastic to mark forehead. Fits all sizes. Colors: **Pink, Blue or Brown. State color.** Shipping weight, 2 ounces.
25 K 9061
Each............ 15c

Triangular Net

Wear it for outdoor sports or to protect your wave at night. Soft woven rayon—ties firmly at back of head or in turban style. **Dark brown only.** Shipping weight, 2 ounces.
25 K 9072
2 for.......... 17c

Handy Curlers
—"Nob-Lock" Wave Setters

Hold firmly—no slipping. For long or bobbed hair. Rustproof metal. Length, about 4½ inches.
Shipping wt., 2 oz.
25 K 9034
6 for........ 9c

HairStraightener

Extra heavy brass comb retains heat. Curved teeth allow treatment close to scalp. Length, about 9½ inches, with wire handle. Shipping weight, 15 ounces.
25 K 9073
Each........ 39c

Curling Iron

Nickel plated metal with thumb button. Enameled wooden handle—stays cool. Strong spring. Length, about 9½ inches. Shipping weight, 8 ounces.
25 K 9042
Each......... 9c

Waves and Curls make your hair beautiful

At Sears You Choose From

HUNDREDS OF HATS!

ALL NEW, INTERESTING FASHIONS

THERE ARE OVER 650 HATS for *you* to choose from—at Sears! Each picture represents not one but a whole family of hats! All the new colors! Wine hats, Brown hats, Rust or Violet hats! These are only a few! Large hats, small hats! Size twenty-one's! And even up to Size twenty-four's! Ever so many colors, shapes and sizes are waiting for you in Sears large millinery department! You've never stepped into a store that offered you so *many* different choices.

AUTOGRAPHED FASHION
Worn in Hollywood by
Adrienne Ames
TRADE MARK
REGISTERED

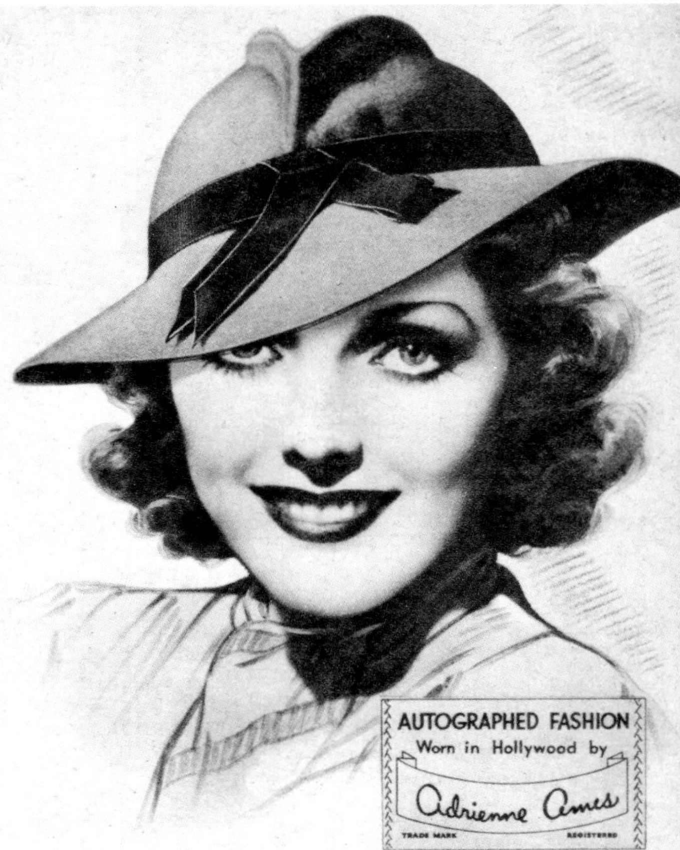

Be Sure to Measure

Adrienne Ames is clever! She puts her autograph on one of the most important, best liked felt hats for Fall! And she wears it in very fine quality felt—a softer, lovelier all wool body. She knows there's nothing smarter than the casual easy lines of the brim, that turns down in front, up in back, the jaunty, soft crease in the crown! And she's right! Sears customers get the benefit of her fashion judgment! The very same hat is yours, at a price far lower than you'd find anywhere for such quality and fashion. You save at Sears.

$1.69

Colors: Lilac with Purple band, Dark Beige with Brown, Chili (dark) Brown with Beige, Dubonnet (dark wine) with deep Rose, Navy Blue with Copen, or Solid Black.
78 K 6020—Fits 21¾ to 22¼ inch headsize.
78 K 6021—Fits 22½ to 23 inch headsize.
Measure your headsize! State color. Shipping weight, 1 lb.

A
B

C
D

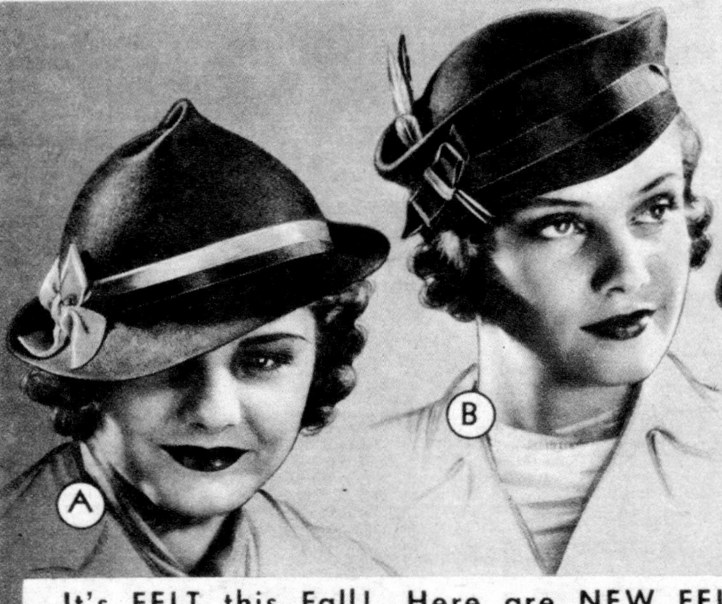

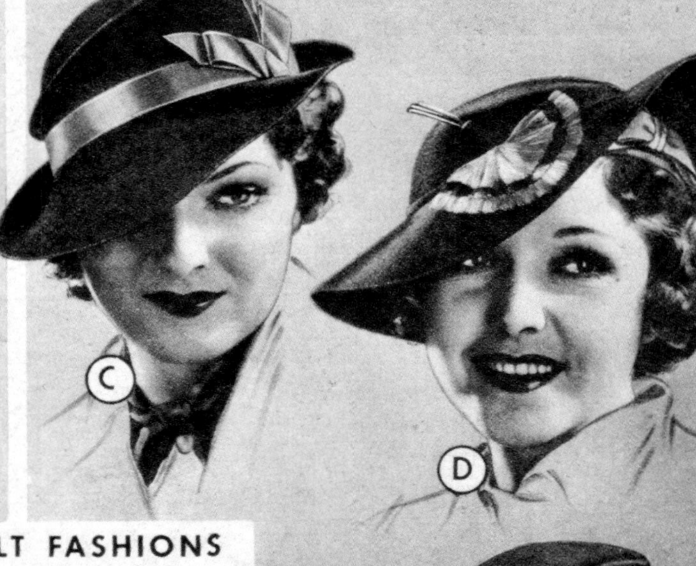

It's FELT this Fall! Here are NEW FELT FASHIONS

(A) Get the gayest — jauntiest fashion! The hat with the peaked crown! All wool body felt with a 2-tone fine quality ribbon and a narrow brim, turned up in back. $1.00
Colors: Chili (dark) Brown, Navy Blue, Kent (dark) Green or Black. *State color.*
78 K 6175—Fits 21¾ to 22¼ in. headsize. *Be sure to measure.*
Shipping weight, 1 lb.

(B) The dressy felt turban looks smartest of all above a big fur collar! Made of good quality, all wool body felt, banded with ribbon and jabbed with a gay feather. $1.00
Colors: Chili (dark) Brown, Dubonnet (dark wine), Navy Blue or Black. *State color.*
78 K 6135—Fits 21¾ to 22¼ in. headsize. *Please measure.*
Shipping weight, 10 oz.

(C) Gracious, modern lines! New forward-swooping brim! Carefree tuck in crown! Ribbon band. Fine all wool body felt. $1.49
Colors: Chili (dark) Brown with Beige ribbon, Navy Blue with Copen, Solid French (deep purple) Violet, or Black.
Measure and state color.
78 K 6205—Fits 21¾ to 22¼ in.
78 K 6206—Fits 22½ to 23 in.
Shipping weight, 1 lb.

(D) Here's the hat that "dresses up" your whole outfit! Very fine all wool body felt! A sweeping brim, set on a ribbon trimmed bandeau. $1.59
Colors: Chili (dark) Brown, Navy Blue, or Black.
78 K 6025—Fits 22 to 22½ in. headsize.
78 K 6026—Fits 22¾ to 23¼ in. headsize.
Measure. State color. Shipping weight, 1 lb.

(E) Rich, soft-hued ribbons, rolled into a thick cord, circle the hat and slip through the brim at the right! Inverted tucking in the crown. Finest all wool body felt. Shipping weight, 1 lb. $1.49
Colors: Chili (dark) Brown, Dubonnet (dark wine), Navy Blue or Black. *Measure, state color.*
78 K 6030—Fits 22 to 22½ in. headsize.
78 K 6031—Fits 22¾ to 23¼ in. headsize.

E

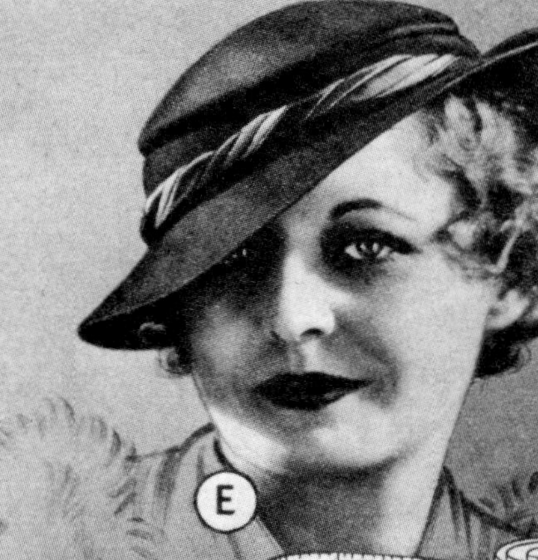

What is your Headsize? — The tape line will tell!

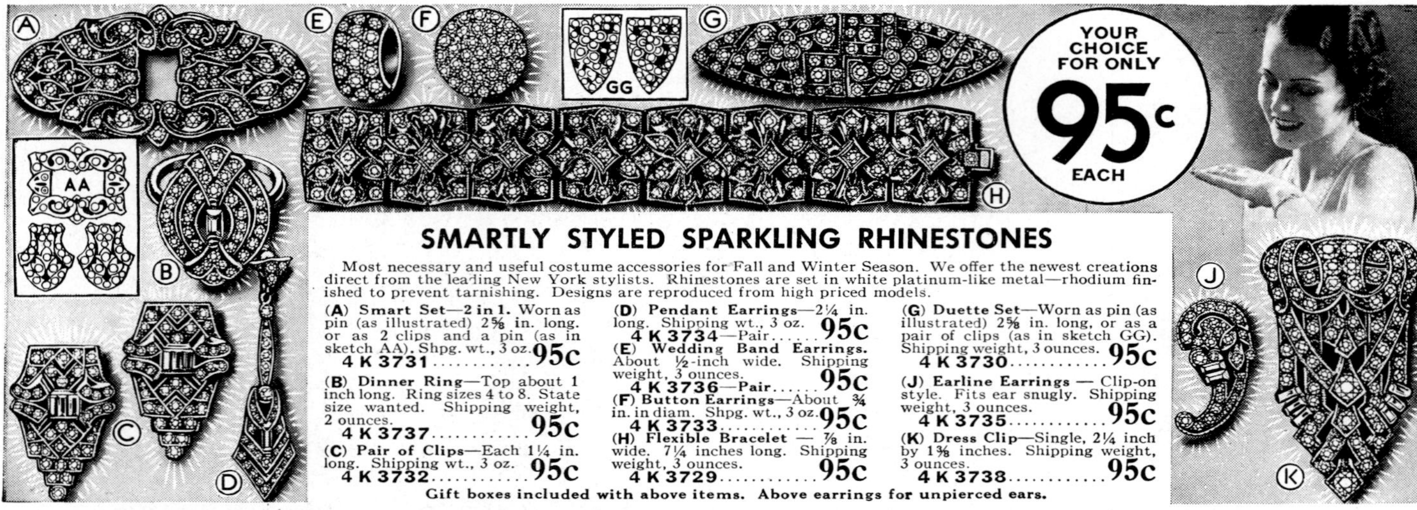

SMARTLY STYLED SPARKLING RHINESTONES

Most necessary and useful costume accessories for Fall and Winter Season. We offer the newest creations direct from the leading New York stylists. Rhinestones are set in white platinum-like metal—rhodium finished to prevent tarnishing. Designs are reproduced from high priced models.

(A) Smart Set—2 in 1. Worn as pin (as illustrated) 2⅝ in. long. or as 2 clips and a pin (as in sketch AA). Shpg. wt., 3 oz.
4 K 3731............95c

(B) Dinner Ring—Top about 1 inch long. Ring sizes 4 to 8. State size wanted. Shipping weight, 2 ounces.
4 K 3737............95c

(C) Pair of Clips—Each 1¼ in. long. Shipping wt., 3 oz.
4 K 3732............95c

(D) Pendant Earrings—2¼ in. long. Shipping wt., 3 oz.
4 K 3734—Pair......95c

(E) Wedding Band Earrings. About ½-inch wide. Shipping weight, 3 ounces.
4 K 3736—Pair......95c

(F) Button Earrings—About ¾ in. in diam. Shpg. wt., 3 oz.
4 K 3733............95c

(H) Flexible Bracelet — ⅞ in. wide. 7¼ inches long. Shipping weight, 3 ounces.
4 K 3729............95c

(G) Duette Set—Worn as pin (as illustrated) 2⅝ in. long, or as a pair of clips (as in sketch GG). Shipping weight, 3 ounces.
4 K 3730............95c

(J) Earline Earrings — Clip-on style. Fits ear snugly. Shipping weight, 3 ounces.
4 K 3735............95c

(K) Dress Clip—Single, 2¼ inch by 1⅜ inches. Shipping weight, 3 ounces.
4 K 3738............95c

Gift boxes included with above items. Above earrings for unpierced ears.

FASHION DICTATES COSTUME JEWELRY

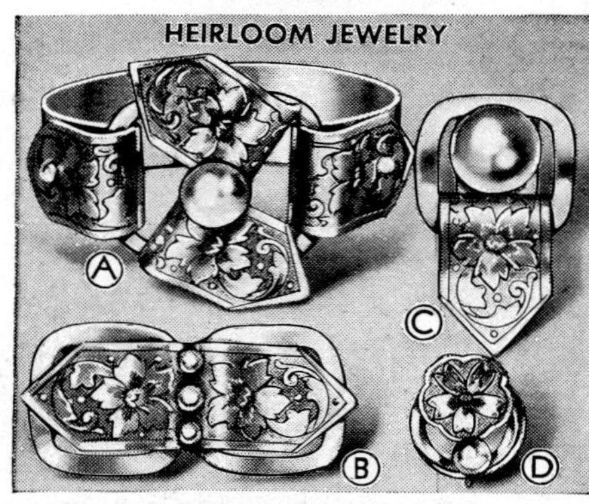

The Kind Grandmother Wore

Antique designs are new again. Modernized into up-to-the minute accessories. Natural gold color metal with just a trace of black enameling outlining the engraved designs. Will give a rich added touch to most any costume. Has the appearance of much more expensive jewelry. So lovely they must be seen to be appreciated

(A) Bracelet—¾ inch wide. Center motif about 1⅞ inches long. Shipping wt., 4 oz.
4 K 3513......95c

(B) Brooch—Size about 2¼ inches long. 1⅛ inches wide. Shipping weight, 3 ounces.
4 K 3515......95c

(C) Dress Clip — Single 1⅞ inches long. 1¹⁄₁₆ inches wide. Shipping wt., 3 ounces.
4 K 3514....95c

(D) Button Earrings. Size about ¾ inches wide. Shipping wt., 3 oz.
4 K 3516....95c

Gift Boxes Included

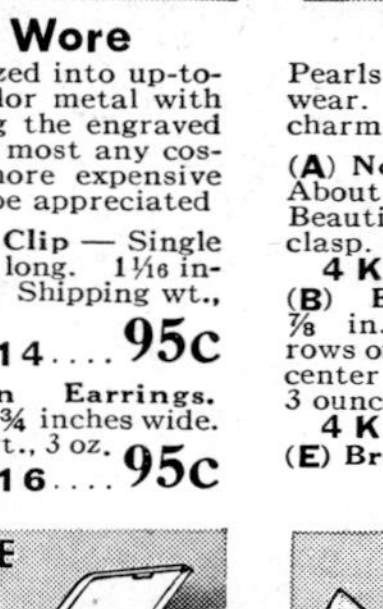

Pearls Are Always in Vogue

Pearls are being worn for all occasions, Daytime, Sports, or Evening wear. These are simulated Pearls of fine lustre that will add to the charm of any costume. Don't be without pearls!

(A) Necklace—Single strand. About 18 in. long. Graduated. Beautiful sparkling rhinestone clasp. Shpg. wt., 5 oz.
4 K 3852.........95c

(B) Earrings—Button style ⅞ in. diameter. Numerous rows of small pearls with larger center pearl. Shipping weight, 3 ounces.
4 K 3856.........95c

(C) Necklace — Two strand. One strand about 16 in. The other about 18 in. long. Bow-knot rhinestone clasp. Shipping weight, 5 ounces.
4 K 3853.........95c

(D) Necklace — Three strand. Uniform size. Choker style. Shortest strand about 15½ in. long. Large pearl clasp.
4 K 3854—Shpg. wt., 7 oz. 95c

(E) Bracelet—Three rows of uniform size. Large pearl clasp.
4 K 3855—Shipping weight, 4 ounces..........95c

Gift Boxes Included

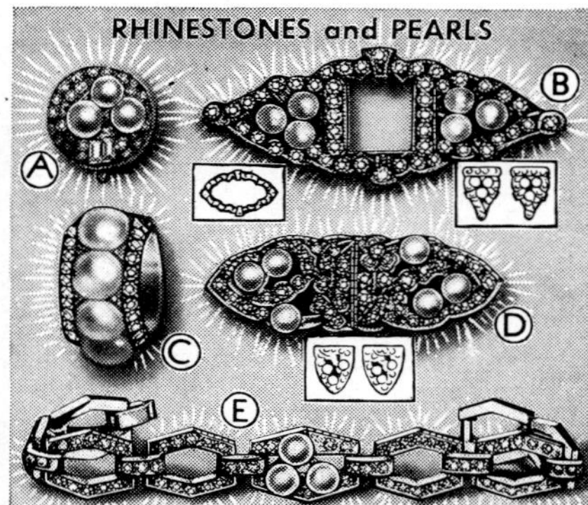

Rhinestones and Simulated Pearls

A most pleasing combination. Mountings in choice of gold or silver color metal. **State choice.** Words cannot express the real beauty of these accessories.

(A) Button Earrings. ⅝ in. diameter. Screw wire fasteners. Shpg. wt., 3 oz.
4 K 3520....95c

(B) Smart Set — Worn as pin 2¾ in. long (as illustrated) or as brooch and clips (as sketched). Shpg. wt., 3 oz.
4 K 3519....95c

(D) Duette Set—Worn as pin 2¼ in. long (as illustrated) or as pair of clips. Shipping weight, 3 ounces.
4 K 3518.95c

(E) Flexible Bracelet—About ½-in. wide. 6¾ inches long. Shipping wt., 3 oz.
4 K 3517.95c

(C) Wedding Band Earrings—Clip-on style. ⅜ inch wide.
4 K 3521—Shipping wt., 3 oz.....95c

Gift Boxes Included

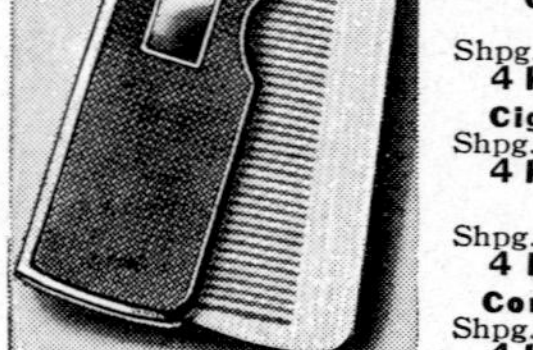

Cigarette Case—Compact—Comb

Beautifully designed in green gold color metal. Cigarette case is thin graceful style. 2⅞x3¾ inches. Holds ten cigarettes. Compact is a double with medium rouge and loose powder compartment, mirror and two puffs. 3¼x1⅞ inches. Comb is of white celluloid with fine teeth. Fits in case snugly. 4⅝ inches long.

Complete Set in Gift Box
Shpg. wt., 1 lb.
4 K 3523...$2.29

Cigarette Case Only
Shpg. wt., 7 oz.
4 K 5501......95c

Compact Only
Shpg. wt., 5 oz.
4 K 4622......95c

Comb and Case Only
Shpg. wt., 4 oz.
4 K 3522......48c

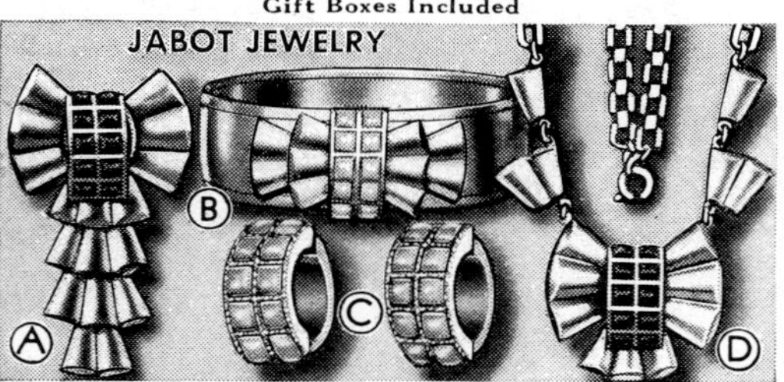

Stone Set — Gold or Silver Color

Stone set metal jewelry is very popular. Comes in choice of Gold color finish with Coral color stones or Silver color finish with Navy Blue or Red color stones. **State stone color.**

(A) Dress Clip—2⅜ in. long. Shipping weight, 3 oz.
4 K 3526.........95c

(B) Bracelet — Hinge type. ¾ inches wide. Shipping weight, 4 ounces.
4 K 3524.........95c

(C) Earrings—Wedding band. Clip-on style. ⅜ in. wide. Shipping weight, 3 ounces.
4 K 3527.........95c

(D) Necklace — About 16 in. long. Shipping wt., 4 oz.
4 K 3525.........95c

Gift Boxes Included

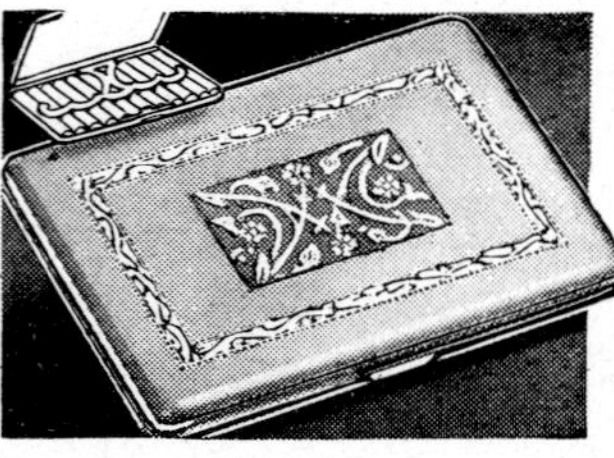

Chantilly Cigarette Case

A real beauty. Gold color brocaded on choice of White or Black enamel. Highly polished silver-like interior. Holds 14 cigarettes. Size 4⅝x3 in. **Be sure to state color wanted.** Shipping weight, 7 ounces.

4 K 5503
In Gift Box....95c

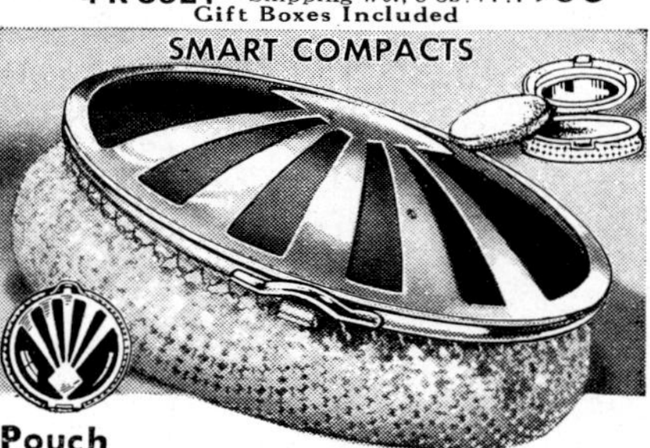

Pouch

Compacts Are Always Smart

Tremendously popular loose powder compact. Silver plated mesh pouch, lined with genuine white leather. Large velour puff, powder sifter and mirror. Top is enameled in choice of Black, White, Navy, Red or Green. **State color.** 2½ in. in diameter.
4 K 4623—Shpg. wt., 5 oz. **In Gift Box.** 95c

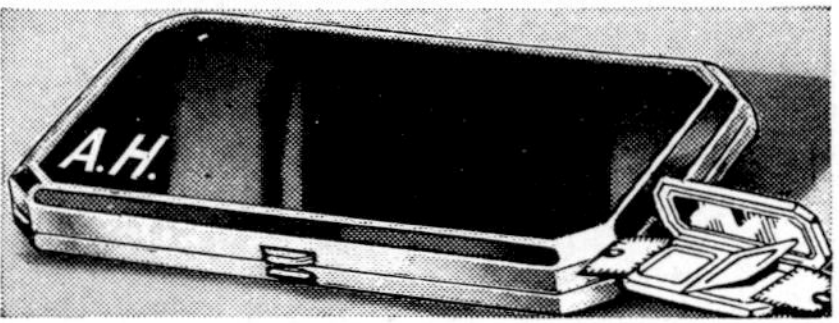

Countess Thin Style Compact

Double compact, with medium rouge, loose powder compartment, mirror and two puffs. Beautifully enameled in choice of Black, White, Navy Blue, Red or Green. Smart thin model. Size, 3¼x1⅞ inches. Any two raised initials applied free. Makes a lovely gift. **Be sure to state color and initials wanted. In gift box.** Shipping weight, 5 ounces.
4 K 4624........................95c

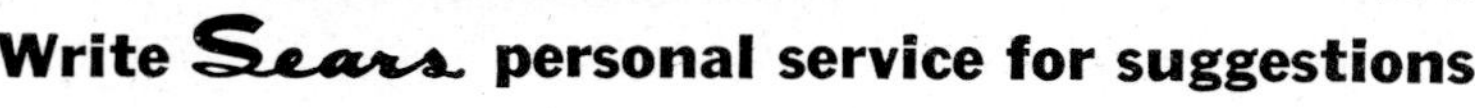

California to Harvard . .

BOND

American Honors!

QUALITY

Long famous for style and wear, GOLD BONDS this season rise to even greater heights of perfection. The styling is smarter—the finishing neater—the quality finer than ever before.

$3.45 A PAIR

Today's Value ~~$4.50~~

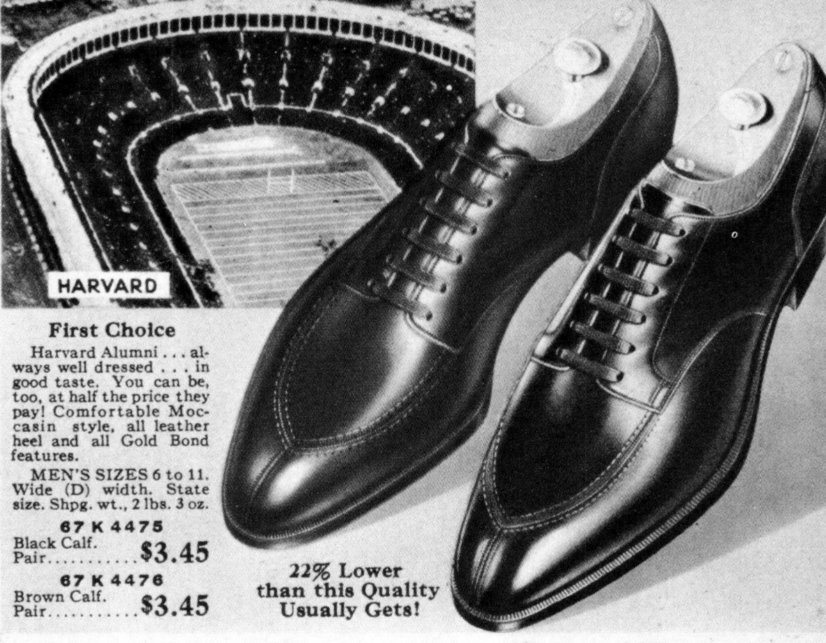

First Choice

Harvard Alumni . . . always well dressed . . . in good taste. You can be, too, at half the price they pay! Comfortable Moccasin style, all leather heel and all Gold Bond features.

MEN'S SIZES 6 to 11. Wide (D) width. State size. Shpg. wt., 2 lbs. 3 oz.

67 K 4475 Black Calf. Pair........... $3.45

67 K 4476 Brown Calf. Pair........... $3.45

22% Lower than this Quality Usually Gets!

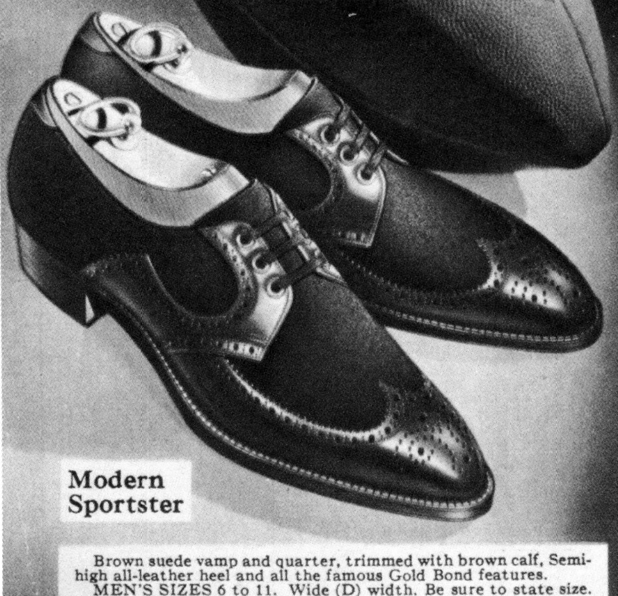

Modern Sportster

Brown suede vamp and quarter, trimmed with brown calf, Semi-high all-leather heel and all the famous Gold Bond features.
MEN'S SIZES 6 to 11. Wide (D) width. Be sure to state size. Shipping weight, 2 pounds 2 ounces.
67 K 4473—Pair.............................. $3.45

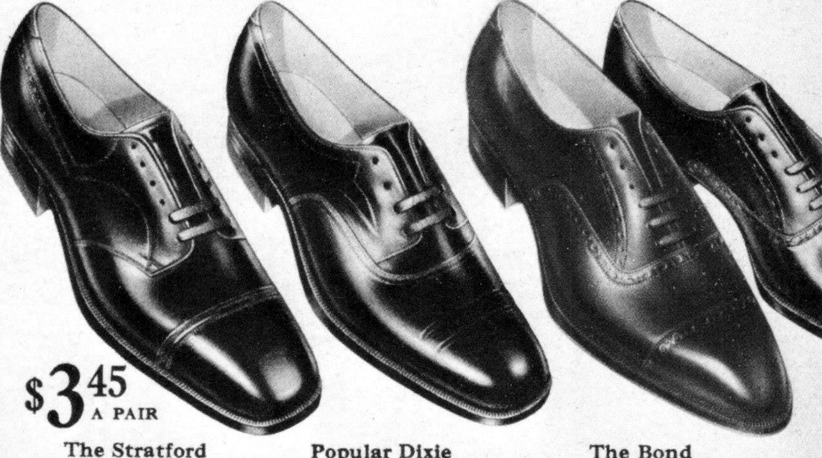

$3.45 A PAIR

The Stratford

Smooth, trim and comfortable Goodyear Wingfoot rubber heels. Finely made with all the Gold Bond features on opposite page.
MEN'S SIZES 6 to 11. Wide (D) width. State size. Shipping wt., 2 lbs. 2 oz.
67 K 4472 Black Calf. Pair............ $3.45

Popular Dixie

Good looks plus comfort. All the Gold Bond features above and Goodyear Wingfoot rubber heels.
MEN'S SIZES 5 to 11. Wide (D) width. State size. Shipping weight, 2 pounds 5 ounces.
67 K 4483 Black Calf. Pair............ $3.45

The Bond

A handsome straight tip. Goodyear Wingfoot rubber heel and the Gold Bond features above at left.
MEN'S SIZES 6 to 11. State size. Shipping weight, 2 lbs. 3 oz.
67 K 4488—Brown, wide (D) width.
67 K 4491—Black, wide (D) width.
67 K 4492—Black, medium (C) width. Pair.................. $3.45

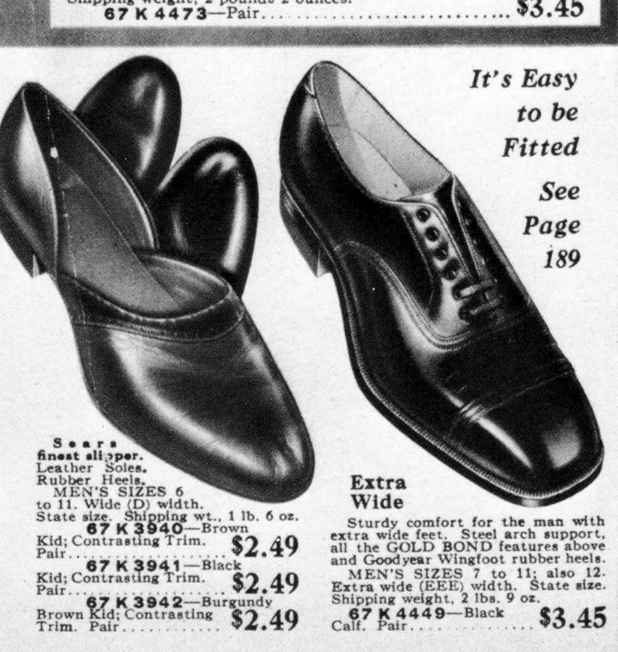

It's Easy to be Fitted

See Page 189

Sears finest slipper. Leather Soles. Rubber Heels.
MEN'S SIZES 6 to 11. Wide (D) width. State size. Shipping wt., 1 lb. 6 oz.
67 K 3940—Brown Kid; Contrasting Trim. Pair.................. $2.49
67 K 3941—Black Kid; Contrasting Trim. Pair.................. $2.49
67 K 3942—Burgundy Brown Kid; Contrasting Trim. Pair........... $2.49

Extra Wide

Sturdy comfort for the man with extra wide feet. Steel arch support, all the GOLD BOND features above and Goodyear Wingfoot rubber heels.
MEN'S SIZES 7 to 11; also 12. Extra wide (EEE) width. State size. Shipping weight, 2 lbs. 9 oz.
67 K 4449—Black Calf. Pair.................. $3.45

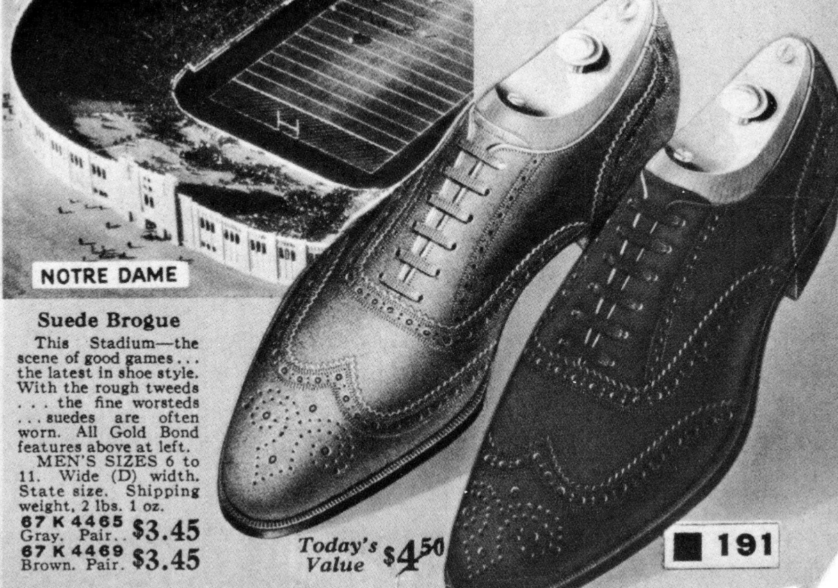

Suede Brogue

This Stadium—the scene of good games . . . the latest in shoe style. With the rough tweeds . . . the fine worsteds . . . suedes are often worn. All Gold Bond features above at left.
MEN'S SIZES 6 to 11. Wide (D) width. State size. Shipping weight, 2 lbs. 1 oz.
67 K 4465 Gray. Pair.. $3.45
67 K 4469 Brown. Pair. $3.45

Today's Value $4.50

191

Pique Coat and Dress
$1.59
Complete
Pique
$1.00
Regulation Middy
75¢
Two-Piece Playsuit
95¢
Pleated Skirt
98¢
For Sports— Middy Slacks and Hat
$1.59
Complete
The Cossack For Sports
$1.25

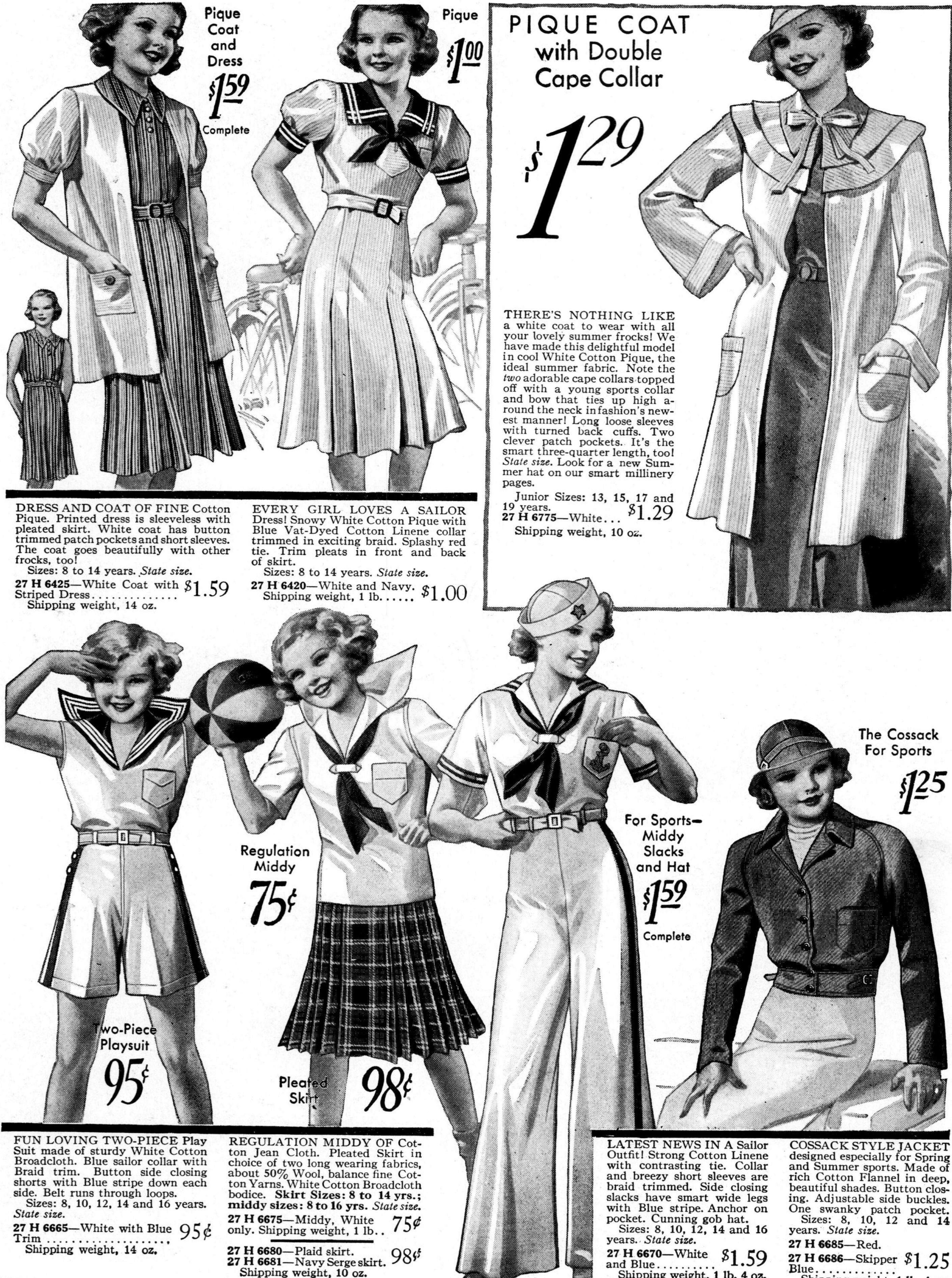

PIQUE COAT with Double Cape Collar

$1.29

THERE'S NOTHING LIKE a white coat to wear with all your lovely summer frocks! We have made this delightful model in cool White Cotton Pique, the ideal summer fabric. Note the *two* adorable cape collars topped off with a young sports collar and bow that ties up high around the neck in fashion's newest manner! Long loose sleeves with turned back cuffs. Two clever patch pockets. It's the smart three-quarter length, too! *State size.* Look for a new Summer hat on our smart millinery pages.

Junior Sizes: 13, 15, 17 and 19 years.
27 H 6775—White... $1.29
Shipping weight, 10 oz.

DRESS AND COAT OF FINE Cotton Pique. Printed dress is sleeveless with pleated skirt. White coat has button trimmed patch pockets and short sleeves. The coat goes beautifully with other frocks, too!
Sizes: 8 to 14 years. *State size.*
27 H 6425—White Coat with Striped Dress.............. $1.59
Shipping weight, 14 oz.

EVERY GIRL LOVES A SAILOR Dress! Snowy White Cotton Pique with Blue Vat-Dyed Cotton Linene collar trimmed in exciting braid. Splashy red tie. Trim pleats in front and back of skirt.
Sizes: 8 to 14 years. *State size.*
27 H 6420—White and Navy. Shipping weight, 1 lb...... $1.00

FUN LOVING TWO-PIECE Play Suit made of sturdy White Cotton Broadcloth. Blue sailor collar with Braid trim. Button side closing shorts with Blue stripe down each side. Belt runs through loops.
Sizes: 8, 10, 12, 14 and 16 years. *State size.*
27 H 6665—White with Blue Trim.................... 95¢
Shipping weight, 14 oz.

REGULATION MIDDY OF Cotton Jean Cloth. Pleated Skirt in choice of two long wearing fabrics, about 50% Wool, balance fine Cotton Yarns. White Cotton Broadcloth bodice. **Skirt Sizes: 8 to 14 yrs.; middy sizes: 8 to 16 yrs.** *State size.*
27 H 6675—Middy, White only. Shipping weight, 1 lb.. 75¢

27 H 6680—Plaid skirt.
27 H 6681—Navy Serge skirt. 98¢
Shipping weight, 10 oz.

LATEST NEWS IN A Sailor Outfit! Strong Cotton Linene with contrasting tie. Collar and breezy short sleeves are braid trimmed. Side closing slacks have smart wide legs with Blue stripe. Anchor on pocket. Cunning gob hat.
Sizes: 8, 10, 12, 14 and 16 years. *State size.*
27 H 6670—White and Blue......... $1.59
Shipping weight, 1 lb. 4 oz.

COSSACK STYLE JACKET designed especially for Spring and Summer sports. Made of rich Cotton Flannel in deep, beautiful shades. Button closing. Adjustable side buckles. One swanky patch pocket.
Sizes: 8, 10, 12 and 14 years. *State size.*
27 H 6685—Red.
27 H 6686—Skipper Blue............. $1.25
Shipping weight, 1 lb. 4 oz.

There's new smartness in Sears playtime fashions

Shirley Temple FASHIONS

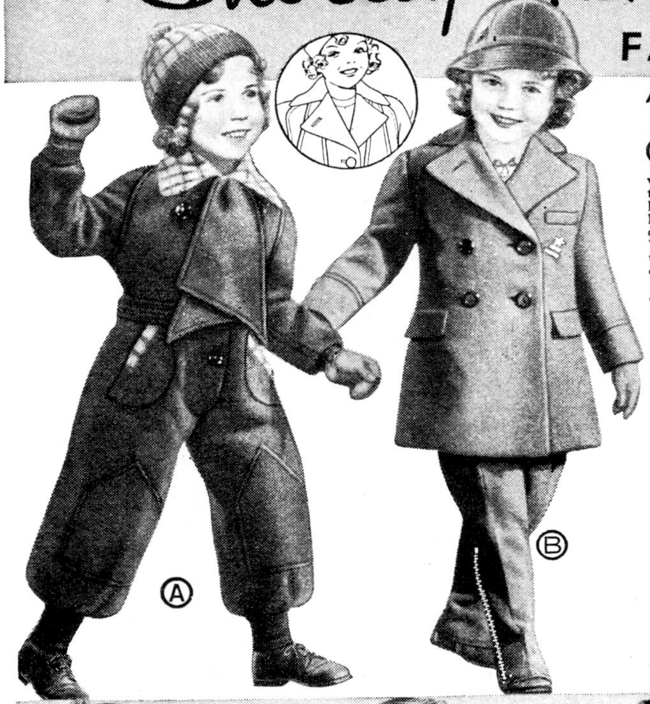

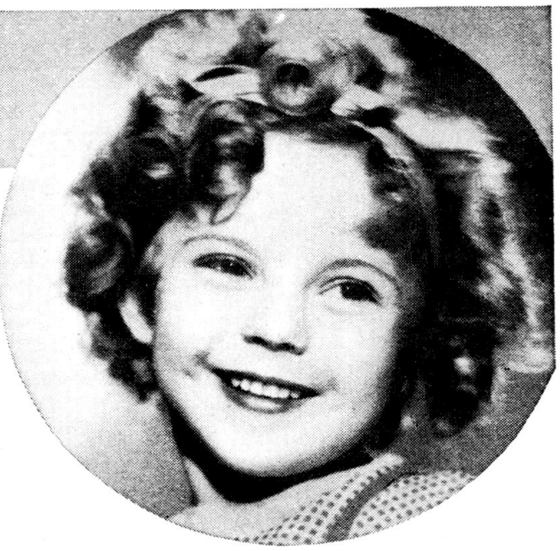

All Wool Fleece Outfit One-Piece Snow Suit with Hat

(A) Hollywood style—at its best! Notice all its brand new fashion points . . . the wide plaid lapels, the ascot-tie, the pocket pipings, the swanky little hat! See how cunning Shirley looks in it! One-piece outdoor suit of heavy weight All Wool Fleece, the fine quality that takes those rich lovely colorings. Expertly tailored.
Ages: 2-3-4-5-6 yrs.
State age-size.
38 K 7932—Blue. $5.95
38 K 7933—Green.
Shipping weight, 2 lbs. 12 oz.

All Wool Fleece Herringbone Coat, Legging and Hat Set

(B) Of course, Shirley's three-piece coat set had to be the very finest quality! It's so soft it feels like velvet, so closely woven it will wear extra long. Beautifully made in every detail. Coat is warmly interlined and lined with Rayon Taffeta. Hat has snap-on earmuffs. Talon slide fastened leggings.
Ages: 2-3-4-5-6 yrs.
State age-size.
38 K 6373—Blue. $10.95
38 K 6374—Red.
Shipping weight, 3 lbs. 14 oz.

A whole page of cunning Shirley Temple Fashions! In big city stores they're going like wildfire! Shirley and her cute clothes have stolen everyone's heart; no wonder every little girl wants to wear the same styles!

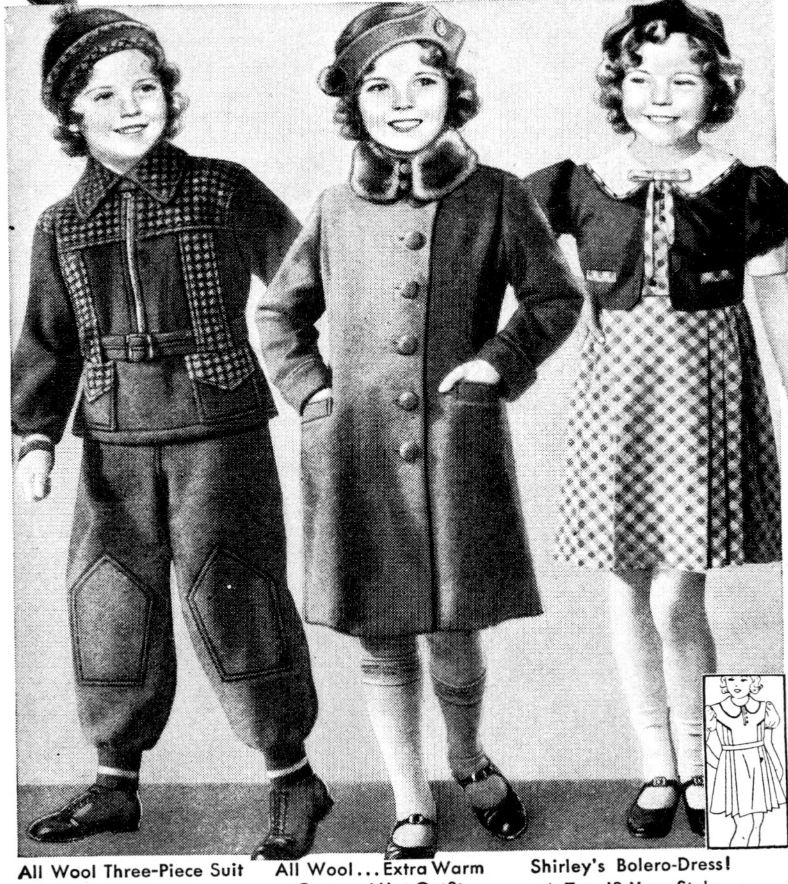

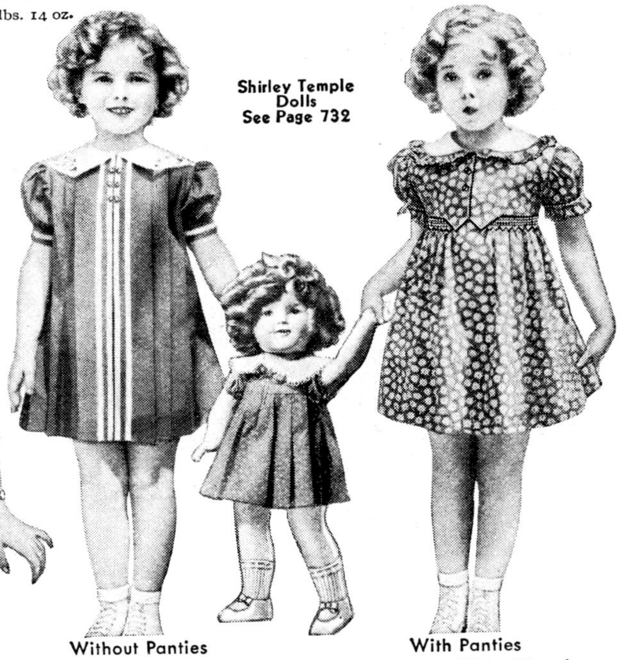

Shirley Temple Dolls See Page 732

Without Panties **With Panties**

These dresses exemplify the beautiful costumes worn by Shirley Temple. The materials are of the finest wash fabrics available. The workmanship is exquisite. The trim is in keeping with the quality of the dresses, and the beautiful styles designed for Shirley. We will send you the dresses shown or equal values developed from Shirley's costumes in her latest pictures.
Ages: 3, 4, 5, 6 and 6½ years. *State age.*
38 K 5942—Blue.
38 K 5943—Red.
Shipping weight, 8 oz.
$1.89 each
38 K 5944—Red.
38 K 5945—Blue.
Shipping weight, 10 oz.

Shirley Temple Hats →

This favorite is made of fine all wool body felt. Stitched brim and fine ribbon bow! Shipping weight, 1 lb.
78 K 6485—Fits 20 to 20½ inch.
78 K 6486—Fits 20¾ to 21¼ inch headsize...... $1.79
Colors: Sand with Brown ribbon or Brown with Sand, Solid Navy or Solid Red. *Measure and state color.*

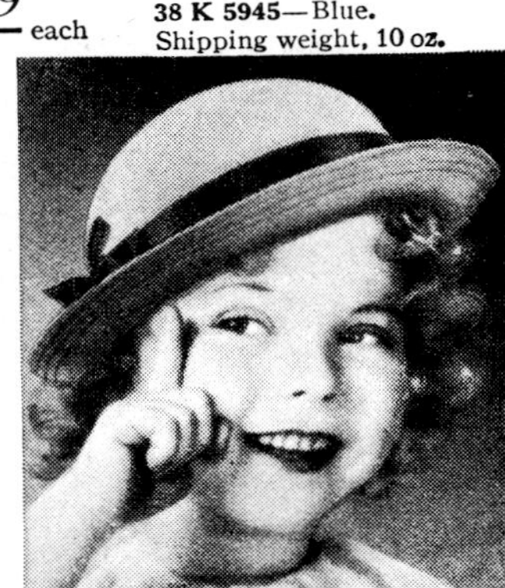

All Wool Three-Piece Suit —Coat, Hat and Pants

One of Shirley's favorites! Zip closing. *State age-size.*
Shipping wt., 3 lbs. 6 oz.
Ages: 7-8-9-10 Years
31 K 2960—Navy with Red and Blue Check.
31 K 2961—Brown with Orange and Brown Check.............. $7.95
Ages: 3-4-5-6 Years
31 K 2963—Navy with Blue and Red Check.
31 K 2964—Brown with Orange and Brown Check.............. $6.95

All Wool . . . Extra Warm Coat and Hat Outfit

Wide turn-back collar is silky-soft Beaver-Dyed Coney Fur! Coat is warm wool, interlined with deep-napped cotton flannel. Has four-button closing with two ornamental buttons. Rayon and cotton taffeta lined. Belted back.
Ages: 7-8-9-10 years. *State size.* $10.95
17 K 4665—Rust.
17 K 4666—Medium Blue.
17 K 4667—Medium Brown.
Shipping wt., 3 lbs. 6 oz.

Shirley's Bolero-Dress! A 7 to 12 Year Style

America's First Lady of Fashion certainly knows a cunning style when she sees it! This "ensemble" would be the prize possession of any lucky little girl who owned it! Washfast percale check dress, pleated at back, too. Vat dyed jacket.
Ages: 7-8-10 and 12 years.
State age-size.
27 K 4296—Red and Navy.
27 K 4297—Copen Blue and Navy.
Shpg. wt., 12 oz. $1.89

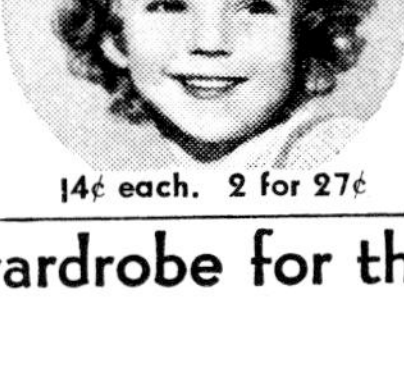

Hair Bow

On band Cameo Center Elastic back.
Colors: Maize, Pink, Lt. Blue, White, Red or Nile. *State Color.*
Shpg. wt., 2 oz.
25 K 1217—Satin
25 K 1218—Rayon Moire.

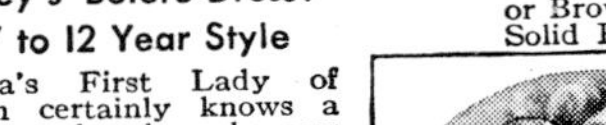
14¢ each. 2 for 27¢

A complete Shirley Temple wardrobe for the little miss

Ingersolls

AMERICA'S LOWEST PRICES

New Deal Watches

Big Hit! Modern! Different!

Buy yourself this good Ingersoll . . . A new Deal Ingersoll! Men, women, boys and girls are wearing them. Made exclusively for Sears; in no other mail order catalog. The New Deal Watches are good timekeepers; sturdy, reliable and an idea as modern as tomorrow.

The Wrist Watch

Chromium plated case, resembles white gold. Capitol dome on dial. Shpg. wt., 6 oz.

4 H 940—With adjustable Safety Clasp Metal Band...**$2.98**

4 H 941—With Genuine Leather Strap **$2.98**

The Pocket Watch

12-size Thin Model Chromium plated case, resembles white gold. Capitol Dome on dial. Back of watch and fob in blue enamel. Genuine leather fob. Shpg. wt., 7 oz.

4 H 1704
With Fob.....**$1.98**

4 H 1705
Watch only...**$1.88**

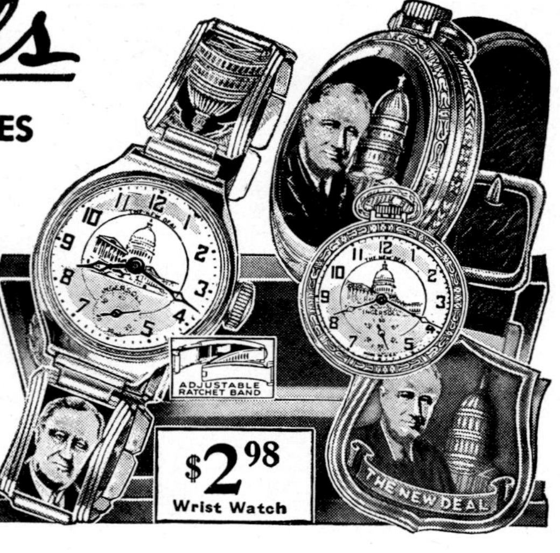

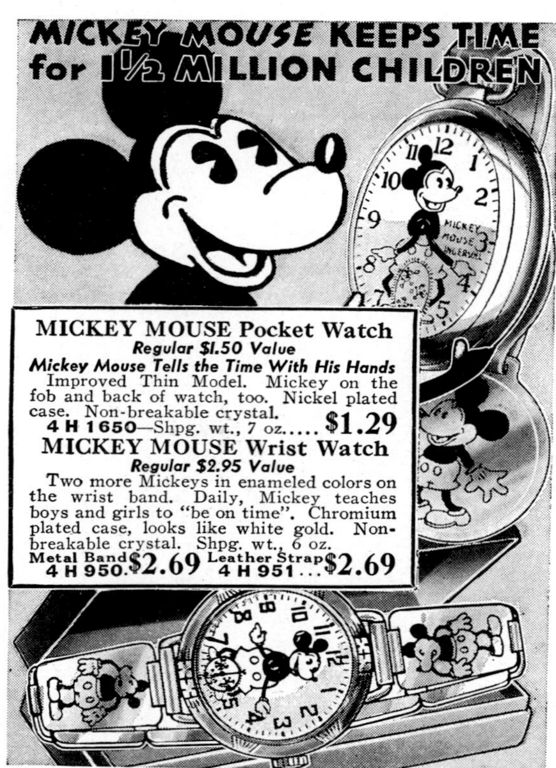

MICKEY MOUSE Pocket Watch

Regular $1.50 Value

Mickey Mouse Tells the Time With His Hands

Improved Thin Model. Mickey on the fob and back of watch, too. Nickel plated case. Non-breakable crystal.

4 H 1650—Shpg. wt., 7 oz..... **$1.29**

MICKEY MOUSE Wrist Watch

Regular $2.95 Value

Two more Mickeys in enameled colors on the wrist band. Daily, Mickey teaches boys and girls to "be on time". Chromium plated case, looks like white gold. Non-breakable crystal. Shpg. wt., 6 oz.

Metal Band 4 H 950..**$2.69** **Leather Strap 4 H 951**...**$2.69**

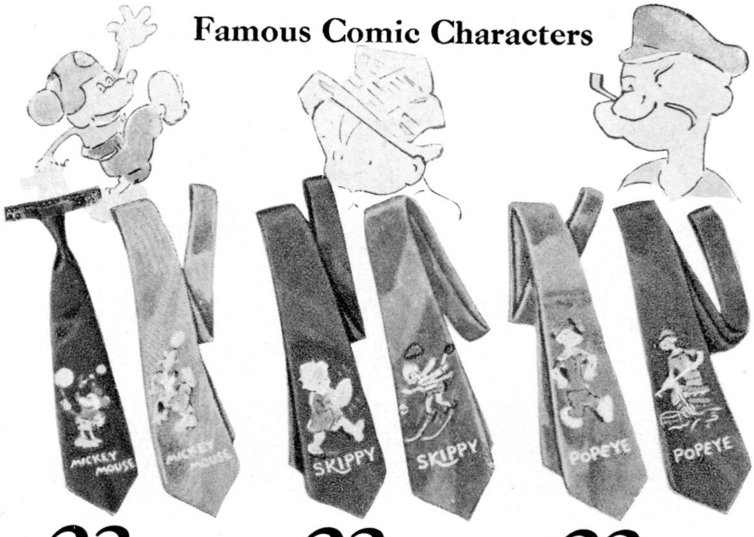

23c EACH

Mickey Mouse painted in colors on this dressy weighted silk crepe tie. Choose a four-in-hand to tie yourself, or a made-up tie, that just hooks around under your collar with a fancy elastic band.

33 K 8550—Four-in-hand.

33 K 8551—Ready tied (elastic band).

Colors: blue, red, light brown or green. State color. Shipping weight, 2 oz.

23c EACH

"Us fellers" are bound to be in style when we wear these ties with the comic figures on them! Skippy is painted in colors on good quality, plain color, weighted silk crepe. Ties up into a dandy knot, wears well. Good colors.

33 K 8553—Colors: Blue, Red, Light Brown or Green. State color. Shipping weight, 2 ounces.

23c EACH

A regular copyrighted Popeye tie, with the genuine Popeye label and a painting in color of "Popeye the Sailor Man" going into action! On good weighted silk crepe, in a practical weave. All the boys wear them.

33 K 8555—Plain colors: Blue, Red, Light Brown or Green. State color. Shipping weight, 2 oz.

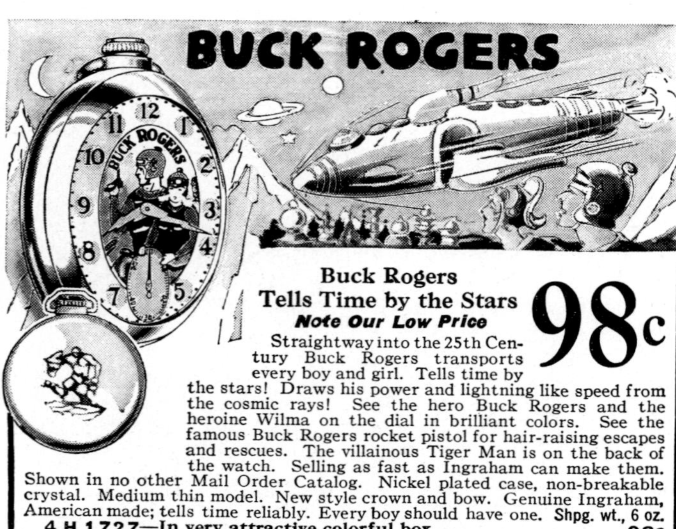

Buck Rogers Tells Time by the Stars

Note Our Low Price

98c

Straightway into the 25th Century Buck Rogers transports every boy and girl. Tells time by the stars! Draws his power and lightning like speed from the cosmic rays! See the hero Buck Rogers and the heroine Wilma on the dial in brilliant colors. See the famous Buck Rogers rocket pistol for hair-raising escapes and rescues. The villainous Tiger Man is on the back of the watch. Selling as fast as Ingraham can make them. Shown in no other Mail Order Catalog. Nickel plated case, non-breakable crystal. Medium thin model. New style crown and bow. Genuine Ingraham, American made; tells time reliably. Every boy should have one. **Shpg. wt., 6 oz.**

4 H 1727—In very attractive colorful box.......................98c

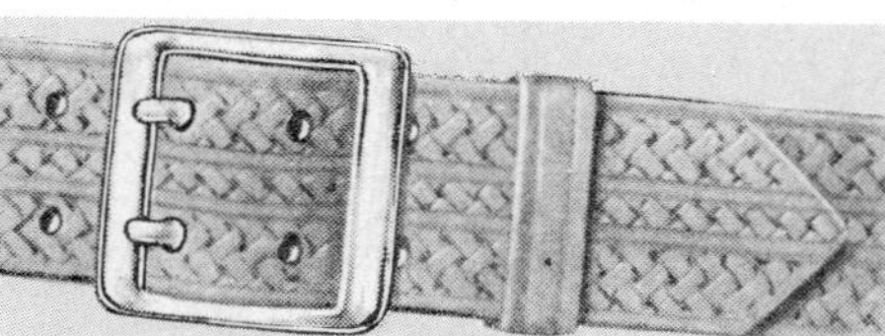

49c

A wide sporty western type belt that boys like to wear with their corduroy trousers. Made of fine 1¾-inch full grain bridle leather in fancy embossed design. Big nickel plated double pronged buckle.

33 K 8880—Black **33 K 8883—Tan**

Even sizes: 24 to 30 inches waist measure.

Shipping weight, 5 ounces.

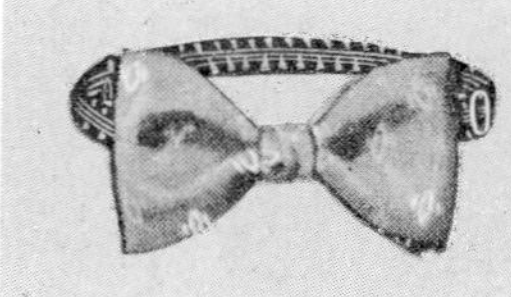

15c

Boys' ready-tied bow. Clever designs in rayon and silk mixed fabrics. Fancy elastic band adjusts to size.

33 K 8572—Colors: Fancy Blue, Red, Brown, Gray, Green Black; also Plain Black. State color. Shipping weight, 2 ounces.

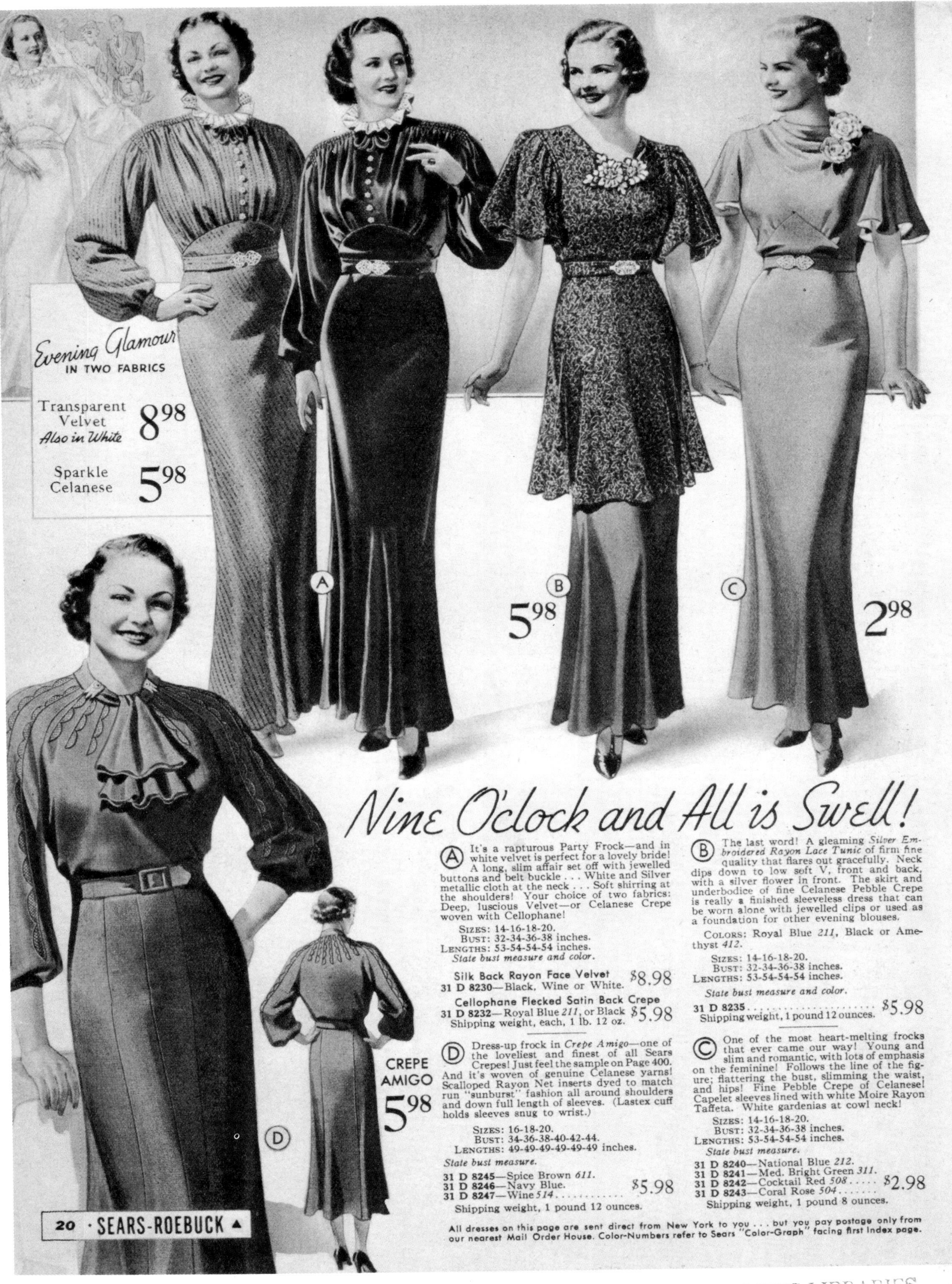

Evening Glamour IN TWO FABRICS

Transparent Velvet *Also in White* 8.98

Sparkle Celanese 5.98

(A) (B) 5.98 (C) 2.98

CREPE AMIGO 5.98

(D)

Nine O'clock and All is Swell!

(A) It's a rapturous Party Frock—and in white velvet is perfect for a lovely bride! A long, slim affair set off with jewelled buttons and belt buckle . . . White and Silver metallic cloth at the neck . . . Soft shirring at the shoulders! Your choice of two fabrics: Deep, luscious Velvet—or Celanese Crepe woven with Cellophane!

SIZES: 14-16-18-20.
BUST: 32-34-36-38 inches.
LENGTHS: 53-54-54-54 inches.
State bust measure and color.

Silk Back Rayon Face Velvet
31 D 8230—Black, Wine or White. $8.98

Cellophane Flecked Satin Back Crepe
31 D 8232—Royal Blue *211*, or Black $5.98
Shipping weight, each, 1 lb. 12 oz.

(D) Dress-up frock in *Crepe Amigo*—one of the loveliest and finest of all Sears Crepes! Just feel the sample on Page 400. And it's woven of genuine Celanese yarns! Scalloped Rayon Net inserts dyed to match run "sunburst" fashion all around shoulders and down full length of sleeves. (Lastex cuff holds sleeves snug to wrist.)

SIZES: 16-18-20.
BUST: 34-36-38-40-42-44.
LENGTHS: 49-49-49-49-49-49 inches.
State bust measure.

31 D 8245—Spice Brown *611*.
31 D 8246—Navy Blue.
31 D 8247—Wine *514*. $5.98
Shipping weight, 1 pound 12 ounces.

(B) The last word! A gleaming *Silver Embroidered Rayon Lace Tunic* of firm fine quality that flares out gracefully. Neck dips down to low soft V, front and back, with a silver flower in front. The skirt and underbodice of fine Celanese Pebble Crepe is really a finished sleeveless dress that can be worn alone with jewelled clips or used as a foundation for other evening blouses.

COLORS: Royal Blue *211*, Black or Amethyst *412*.

SIZES: 14-16-18-20.
BUST: 32-34-36-38 inches.
LENGTHS: 53-54-54-54 inches.
State bust measure and color.

31 D 8235. $5.98
Shipping weight, 1 pound 12 ounces.

(C) One of the most heart-melting frocks that ever came our way! Young and slim and romantic, with lots of emphasis on the feminine! Follows the line of the figure; flattering the bust, slimming the waist, and hips! Fine Pebble Crepe of Celanese! Capelet sleeves lined with white Moire Rayon Taffeta. White gardenias at cowl neck!

SIZES: 14-16-18-20.
BUST: 32-34-36-38 inches.
LENGTHS: 53-54-54-54 inches.
State bust measure.

31 D 8240—National Blue *212*.
31 D 8241—Med. Bright Green *311*.
31 D 8242—Cocktail Red *508* $2.98
31 D 8243—Coral Rose *504* . . . . . .
Shipping weight, 1 pound 8 ounces.

All dresses on this page are sent direct from New York to you . . . but you pay postage only from our nearest Mail Order House. Color-Numbers refer to Sears "Color-Graph" facing first Index page.

20 · SEARS-ROEBUCK ▲

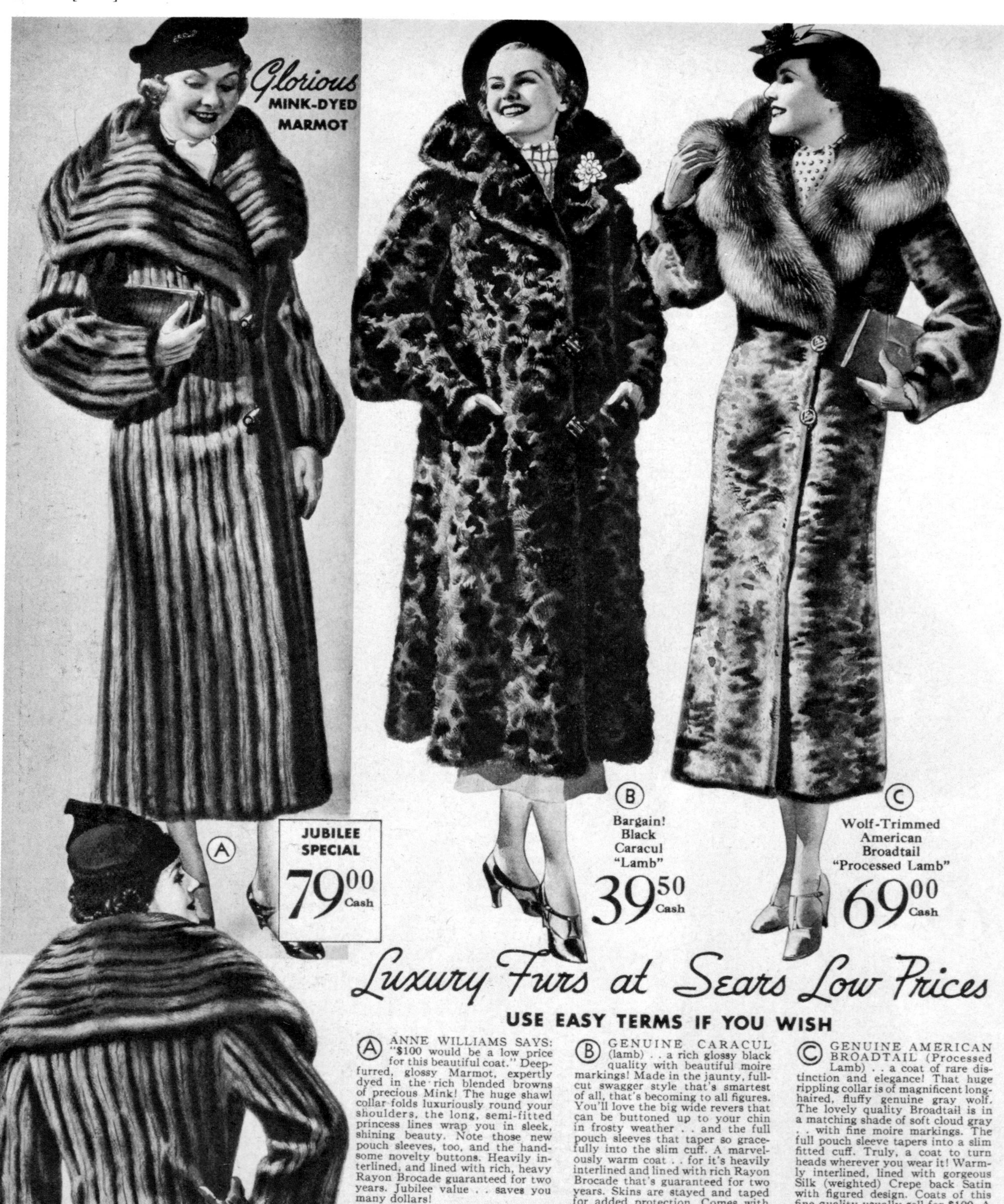

Luxury Furs at Sears Low Prices

USE EASY TERMS IF YOU WISH

(A) ANNE WILLIAMS SAYS: "$100 would be a low price for this beautiful coat." Deep-furred, glossy Marmot, expertly dyed in the rich blended browns of precious Mink! The huge shawl collar folds luxuriously round your shoulders, the long, semi-fitted princess lines wrap you in sleek, shining beauty. Note those new pouch sleeves, too, and the handsome novelty buttons. Heavily interlined, and lined with rich, heavy Rayon Brocade guaranteed for two years. Jubilee value . . saves you many dollars!

SIZES: 14-16-18-20-22.
BUST: 32-34-36-38-40-42-44 in.
LENGTHS: 48-48-49-49-49-49-49 in.
State bust measure.

17 D 7577—Mink Brown.
Cash Price **$79.00**
Easy Payment Price ($17.50 down, $17.50 a month) **$86.90**
Shipping weight, 6 lbs. 10 oz.

(B) GENUINE CARACUL (lamb) . . a rich glossy black quality with beautiful moire markings! Made in the jaunty, full-cut swagger style that's smartest of all, that's becoming to all figures. You'll love the big wide revers that can be buttoned up to your chin in frosty weather . . and the full pouch sleeves that taper so gracefully into the slim cuff. A marvelously warm coat . . for it's heavily interlined and lined with rich Rayon Brocade that's guaranteed for two years. Skins are stayed and taped for added protection. Comes with smart gold-like finished gardenia.

SIZES: 14-16-18-20-22.
BUST: 32-34-36-38-40 inches.
LENGTHS: 45-45-46-46-46 inches.
State bust measure.

17 D 7575—Rich Black.
Cash Price **$39.50**
Easy Payment Price ($9.50 down, $8.50 a month) **$43.45**
Shipping weight, 6 lbs. 10 oz.

Use Easy Payment Order Blank in back of Catalog.

(C) GENUINE AMERICAN BROADTAIL (Processed Lamb) . . a coat of rare distinction and elegance! That huge rippling collar is of magnificent long-haired, fluffy genuine gray wolf. The lovely quality Broadtail is in a matching shade of soft cloud gray . . with fine moire markings. The full pouch sleeve tapers into a slim fitted cuff. Truly, a coat to turn heads wherever you wear it! Warmly interlined, lined with gorgeous Silk (weighted) Crepe back Satin with figured design. Coats of this fine quality usually sell for $100. A rare value!

SIZES: 14-16-18-20-22.
BUST: 32-34-36-38-40-42 in.
LENGTHS: 48-48-49-49-49-49 in.
State bust measure.

17 D 7578—Silvery Gray.
Cash Price **$69.00**
Easy Payment Price ($16.00 down, $15.00 a month) **$75.90**
Shipping weight, 8 pounds.
Use Easy Payment Order Blank in back of Catalog.

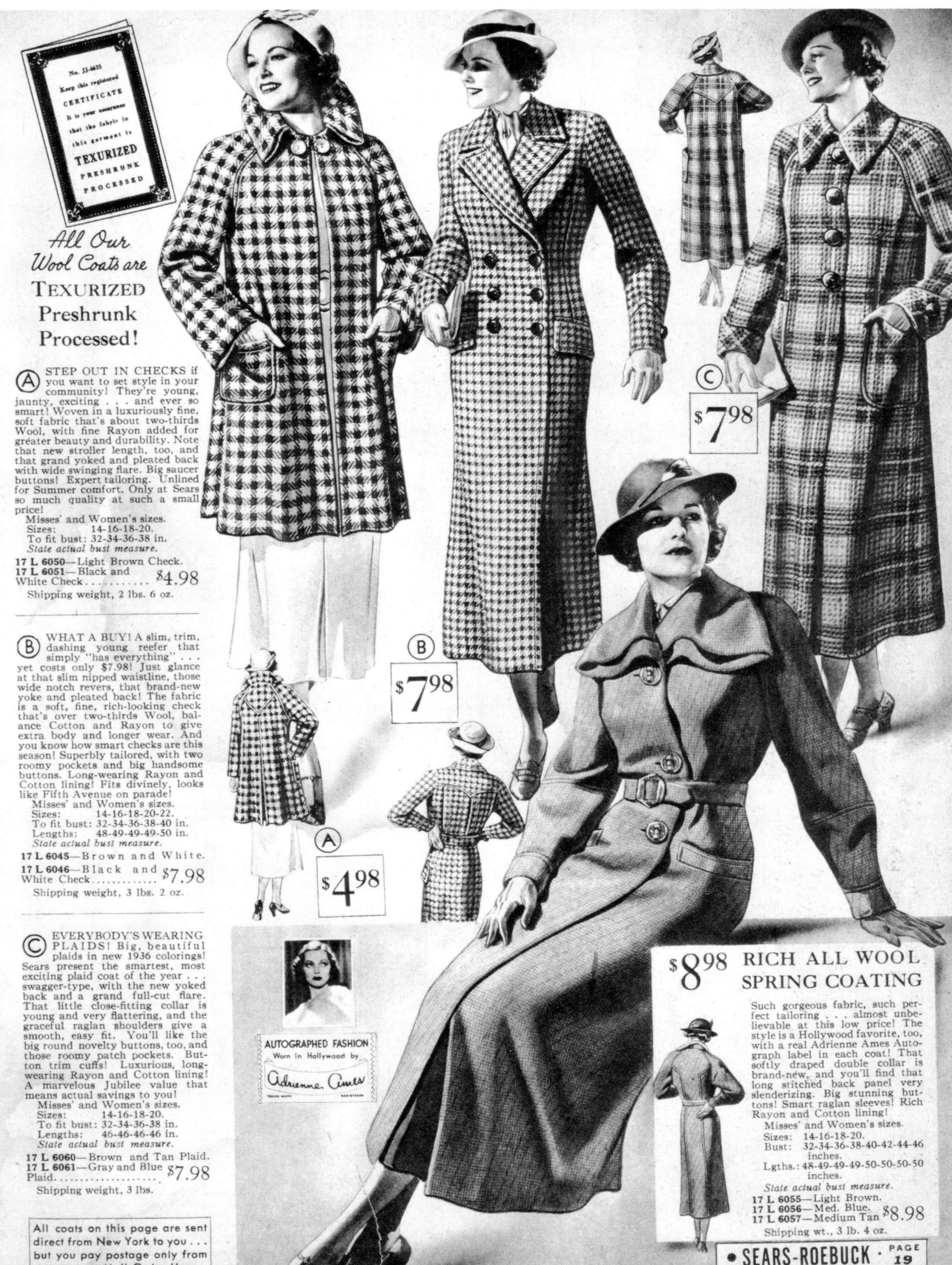

Keep this registered CERTIFICATE It is your assurance that the fabric in this garment is TEXURIZED PRESHRUNK PROCESSED

All Our Wool Coats are TEXURIZED Preshrunk Processed!

(A) STEP OUT IN CHECKS if you want to set style in your community! They're young, jaunty, exciting . . . and ever so smart! Woven in a luxuriously fine, soft fabric that's about two-thirds Wool, with fine Rayon added for greater beauty and durability. Note that new stroller length, too, and that grand yoked and pleated back with wide swinging flare. Big saucer buttons! Expert tailoring. Unlined for Summer comfort. Only at Sears so much quality at such a small price!
Misses' and Women's sizes.
Sizes: 14-16-18-20.
To fit bust: 32-34-36-38 in.
State actual bust measure.
17 L 6050—Light Brown Check.
17 L 6051—Black and White Check $4.98
Shipping weight, 2 lbs. 6 oz.

(B) WHAT A BUY! A slim, trim, dashing young reefer that simply "has everything" . . . yet costs only $7.98! Just glance at that slim nipped waistline, those wide notch revers, that brand-new yoke and pleated back! The fabric is a soft, fine, rich-looking check that's over two-thirds Wool, balance Cotton and Rayon to give extra body and longer wear. And you know how smart checks are this season! Superbly tailored, with two roomy pockets and big handsome buttons. Long-wearing Rayon and Cotton lining! Fits divinely, looks like Fifth Avenue on parade!
Misses' and Women's sizes.
Sizes: 14-16-18-20-22.
To fit bust: 32-34-36-38-40 in.
Lengths: 48-49-49-49-50 in.
State actual bust measure.
17 L 6045—Brown and White.
17 L 6046—Black and White Check $7.98
Shipping weight, 3 lbs. 2 oz.

(C) EVERYBODY'S WEARING PLAIDS! Big, beautiful plaids in new 1936 colorings! Sears present the smartest, most exciting plaid coat of the year . . . swagger-type, with the new yoked back and a grand full-cut flare. That little close-fitting collar is young and very flattering, and the graceful raglan shoulders give a smooth, easy fit. You'll like the big round novelty buttons, too, and those roomy patch pockets. Button trim cuffs! Luxurious, long-wearing Rayon and Cotton lining! A marvelous Jubilee value that means actual savings to you!
Misses' and Women's sizes.
Sizes: 14-16-18-20.
To fit bust: 32-34-36-38 in.
Lengths: 46-46-46-46 in.
State actual bust measure.
17 L 6060—Brown and Tan Plaid.
17 L 6061—Gray and Blue Plaid $7.98
Shipping weight, 3 lbs.

All coats on this page are sent direct from New York to you . . . but you pay postage only from our nearest Mail Order House.

(C) $7.98

(B) $7.98

(A) $4.98

AUTOGRAPHED FASHION
Worn in Hollywood by
Adrienne Ames

$8.98 RICH ALL WOOL SPRING COATING

Such gorgeous fabric, such perfect tailoring . . . almost unbelievable at this low price! The style is a Hollywood favorite, too, with a real Adrienne Ames Autograph label in each coat! That softly draped double collar is brand-new, and you'll find that long stitched back panel very slenderizing. Big stunning buttons! Smart raglan sleeves! Rich Rayon and Cotton lining!
Misses' and Women's sizes.
Sizes: 14-16-18-20.
Bust: 32-34-36-38-40-42-44-46 inches.
Lgths.: 48-49-49-49-50-50-50-50 inches.
State actual bust measure.
17 L 6055—Light Brown.
17 L 6056—Med. Blue.
17 L 6057—Medium Tan $8.98
Shipping wt., 3 lb. 4 oz.

• SEARS-ROEBUCK • PAGE 19

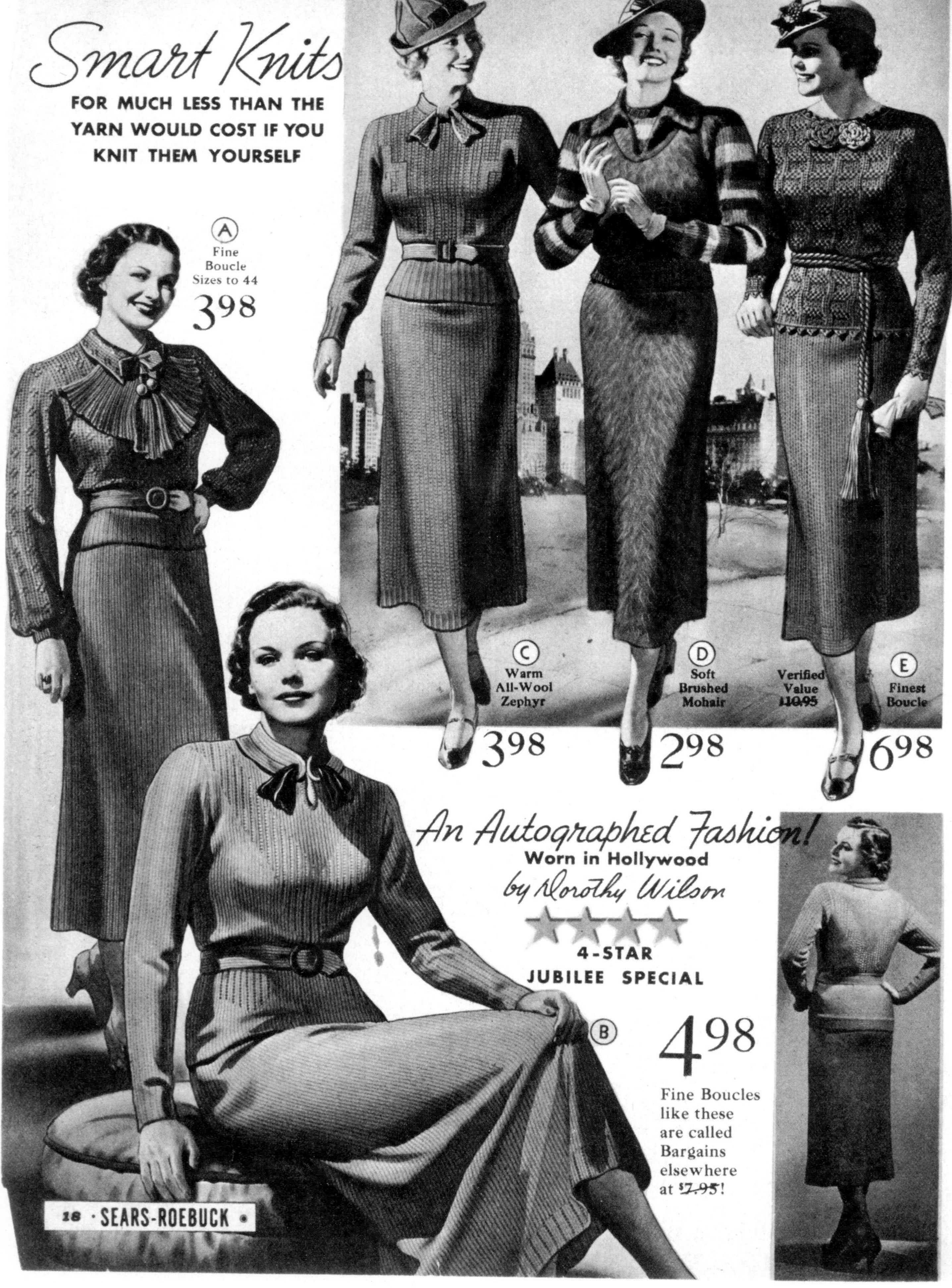

Smart Knits
FOR MUCH LESS THAN THE YARN WOULD COST IF YOU KNIT THEM YOURSELF
A
Fine Boucle Sizes to 44
3.98
C
Warm All-Wool Zephyr
3.98
D
Soft Brushed Mohair
2.98
Verified Value $10.95
E
Finest Boucle
6.98
An Autographed Fashion!
Worn in Hollywood
by Dorothy Wilson
4-STAR JUBILEE SPECIAL
B
4.98
Fine Boucles like these are called Bargains elsewhere at $7.95!
18 · SEARS-ROEBUCK ·

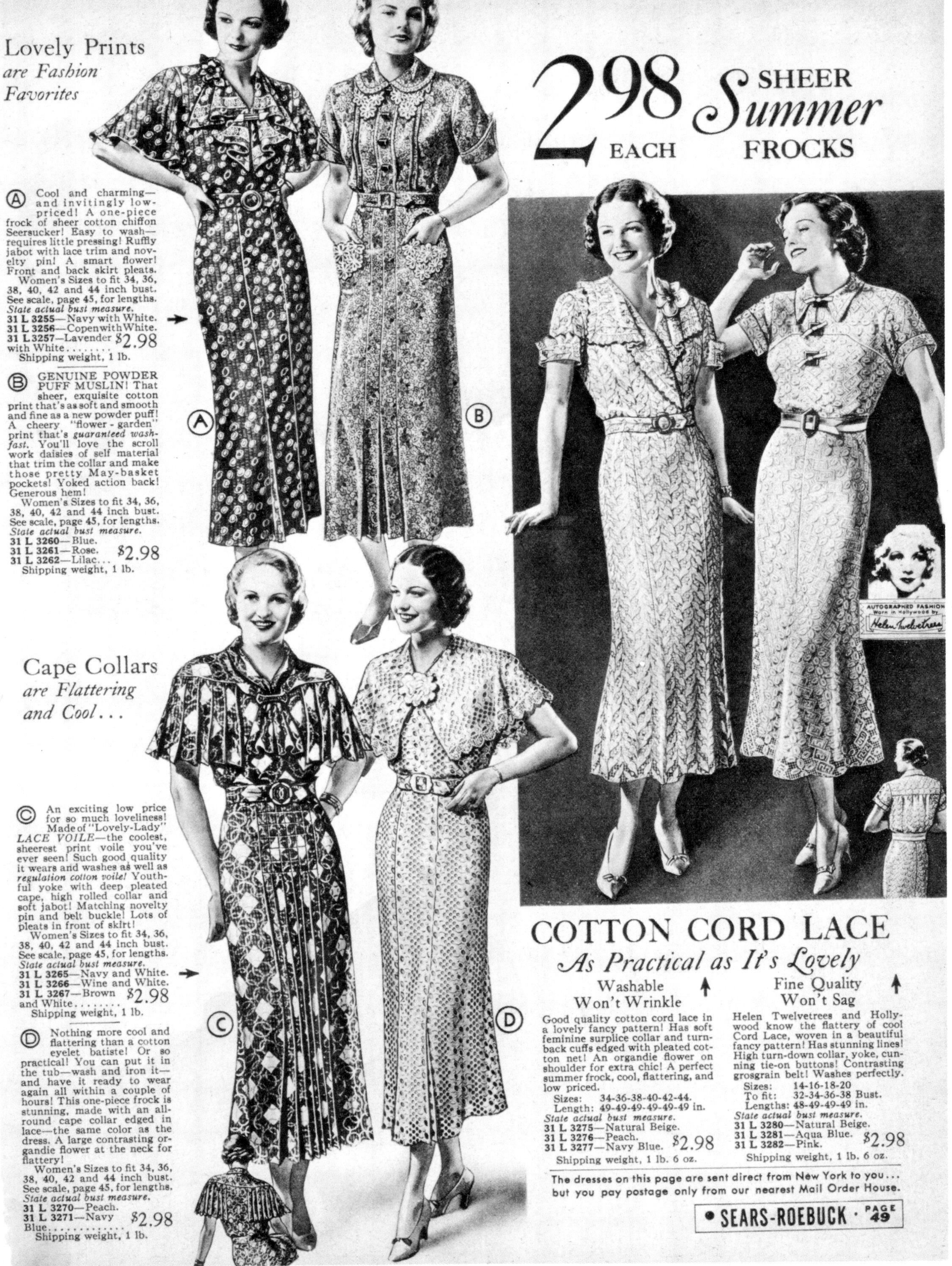

Lovely Prints
are Fashion Favorites

(A) Cool and charming—and invitingly low-priced! A one-piece frock of sheer cotton chiffon Seersucker! Easy to wash—requires little pressing! Ruffly jabot with lace trim and novelty pin! A smart flower! Front and back skirt pleats.
Women's Sizes to fit 34, 36, 38, 40, 42 and 44 inch bust. See scale, page 45, for lengths.
State actual bust measure.
31 L 3255—Navy with White.
31 L 3256—Copen with White.
31 L 3257—Lavender with White........ $2.98
Shipping weight, 1 lb.

(B) GENUINE POWDER PUFF MUSLIN! That sheer, exquisite cotton print that's as soft and smooth and fine as a new powder puff! A cheery "flower-garden" print that's *guaranteed wash-fast.* You'll love the scroll work daisies of self material that trim the collar and make those pretty May-basket pockets! Yoked action back! Generous hem!
Women's Sizes to fit 34, 36, 38, 40, 42 and 44 inch bust. See scale, page 45, for lengths.
State actual bust measure.
31 L 3260—Blue.
31 L 3261—Rose.
31 L 3262—Lilac... $2.98
Shipping weight, 1 lb.

2.98 EACH SHEER *Summer* FROCKS

AUTOGRAPHED FASHION Worn in Hollywood by Helen Twelvetrees

Cape Collars
are Flattering and Cool...

(C) An exciting low price for so much loveliness! Made of "Lovely-Lady" *LACE VOILE*—the coolest, sheerest print voile you've ever seen! Such good quality it wears and washes as well as *regulation cotton voile!* Youthful yoke with deep pleated cape, high rolled collar and soft jabot! Matching novelty pin and belt buckle! Lots of pleats in front of skirt!
Women's Sizes to fit 34, 36, 38, 40, 42 and 44 inch bust. See scale, page 45, for lengths.
State actual bust measure.
31 L 3265—Navy and White.
31 L 3266—Wine and White.
31 L 3267—Brown and White........ $2.98
Shipping weight, 1 lb.

(D) Nothing more cool and flattering than a cotton eyelet batiste! Or so practical! You can put it in the tub—wash and iron it—and have it ready to wear again all within a couple of hours! This one-piece frock is stunning, made with an all-round cape collar edged in lace—the same color as the dress. A large contrasting organdie flower at the neck for flattery!
Women's Sizes to fit 34, 36, 38, 40, 42 and 44 inch bust. See scale, page 45, for lengths.
State actual bust measure.
31 L 3270—Peach.
31 L 3271—Navy Blue.............. $2.98
Shipping weight, 1 lb.

COTTON CORD LACE
As Practical as It's Lovely

Washable
Won't Wrinkle

Good quality cotton cord lace in a lovely fancy pattern! Has soft feminine surplice collar and turn-back cuffs edged with pleated cotton net! An organdie flower on shoulder for extra chic! A perfect summer frock, cool, flattering, and low priced.
Sizes: 34-36-38-40-42-44.
Length: 49-49-49-49-49-49 in.
State actual bust measure.
31 L 3275—Natural Beige.
31 L 3276—Peach.
31 L 3277—Navy Blue. $2.98
Shipping weight, 1 lb. 6 oz.

Fine Quality
Won't Sag

Helen Twelvetrees and Hollywood know the flattery of cool Cord Lace, woven in a beautiful fancy pattern! Has stunning lines! High turn-down collar, yoke, cunning tie-on buttons! Contrasting grosgrain belt! Washes perfectly.
Sizes: 14-16-18-20
To fit: 32-34-36-38 Bust.
Lengths: 48-49-49-49 in.
State actual bust measure.
31 L 3280—Natural Beige.
31 L 3281—Aqua Blue.
31 L 3282—Pink. $2.98
Shipping weight, 1 lb. 6 oz.

The dresses on this page are sent direct from New York to you... but you pay postage only from our nearest Mail Order House.

• SEARS-ROEBUCK • PAGE 49

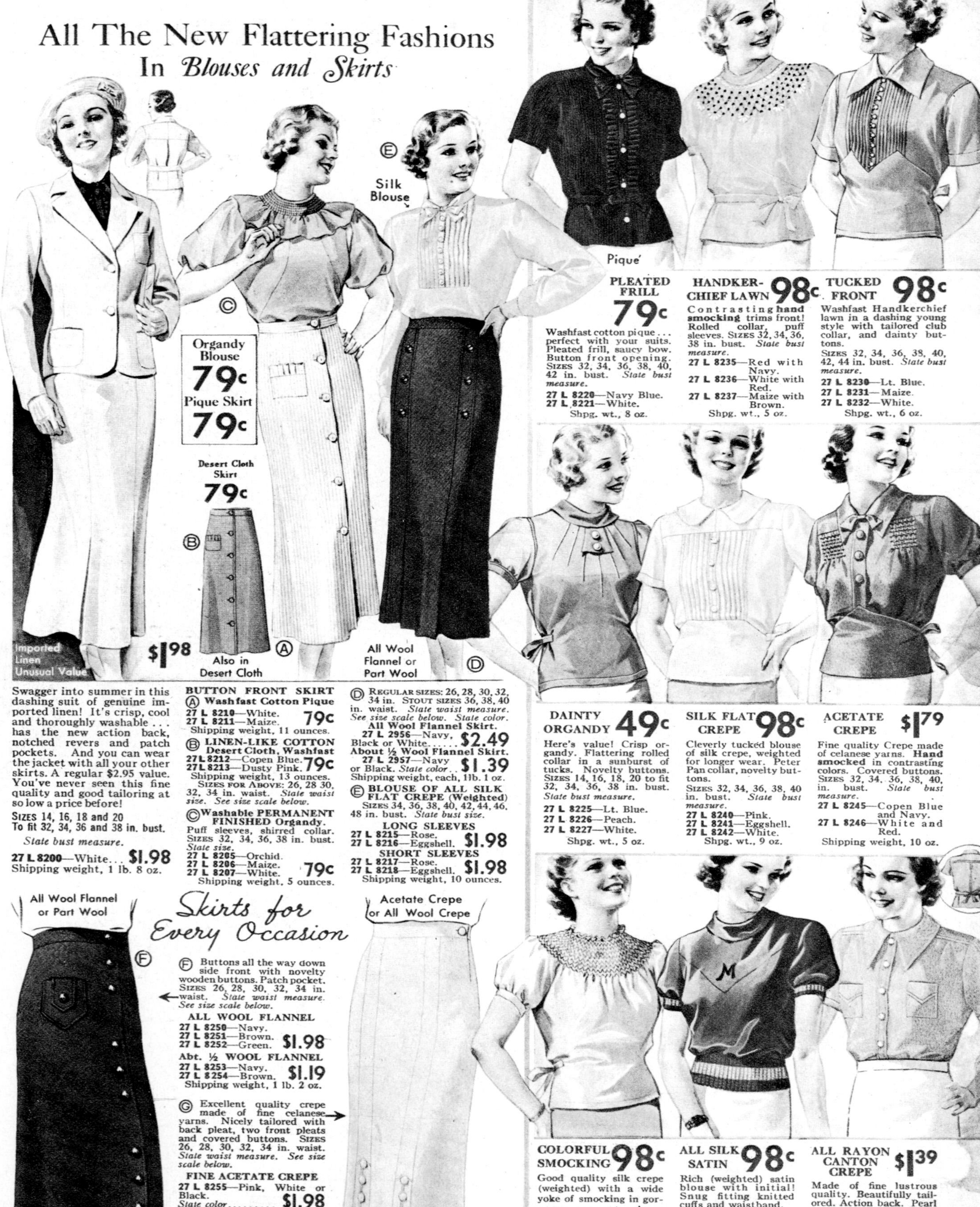
All The New Flattering Fashions
In Blouses and Skirts
Silk Blouse
Ⓔ
Ⓒ
Organdy Blouse
79c
Pique Skirt
79c
Desert Cloth Skirt
79c
Ⓑ
Imported Linen Unusual Value
$1.98
Also in Desert Cloth
Ⓐ
All Wool Flannel or Part Wool
Ⓓ
Pique'
PLEATED FRILL 79c
Washfast cotton pique . . . perfect with your suits. Pleated frill, saucy bow. Button front opening. SIZES 32, 34, 36, 38, 40, 42 in. bust. State bust measure.
27 L 8220—Navy Blue.
27 L 8221—White.
Shpg. wt., 8 oz.
HANDKERCHIEF LAWN 98c
Contrasting hand smocking trims front! Rolled collar, puff sleeves. SIZES 32, 34, 36, 38 in. bust. State bust measure.
27 L 8235—Red with Navy.
27 L 8236—White with Red.
27 L 8237—Maize with Brown.
Shpg. wt., 5 oz.
TUCKED FRONT 98c
Washfast Handkerchief lawn in a dashing young style with tailored club collar, and dainty buttons.
SIZES 32, 34, 36, 38, 40, 42, 44 in. bust. State bust measure.
27 L 8230—Lt. Blue.
27 L 8231—Maize.
27 L 8232—White.
Shpg. wt., 6 oz.
Swagger into summer in this dashing suit of genuine imported linen! It's crisp, cool and thoroughly washable . . . has the new action back, notched revers and patch pockets. And you can wear the jacket with all your other skirts. A regular $2.95 value. You've never seen this fine quality and good tailoring at so low a price before!
SIZES 14, 16, 18 and 20
To fit 32, 34, 36 and 38 in. bust.
State bust measure.
27 L 8200—White. . . $1.98
Shipping weight, 1 lb. 8 oz.
BUTTON FRONT SKIRT
Ⓐ Washfast Cotton Pique
27 L 8210—White.
27 L 8211—Maize. 79c
Shipping weight, 11 ounces.
Ⓑ LINEN-LIKE COTTON Desert Cloth, Washfast
27 L 8212—Copen Blue.
27 L 8213—Dusty Pink. 79c
Shipping weight, 13 ounces.
SIZES FOR ABOVE: 26, 28 30, 32, 34 in. waist. State waist size. See size scale below.
Ⓒ Washable PERMANENT FINISHED Organdy.
Puff sleeves, shirred collar. SIZES 32, 34, 36, 38 in. bust. State size.
27 L 8205—Orchid.
27 L 8206—Maize.
27 L 8207—White. 79c
Shipping weight, 5 ounces.
Ⓓ REGULAR SIZES: 26, 28, 30, 32, 34 in. STOUT SIZES 36, 38, 40 in. waist. State waist measure. See size scale below. State color.
All Wool Flannel Skirt.
27 L 2956—Navy, Black or White. $2.49
About ½ Wool Flannel Skirt.
27 L 2957—Navy or Black. State color. . $1.39
Shipping weight, each, 1lb. 1 oz.
Ⓔ BLOUSE OF ALL SILK FLAT CREPE (Weighted)
SIZES 34, 36, 38, 40, 42, 44, 46, 48 in. bust. State bust size.
LONG SLEEVES
27 L 8215—Rose.
27 L 8216—Eggshell. $1.98
SHORT SLEEVES
27 L 8217—Rose.
27 L 8218—Eggshell. $1.98
Shipping weight, 10 ounces.
DAINTY ORGANDY 49c
Here's value! Crisp organdy. Flattering rolled collar in a sunburst of tucks. Novelty buttons. SIZES 14, 16, 18, 20 to fit 32, 34, 36, 38 in. bust. State bust measure.
27 L 8225—Lt. Blue.
27 L 8226—Peach.
27 L 8227—White.
Shpg. wt., 5 oz.
SILK FLAT CREPE 98c
Cleverly tucked blouse of silk crepe, weighted for longer wear. Peter Pan collar, novelty buttons.
SIZES 32, 34, 36, 38, 40 in. bust. State bust measure.
27 L 8240—Pink.
27 L 8241—Eggshell.
27 L 8242—White.
Shpg. wt., 9 oz.
ACETATE CREPE $1.79
Fine quality Crepe made of celanese yarns. Hand smocked in contrasting colors. Covered buttons. SIZES 32, 34, 36, 38, 40, in. bust. State bust measure.
27 L 8245—Copen Blue and Navy.
27 L 8246—White and Red.
Shipping weight, 10 oz.
All Wool Flannel or Part Wool
Skirts for Every Occasion
Acetate Crepe or All Wool Crepe
Ⓕ
Ⓕ Buttons all the way down side front with novelty wooden buttons. Patch pocket. SIZES 26, 28, 30, 32, 34 in. waist. State waist measure. See size scale below.
ALL WOOL FLANNEL
27 L 8250—Navy.
27 L 8251—Brown.
27 L 8252—Green. $1.98
Abt. ½ WOOL FLANNEL
27 L 8253—Navy.
27 L 8254—Brown. $1.19
Shipping weight, 1 lb. 2 oz.
Ⓖ Excellent quality crepe made of fine celanese yarns. Nicely tailored with back pleat, two front pleats and covered buttons. SIZES 26, 28, 30, 32, 34 in. waist. State waist measure. See size scale below.
FINE ACETATE CREPE
27 L 8255—Pink, White or Black.
State color. $1.98
ALL WOOL CREPE
27 L 8256—Navy or Brown. State color. $1.98
Shipping weight, 13 oz.
SIZE SCALE FOR SKIRTS
Waist : 26-28-30-32-34-36-38-40 in.
Hips : 37-39-41-43-45-47-49-51 in.
Lgths.: 32-33-33-33-33-35-35-35 in.
Ⓖ
COLORFUL SMOCKING 98c
Good quality silk crepe (weighted) with a wide yoke of smocking in gorgeous peasant colors. Puffed sleeves.
SIZES 14, 16, 18, 20 to fit 32, 34, 36, 38 in. bust.
State bust measure.
27 L 2884—White.
27 L 2885—Tea Rose.
Shipping weight, 8 oz.
ALL SILK SATIN 98c
Rich (weighted) satin blouse with initial! Snug fitting knitted cuffs and waistband. SIZES 14, 16, 18, 20 to fit 32, 34, 36, 38 in. bust.
State bust measure.
Print initial desired.
27 L 8260—Copen Blue.
27 L 8261—Eggshell.
Shipping weight, 9 oz.
ALL RAYON CANTON CREPE $1.39
Made of fine lustrous quality. Beautifully tailored. Action back. Pearl buttons. SIZES 32, 34, 36, 38, 40 in. bust. State bust measure.
27 L 8265—Tile Red.
27 L 8266—White.
Shipping weight, 11 oz.
• SEARS-ROEBUCK • PAGE 65

B
Extra Warm Wool
7.95
C
Suit with Cap and Vestee
9.95 SET
D
Plaid for Swank!
7.95
E
Jubilee Value!
6.75
Outdoor Sports Suits
WATER-REPELLENT, WINTER-WARM—FOR SKIING, SKATING, DRIVING, PLAYING!
A
ST. MORITZ SPECIAL
Our Best
Suit with Cap
10.95 SET

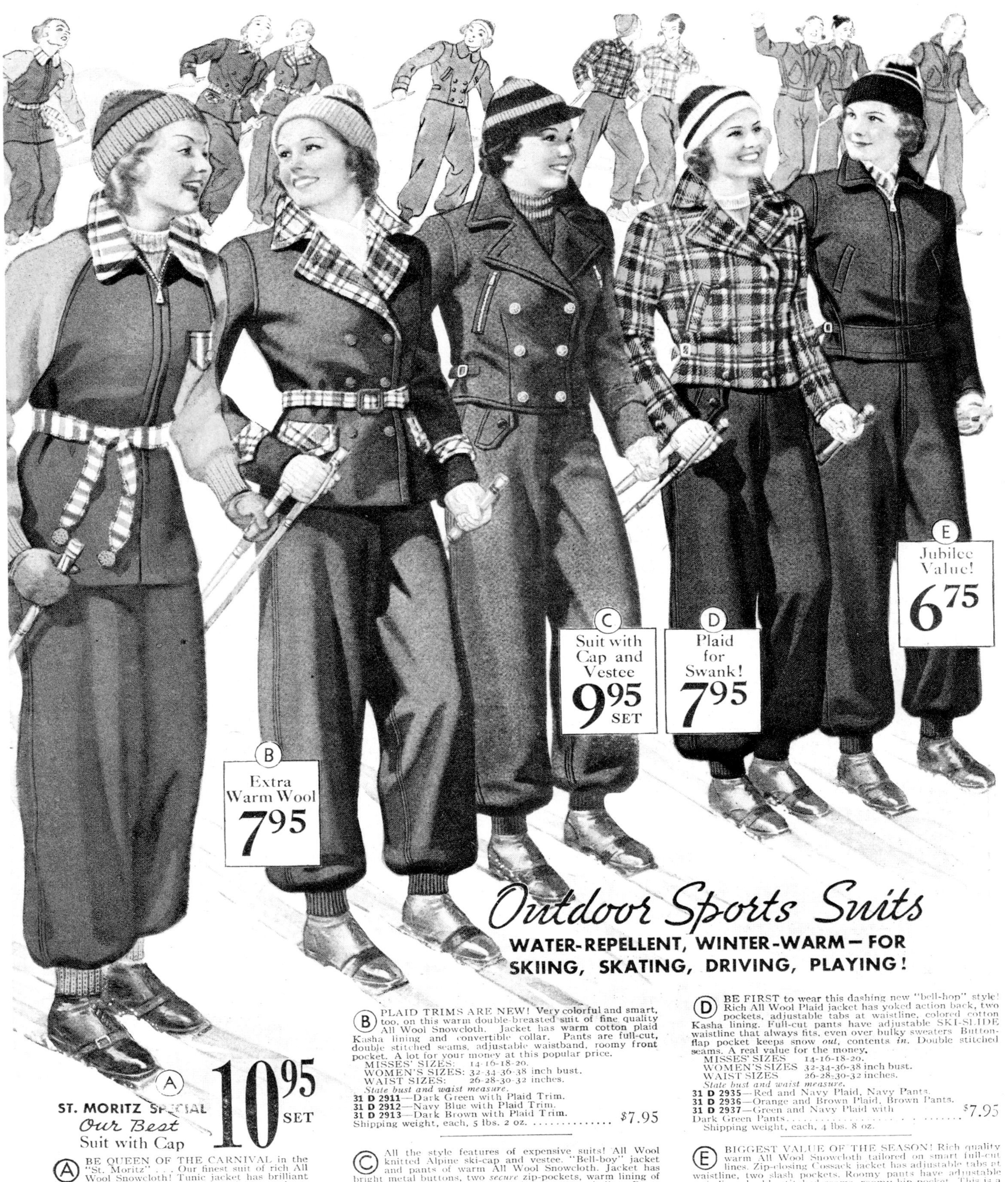

(A) BE QUEEN OF THE CARNIVAL in the "St. Moritz" . . . Our finest suit of rich All Wool Snowcloth! Tunic jacket has brilliant color contrast, Zip front, pleated button-down pocket. Pants are extra full-cut for comfort, with adjustable waistband. Double-stitched seams. Hockey cap to match fits all headsizes.

MISSES' SIZES. 14-16-18-20.
WOMEN'S SIZES 32-34-36-38 inch bust.
WAIST SIZES 26-28-30-32 ins.
State bust and waist measure.

31 D 2909—Royal Blue and Red Trim.
31 D 2910—Dk. Green with Brt. Green.
Shipping weight, 5 lbs. 8 oz. \$10.95 Set

(B) PLAID TRIMS ARE NEW! Very colorful and smart, too, on this warm double-breasted suit of fine quality All Wool Snowcloth. Jacket has warm cotton plaid Kasha lining and convertible collar. Pants are full-cut, double stitched seams, adjustable waistband, roomy front pocket. A lot for your money at this popular price.

MISSES' SIZES: 14-16-18-20.
WOMEN'S SIZES: 32-34-36-38 inch bust.
WAIST SIZES: 26-28-30-32 inches.
State bust and waist measure.

31 D 2911—Dark Green with Plaid Trim.
31 D 2912—Navy Blue with Plaid Trim.
31 D 2913—Dark Brown with Plaid Trim.
Shipping weight, each, 5 lbs. 2 oz. \$7.95

(C) All the style features of expensive suits! All Wool knitted Alpine ski-cap and vestee. "Bell-boy" jacket and pants of warm All Wool Snowcloth. Jacket has bright metal buttons, two *secure* zip-pockets, warm lining of colored cotton Kasha. Adjustable tabs at waistline. Pants have adjustable SKI-SLIDE waist fastening, button-flap pocket. Double stitched seams!

MISSES' SIZES: 14-16-18-20.
WOMEN'S SIZES. 32-34-36-38 inch bust.
WAIST SIZES: 26-28-30-32 inches.
State bust and waist measure.

31 D 2932—Dark Brown.
31 D 2933—Navy Blue.
31 D 2934—Dark Green.. .... Complete Set \$9.95
Shipping weight, each, 5 lbs. 7 oz.

(D) BE FIRST to wear this dashing new "bell-hop" style! Rich All Wool Plaid jacket has yoked action back, two pockets, adjustable tabs at waistline, colored cotton Kasha lining. Full-cut pants have adjustable SKI-SLIDE waistline that always fits, even over bulky sweaters Button-flap pocket keeps snow *out*, contents *in*. Double stitched seams. A real value for the money.

MISSES' SIZES 14-16-18-20.
WOMEN'S SIZES 32-34-36-38 inch bust.
WAIST SIZES 26-28-30-32 inches.
State bust and waist measure.

31 D 2935—Red and Navy Plaid, Navy Pants.
31 D 2936—Orange and Brown Plaid, Brown Pants.
31 D 2937—Green and Navy Plaid with Dark Green Pants.......................... \$7.95
Shipping weight, each, 4 lbs. 8 oz.

(E) BIGGEST VALUE OF THE SEASON! Rich quality warm All Wool Snowcloth tailored on smart full-cut lines. Zip-closing Cossack jacket has adjustable tabs at waistline, two slash pockets. Roomy pants have adjustable waistline, double-stitched seams, roomy hip pocket This is a real Jubilee value at this very low price for fine quality.

MISSES' SIZES 14-16-18-20.
WOMEN'S SIZES 32-34-36-38 inch bust
WAIST SIZES 26-28-30-32 inches.
State bust and waist measure.

31 D 2905—Navy Blue.
31 D 2906—Winetone.
31 D 2907—Dark Green.
31 D 2908—Dark Brown.
Shipping weight, 4 lbs. 8 oz.. .... \$6.75

All snow suits on this page are sent direct from New York to you .. but you pay postage only from our nearest Mail Order House. Ideal undies for winter sports. See page 215.

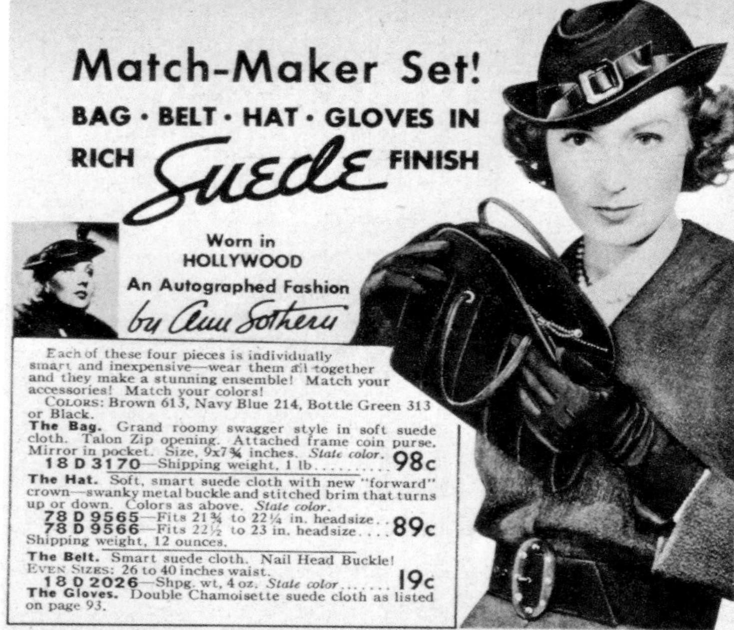

Match-Maker Set!

BAG · BELT · HAT · GLOVES IN RICH *Suede* FINISH

Worn in HOLLYWOOD
An Autographed Fashion
by Ann Sothern

Each of these four pieces is individually smart and inexpensive—wear them all together and they make a stunning ensemble! Match your accessories! Match your colors!

COLORS: Brown 613, Navy Blue 214, Bottle Green 313 or Black.

The Bag. Grand roomy swagger style in soft suede cloth. Talon Zip opening. Attached frame coin purse. Mirror in pocket. Size, 9x7¾ inches. *State color.*
18 D 3170—Shipping weight, 1 lb.......... **98c**

The Hat. Soft, smart suede cloth with new "forward" crown—swanky metal buckle and stitched brim that turns up or down. Colors as above. *State color.*
78 D 9565—Fits 21¾ to 22¼ in. headsize..
78 D 9566—Fits 22½ to 23 in. headsize.... **89c**
Shipping weight, 12 ounces.

The Belt. Smart suede cloth. Nail Head Buckle! EVEN SIZES: 26 to 40 inches waist.
18 D 2026—Shpg. wt., 4 oz. *State color*....... **19c**

The Gloves. Double Chamoisette suede cloth as listed on page 93.

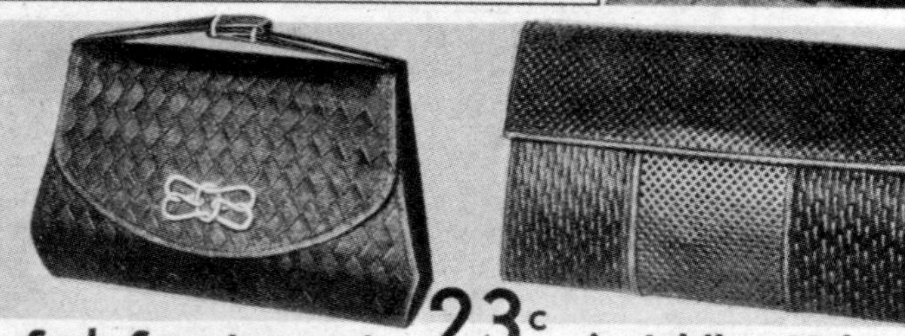

Such Smartness at 23c is Jubilee Value!

Convertible handle lengthens for use or fits flat against top! Good quality artificial leather. Size, 9x5¼ in. COLORS: Black or Brown 613. *State color.*

18 D 3171—Shipping weight, 8 oz...**23c**

Envelope type of artificial leather with cleverly contrasted graining. Gusseted sides. Mirror. Large size, 10x6¾ in. COLORS: Black, Brown 614, or Navy Blue. *State color.*

18 D 3172—Shipping weight, 9 oz....**23c**

Genuine Leather GRAND HAND BRAIDED "SOFTEES"!

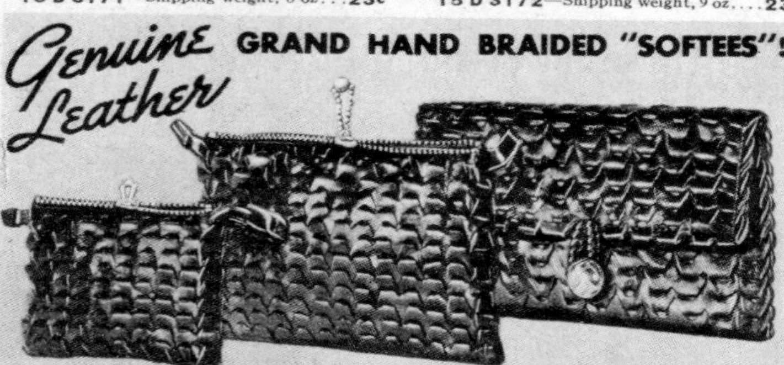

55c **Misses' Size**
Genuine Calf leather! Soft pliable braided style keeps its shape. Zip top. Rayon lining. Handy for women, too. Size, 6x4½ in. COLORS: Red 511, Navy Blue 214, or Brown 614. *State color.*
18 D 3173........**55c**
Shipping weight, 5 ounces.

89c **Women's Size**
Genuine braided Calfskin. Splendid value! Genuine Talon Zip top. Attached genuine leather coin purse. Mirror. Size, 8¼x6 in. COLORS: Black, Brown 613 or Navy Blue 214. *State color.*
18 D 3174..........**89c**
Shipping weight, 7 ounces.

59c **Envelope style.** Braided genuine Calf leather! Self-back strap. Sturdy, lasting artificial leather lining **adds** to wear. Double faced mirror. Size, 9½x5¾ inches. COLORS: Black or Brown 613. *State color.*
18 D 3175........**59c**
Shipping weight, 12 ounces.

Spanish Craft Bags

GENUINE STEERHIDE NEVER WEARS SHABBY!

Usually $4.00 Elsewhere

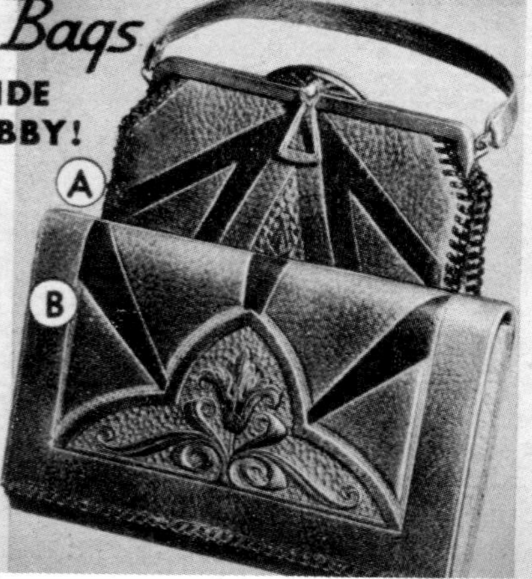

Ⓐ **18 D 3177**—Fine quality, scuffless Steerhide in popular handle style! Shaded, embossed design. Double hand laced edges of India Goat Leather. Gunmetal turn-lock top. Suedine lined. Leather backed mirror. Leather coin purse. Identification card. Shaded Brown only. Size 7½x6¼ inches. **$2.95**
Shipping weight, 15 oz.

Ⓑ **18 D 3178**—Fine Steerhide envelope with handsome deeply embossed design. Talon Zip pocket. Hand laced leather edge. Flap lined with suedine, the interior is rayon moire. Identification card in pocket. Size, 8¾x6 inches. Shaded Brown only. A typical Sears saving. Compare with usual $4.00 values. Shipping weight, 15 oz. **$2.95**

BELTS ARE SMARTER THAN EVER!

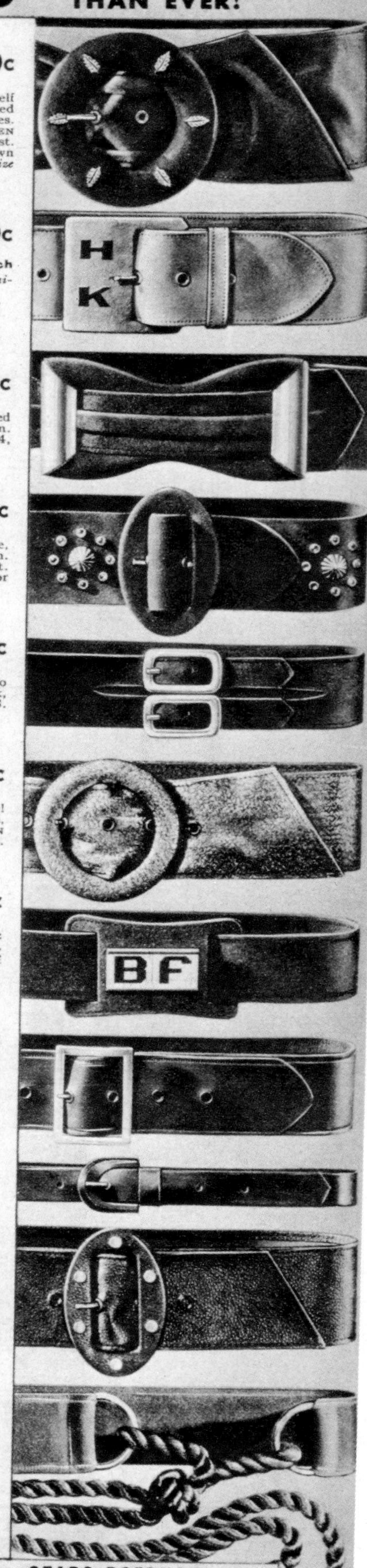

Wide and Metal Studded
18 D 2013—3 inches wide, and the wide belts are smartest this year! Stunning, crushable artificial Suede with a self covered buckle brightly studded with tiny metal autumn leaves. Sateen lined. Adjustable. EVEN SIZES: 26 to 40 inches waist. COLORS: Black, Red 514, Brown 613, Navy Blue 214. *State size and color.* **29c**
Shipping weight, 5 ounces.

Real Suede! Initialed
Fine quality suede leather. EVEN SIZES: 26 to 40 in. waist. COLORS: Black, British Tan 608, Navy Blue 214, Green 314. *State size and color. Print initials plainly.* **39c** 1½-inch
18 D 2015 2-in. width **49c**
18 D 2014 1½-in. width **39c**
Shipping weight, each, 4 ounces.

Suede! New Long Buckle!
18 D 2016—Stunning new Suede covered buckle with burnished metal ends. Fine suede leather belt, 2¼ in. wide, stitched edges. EVEN SIZES: 26 to 40 in. waist. COLORS: Black, Brown 614, or Wine 514. *State size, color.* **89c**
Shipping weight, 5 ounces.

Jewel Studded
18D2017—Studded with sparkling, multicolored stones in front and back! Unbelievably rich and beautiful. Artificial suede, self covered buckle. Width, 2 in. EVEN SIZES: 26 to 40 inch waist. COLORS: Black, Brown 613, or Red 511. *State size and color.* **29c**
Shipping weight, 4 ounces.

Suede! Twin Metal Buckles!
18 D 2018—"Saddle Sport Style." Genuine suede leather, stitched edges. Fine quality. Width, 1½ in. EVEN SIZES: 26 to 40 in. waist. COLORS: Black, Brown 613, or British Tan 608. *State size and color.* **49c**
Shipping weight, 3 ounces.

Glittering Metal Cloth
18 D 2019—Lasting, non-cracking gold-color finish on embossed artificial leather! Adds dollars to the richness of your dress! 2½ in. wide with self covered buckle, moire lining. Gold color only. EVEN SIZES: 26 to 40 in. waist. *State size.* **39c**
Shipping weight, 4 ounces.

Suedine! Initialed!
18 D 2020—Stunning gold colored metal plaque buckle with *your* initials. Suede-like cloth belt. 1½ in. wide. EVEN SIZES: 26 to 40 in. waist. COLORS: Black, Brown 613, Navy Blue 214, Wine 514. *State color. All letters except X and Q. Print initials.* **25c**
Shipping weight, 4 ounces.

Real Leather
COLORS: Black, Red 511, Brown 614, or Navy Blue 214. EVEN SIZES: 26 to 40 in. *State size, color.* Shpg. wt., each, 4 oz. **15c** 1 inch
Calf Finish
18 D 2004—1 in.........**15c**
18 D 2006—1¾ in.......**29c**
Suede Finish
18 D 2023—1¾ in.......**29c**

Tubular! ¾ Inches Wide! →
18 D 2024—Artificial leather. Composition buckle. EVEN SIZES: 26 to 40 in. waist. COLORS: Black, Brown 613 or British Tan 608. *State size and color.* **10c**
Shipping weight, 3 ounces.

Nail Heads on Buckle! →
Artificial leather. Turned edges! 2 inches wide. Choice of 2 finishes! EVEN SIZES: 26 to 40 in. waist. COLORS: Black, Brown 613, Bottle Green 313, Navy 214. *State size, color.* **19c** each
18 D 2025—Pin Grain.....**19c**
18 D 2026—Suede Finish...**19c**
Shipping weight, each, 4 ounces.

Graceful Cord Belt
18 D 2027—Thick, lustrous rayon cords with full graceful tassels hang from metal loops and tie this adjustable artificial suede belt. A semi-dress belt that brightens up your outfit! 1½ inches wide. EVEN SIZES: 26 to 40 inches waist. COLORS: Red 511, Brown 614, Navy Blue 214. *State color and size.* **23c**
Shipping weight, 4 ounces.

Color-numbers refer to Sears "COLOR-GRAPH" facing first Pink Index Page.

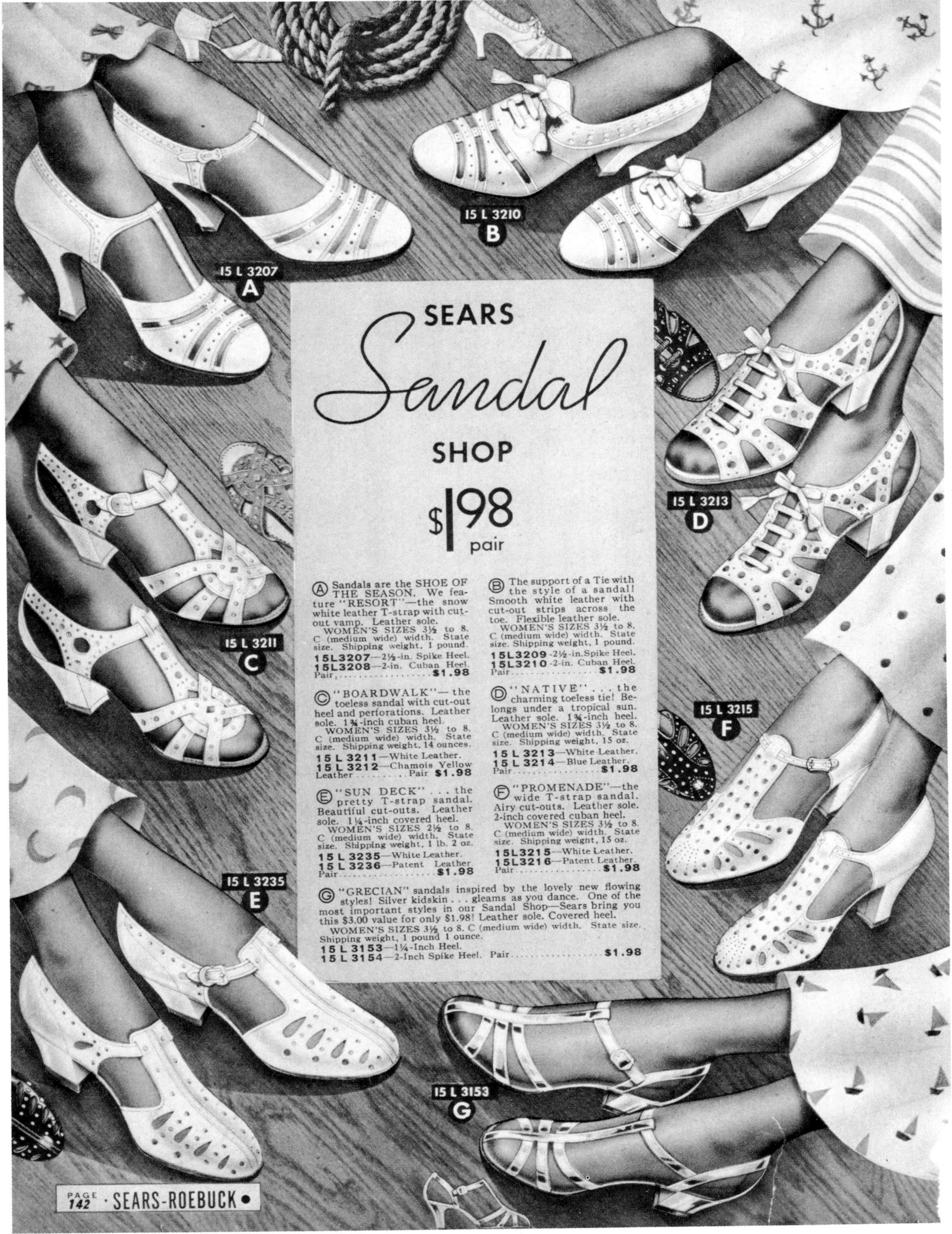
15 L 3207
A
15 L 3210
B
15 L 3211
C
15 L 3213
D
15 L 3235
E
15 L 3215
F
15 L 3153
G
SEARS
Sandal
SHOP
$1.98 pair
(A) Sandals are the SHOE OF THE SEASON. We feature "RESORT"—the snow white leather T-strap with cut-out vamp. Leather sole.
WOMEN'S SIZES 3½ to 8. C (medium wide) width. State size. Shipping weight, 1 pound.
15L3207—2½-in. Spike Heel.
15L3208—2-in. Cuban Heel.
Pair. $1.98
(B) The support of a Tie with the style of a sandal! Smooth white leather with cut-out strips across the toe. Flexible leather sole.
WOMEN'S SIZES 3½ to 8. C (medium wide) width. State size. Shipping weight, 1 pound.
15L3209-2½-in. Spike Heel.
15L3210-2-in. Cuban Heel.
Pair. $1.98
(C) "BOARDWALK"—the toeless sandal with cut-out heel and perforations. Leather sole. 1¾-inch cuban heel.
WOMEN'S SIZES 3½ to 8. C (medium wide) width. State size. Shipping weight, 14 ounces.
15 L 3211—White Leather.
15 L 3212—Chamois Yellow Leather. . . . . . Pair $1.98
(D) "NATIVE" . . . the charming toeless tie! Belongs under a tropical sun. Leather sole. 1¾-inch heel.
WOMEN'S SIZES 3½ to 8. C (medium wide) width. State size. Shipping weight, 15 oz.
15 L 3213—White Leather.
15 L 3214—Blue Leather.
Pair. $1.98
(E) "SUN DECK" . . . the pretty T-strap sandal. Beautiful cut-outs. Leather sole. 1¼-inch covered heel.
WOMEN'S SIZES 2½ to 8. C (medium wide) width. State size. Shipping weight, 1 lb. 2 oz.
15 L 3235—White Leather.
15 L 3236—Patent Leather
Pair. $1.98
(F) "PROMENADE"—the wide T-strap sandal. Airy cut-outs. Leather sole. 2-inch covered cuban heel.
WOMEN'S SIZES 3½ to 8. C (medium wide) width. State size. Shipping weight, 15 oz.
15L3215—White Leather.
15L3216—Patent Leather.
Pair. $1.98
(G) "GRECIAN" sandals inspired by the lovely new flowing styles! Silver kidskin . . . gleams as you dance. One of the most important styles in our Sandal Shop—Sears bring you this $3.00 value for only $1.98! Leather sole. Covered heel.
WOMEN'S SIZES 3½ to 8. C (medium wide) width. State size. Shipping weight, 1 pound 1 ounce.
15 L 3153—1¼-Inch Heel.
15 L 3154—2-Inch Spike Heel. Pair. $1.98
PAGE 142 · SEARS-ROEBUCK

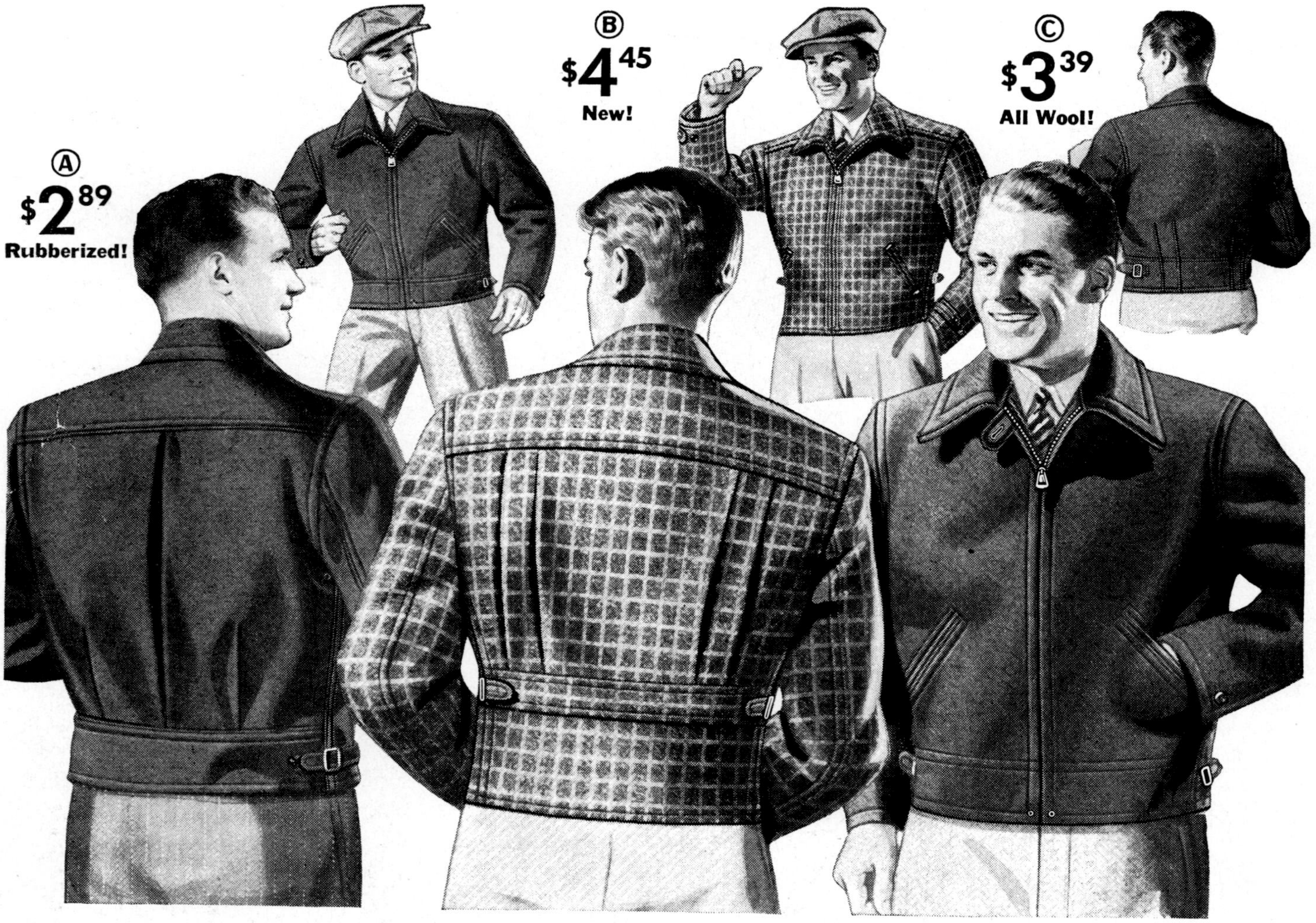

Ⓐ $2.89 Rubberized!

Ⓑ $4.45 New!

Ⓒ $3.39 All Wool!

EVERYBODY WEARS 'EM EVERYWHERE

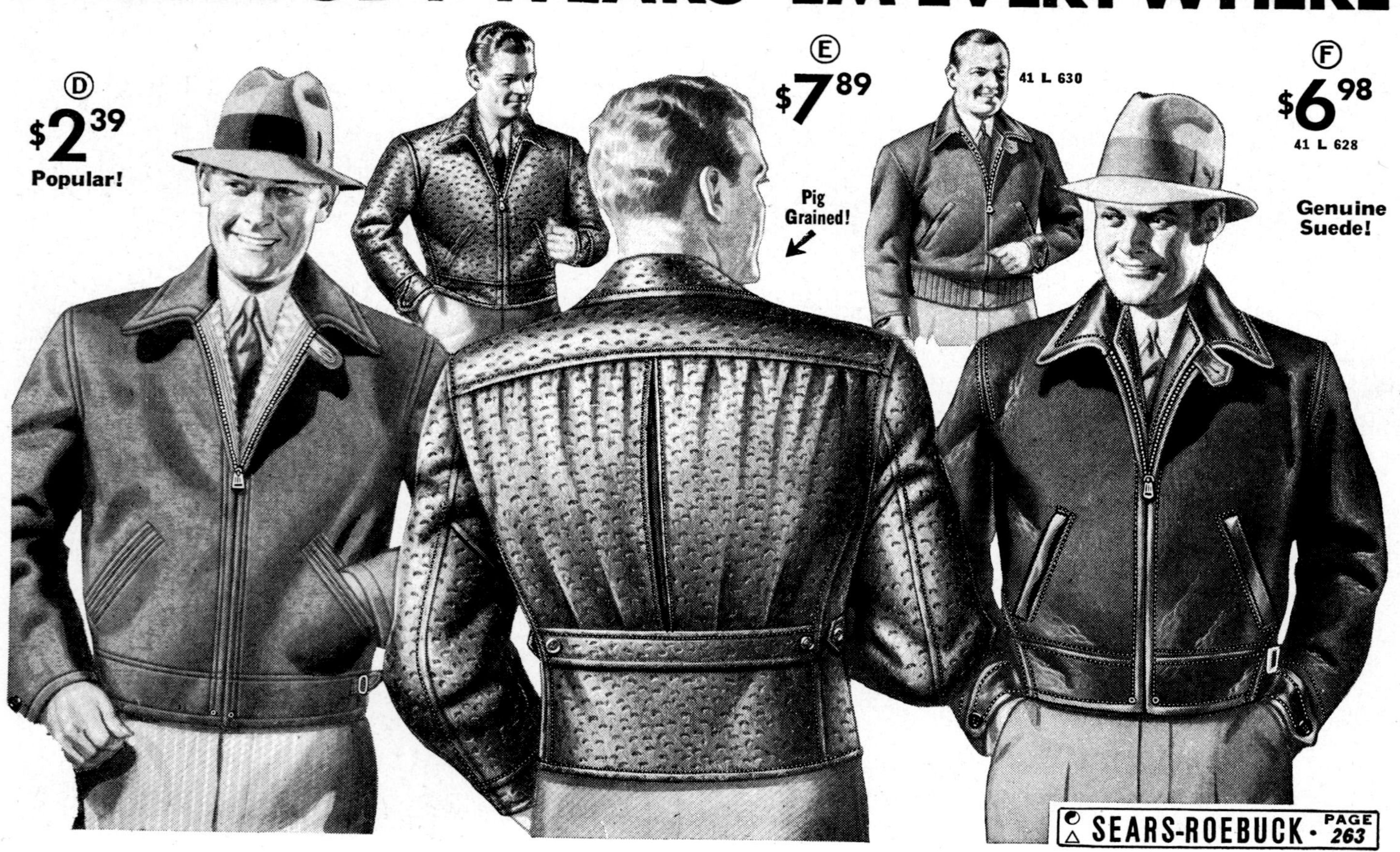

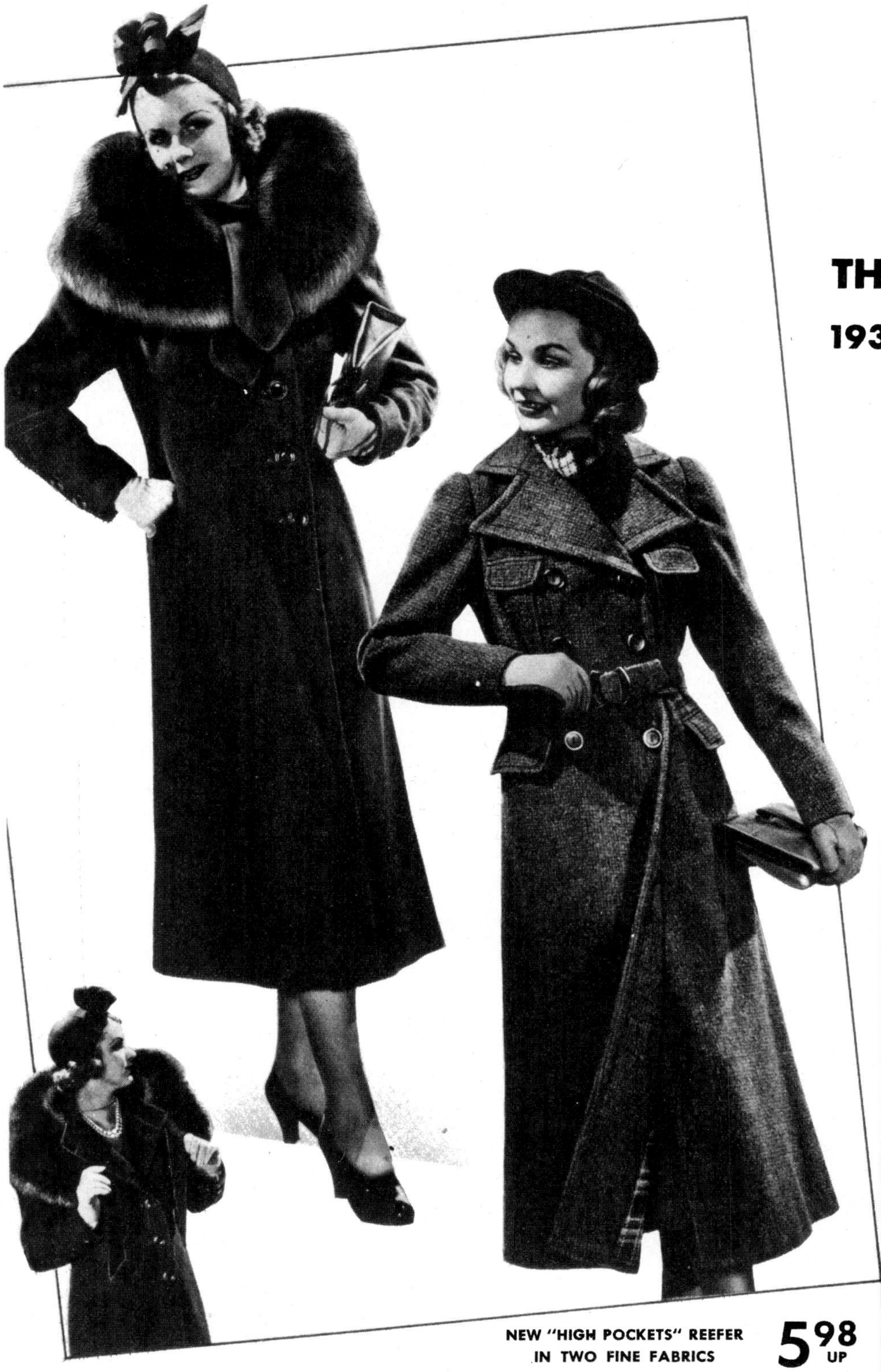

Style

THE MOST DRAMATIC

1938's Favorite Fashions

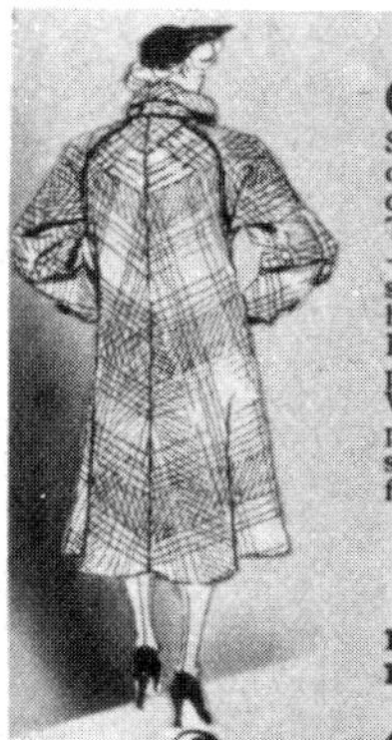

Ⓐ THE BUY OF THE YEAR! A gallant young Swagger coat in one of the glorious new SHADOW PLAID coatings that are all the rage! Three-fourths fine wool! Thicker—warmer—with richer, softer colorings than you would believe possible at this price! Full swinging flare. Slash pockets. Big novelty buttons. Warmly lined with colorful plaid cotton . . . sateen yoke and sleeves. Just try to equal this for less than $8.00!

SIZES: 12-14-16-18-20.
BUST: 30-32-34-36-38 in.
LENGTHS: 45-46-46-47-47 in.
State bust measure.

17 F 2195—Dark Brown.
17 F 2196—Lt. Navy Blue.

Shipping weight, 4 lbs. 14 oz. $6.98

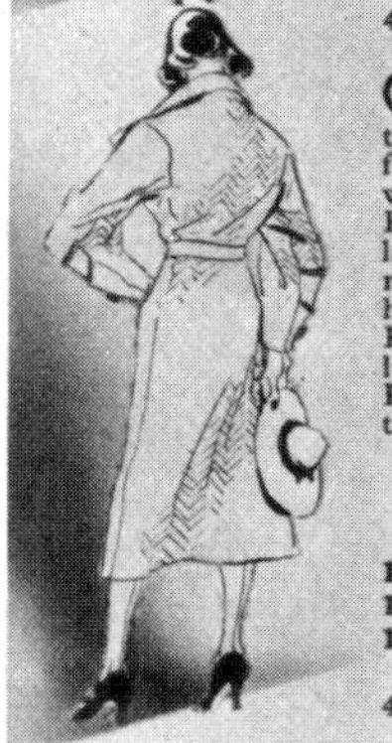

Ⓑ A thrilling low price—on a really GOOD coat! From the minute you put it on, and for many seasons after, you'll wear it with proud satisfaction! Has a stunning wide collar, lavishly stitched. Winter-weight novelty Wool Crepe coating, half wool for warmth, half Rayon and Cotton for a more luxurious look, longer wear. Rayon Taffeta lining, with toasty-warm interlining.

SIZES: 14-16-18-20-22.
BUST: 32-34-36-38-40 in.
LENGTHS: 47-48-49-49-49 in.
State bust measure.

17 F 2200—Navy Blue.
17 F 2201—Black.
17 F 2202—Dark Brown *613*.

Shipping weight, 4 lbs. 9 oz. $5.98

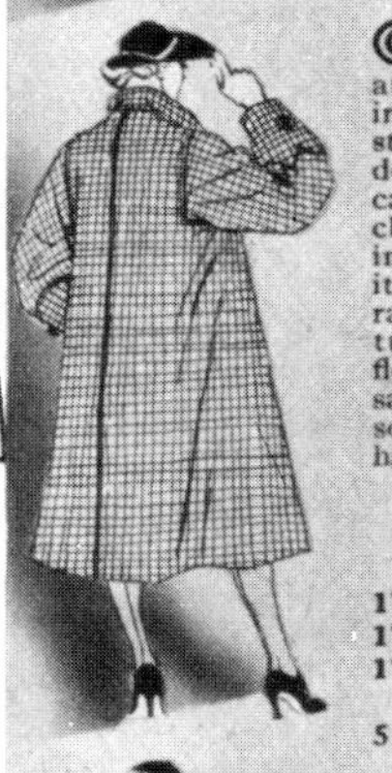

Ⓒ WHAT A BUY! A dashing *plaid lined* Swagger coat . . . at a price that puts a big saving into your pocket! The latest style! Full length slot seam down the back, wide lapels you can button up snug under your chin! Rich novelty fleecy coating, three-fourths wool to make it good and warm, balance rayon and cotton for rich texture and firm weave. Soft, warm fleecy Plaid Cotton lining, with sateen yoke and sleeve linings so it will slide on easily. Yoke has *extra* interlining.

SIZES: 14-16-18-20-22.
BUST: 32-34-36-38-40 in.
LENGTHS: 45-45-46-47-47 in.
State bust measure.

17 F 2205—Navy Blue.
17 F 2206—Oxford Gray.
17 F 2207—Winetone.

Shipping weight, 5 lbs. 6 oz. $6.98

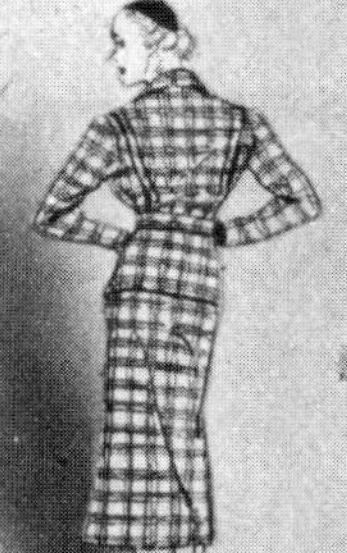

Ⓓ OF COURSE you must have a tailored suit this season! Here's a value you can't beat in a rich, subdued Plaid Tweed! It has 16% good warm wool, balance rayon for that unusual brilliance of texture. Unlined jacket has tucked back with half-belt—smart with other skirts too. Kick-pleated skirt. Wear it all Winter under your coat!

SIZES: 12-14-16-18-20.
BUST: 30-32-34-36-38 in.
State bust measure.

17 F 2480—Medium Gray.
17 F 2481—Medium Brown.

Shipping weight, 3 lbs. 7 oz. $3.98

BIG FUR COLLAR BUTTONS ON AND OFF! 7.98

Just like having *two* coats . . . whisk off that button-on collar of fluffy genuine Manchurian Wolf-dyed Dog Fur and you have a handsome tailored coat you can wear all Fall and next Spring too! The fabric is luxuriously soft Novelty Crepe Coating that's two-fifths fine Wool . . . and is warm and durable. A lot of flattering swank in those slim young princess lines, that new softly flaring skirt! Lustrous Rayon Taffeta lining; warm interlining. A low price for a big Value!

SIZES: 14-16-18-20.
BUST: 32-34-36-38 inches.
LENGTHS: 47-47-48-48 inches. *State bust measure.*

17 F 2180—Black with Black Fur.
17 F 2181—Navy Blue with Black Fur.
17 F 2182—Winetone *514* with Black Fur.

Shipping weight, 6 lbs. 6 oz.

NEW "HIGH POCKETS" REEFER IN TWO FINE FABRICS 5.98 UP

Paris does love pockets this season! Places them high and handsome on the sportiest reefer of the year . . . which we've copied for you in extra-warm, extra-thick Checked Fleece Coating! It's three-fifths warm, sturdy Wool . . . shock-proof against icy winds. Fleecy cotton plaid lining, with deep sateen yoke and sleeve linings. A REAL BARGAIN!

SIZES: 14-16-18-20-22.
BUST: 32-34-36-38-40 inches.
LENGTHS: 46-47-47-48-48 inches. *State bust measure.*

17 F 2185—Oakleaf Brown.
17 F 2186—Oxford Gray.
17 F 2187—Heather Green. $7.98

SAME STYLE IN STUNNING HERRINGBONE TWEED, FOUR-FIFTHS WARM, STURDY WOOL

17 F 2190—Dark Brown.
17 F 2191—Dark Green.
17 F 2192—Navy Blue. $5.98

Shipping weight, each, 5 lbs. 6 oz.

These coats are sent from New York direct to you. You pay postage only from our nearest Mail Order House. Numbers after color names refer to Sears COLOR-GRAPH facing first index page in back of book.

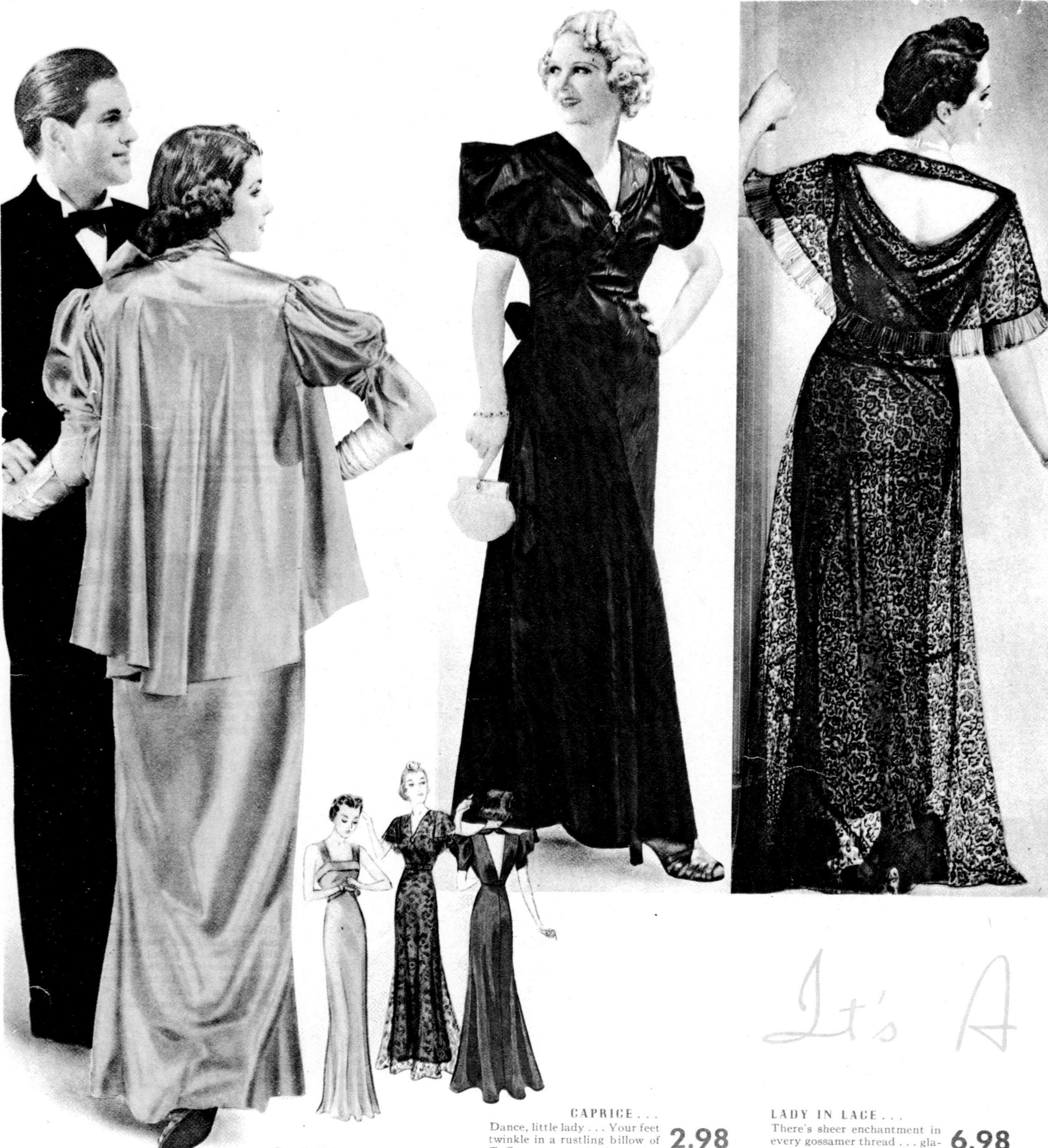

See Full Back View of this Dress on Page 133

EVENING STAR . . . Just imagine how glamorous you'll look! It's really glorious Satin, the heavy, luxurious, softly gleaming quality, woven of genuine Celanese yarns. Puff-sleeved jacket ties under your chin with a big flattering bow. Dress has the new square cut top, softened with graceful bias folds. Bias-cut, flaring skirt. Nevagape adjustable placket smooths your waistline. (See illustration on page 12). Grand value at this price! **5.98**

SIZES: 14, 16, 18, 20, to fit bust 32, 34, 36, 38 in. Lengths, 59 inches. *See size scale on Page 8. State bust measure and color.*

COLORS: American Beauty Rose, Royal Blue *218*, Black or White.

31 F 4045 . . . . Shipping weight, 1 lb. 14 oz.

CAPRICE . . .
Dance, little lady . . . Your feet twinkle in a rustling billow of Taffeta, your waist is molded and slim, there's something about those angel-wing sleeves that goes straight to a man's heart. No one dreams the cost was so little! The rich All Rayon Moire Taffeta is very expensive-looking; fine shirring gives you that lovely bustline. The sash tied in back and the Nevagape placket (see illustration on Page 12) assure a trim, perfect fit. **2.98**

JUNIOR SIZES: 13 to 19, MISSES' SIZES: 12 to 20. Lengths, about 55 inches. *See size scale on Page 8. State bust measure and color.*

COLORS: Royal Blue *218*, Peacock Blue *320*, Cocktail Red *508* or Black.

31 F 4050 . . . . Shipping weight, 1 lb. 10 oz.

LADY IN LACE . . .
There's sheer enchantment in every gossamer thread . . . glamour and *chic* in every ripple of that full, fluttering skirt! Exquisitely made of our finest quality, beautifully patterned All Rayon Lace. Matching slip of gleaming Rayon Taffeta. Draped capelet edged with finely pleated net, cowled in back to give you a graceful shoulder line. Smooth Nevagape placket (see Page 12). A real $10.95 value! **6.98**

SIZES: 34, 36, 38, 40, 42, 44 inches bust measure. Lengths, about 59 inches. *State bust measure and color.*

COLORS: Ruby Wine *514*, Black or Royal Blue *218*.

31 F 4055 . . . . Shipping weight, 1 lb. 12 oz.

The dresses on this page shipped from New York to you. You pay postage only from our nearest Mail Order House.
Numbers after color names refer to Sears Color-Graph facing first index page in back of book.

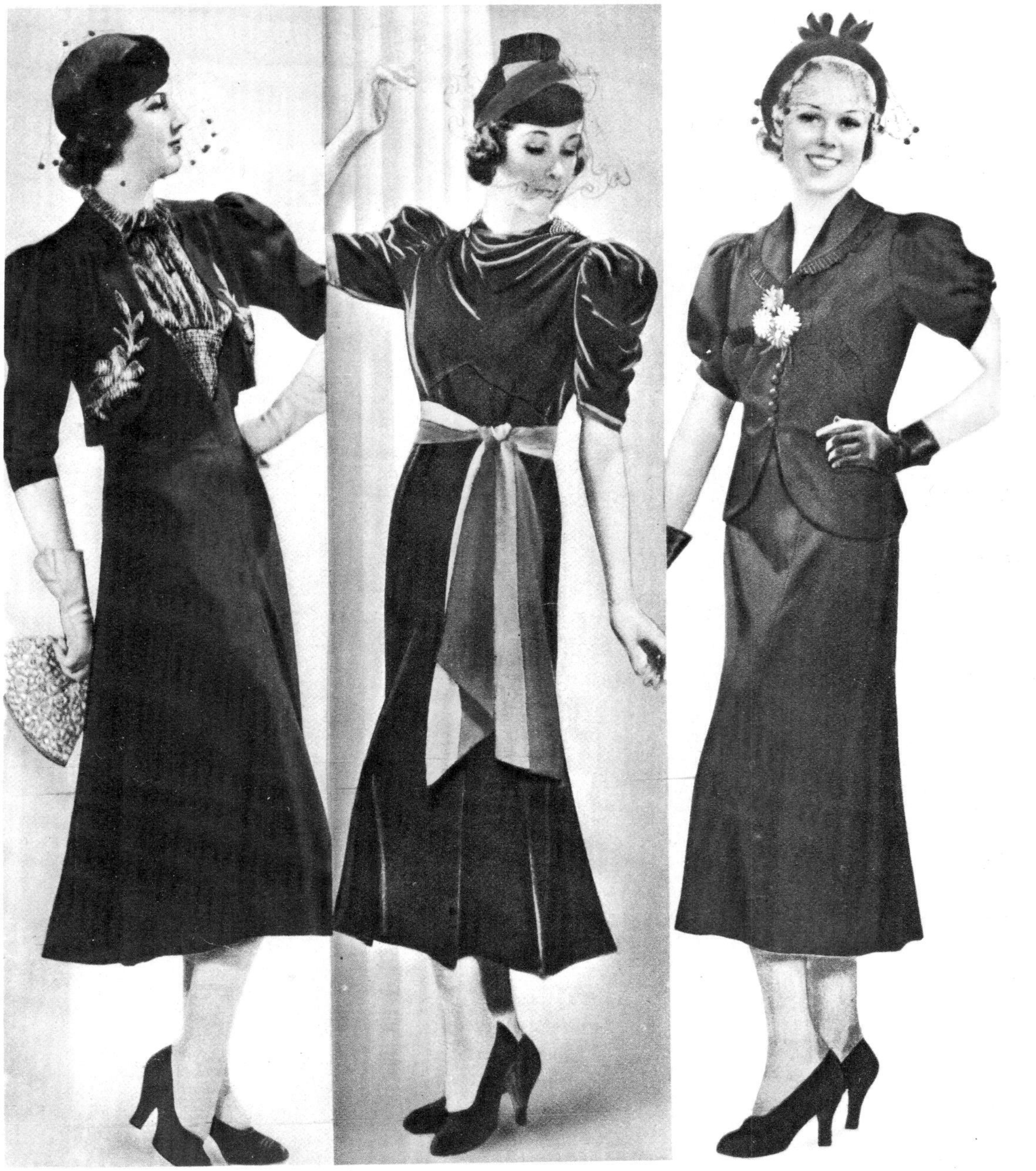

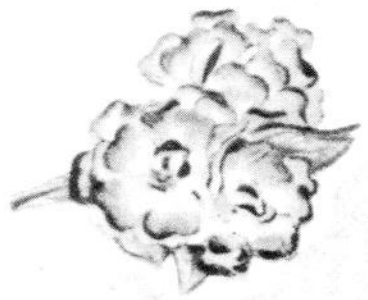

GATHER YE ROSES—these three are Chiffon; they cover at least 7 x 9 inches of your evening dress. Red only.
18 F 4334—Shipping weight, 5 ounces **49c**

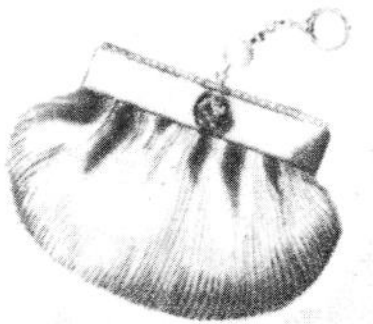

MAD MONEY "stays put" in this pleated Acetate Crepe bag with "jools" on top and the right fixin's inside. Gold, White or Black. *State color.*
18 F 3324—Shipping weight, 10 ounces **94c**

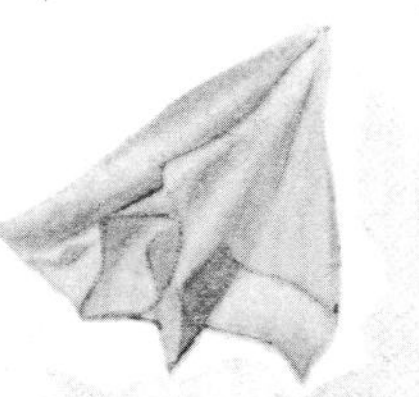

THIS CHIFFON HANKIE is 19 inches square but wins attention many yards away. Comes in Red, Royal Blue, Kelly Green. *State color.*
18 F 4337—Shipping weight, 5 ounces **25c**

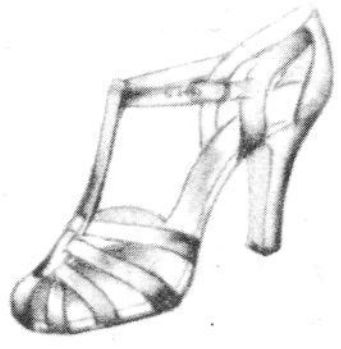

Gleaming silver fabric . . . looks just like silver kid but is softer, easier to wear. The soles are durable leather.
WOMEN'S SIZES: 2½ to 8. C (medium wide) width. *State size.* Shpg. wt., 1 lb. 2 oz.
15 F 2185—2½-in. Spike Heel. Pair **$1.98**

Gay Life

ENJOY IT IN STYLE

LUXURY . . .

5.98

A world of chic . . . Gay young bolero effect. Glittering Metal Lame, the really expensive quality, makes that flattering vestee and the lovely appliqued flowers. The body of the dress is our very finest Satin-back Crepe Amigo of Celanese . . . "*Aqua-Sec*" Rain-Away finish resists spotting. Graceful flared skirt. Nevagape placket (see Page 12).

SIZES: 14 to 20, to fit bust 32 to 38 inches. *See size scale on Page 8. State bust measure and color.*

COLORS: Royal Blue *218* with Wine, Black with Royal Blue or Peacock Blue *320* with Gold.
31 F 4060 . . . . . . Shpg. wt., 1 lb., 14 oz.

RHYTHM IN VELVET . . .

7.98

That new gored skirt fairly flutters when she walks, floats when she dances . . . and those big jeweled butterflies (like the ones Schiaparelli uses in Paris) put a devastating sparkle in her eye. And such fabric! Luxurious, shimmering Transparent Velvet, silk-backed with rich Rayon pile. Two-tone girdle and sleeve bandings are of lovely sheer Chiffon. Intricately shirred sleeves. Nevagape placket (see Page 12).

SIZES: 14 to 20, to fit bust 32 to 38 inches. *See size scale on Page 8. State bust measure and color.*

COLORS: Ruby Wine *514* or Black.
31 F 4065 . . . . . . Shpg. wt., 1 lb., 12 oz.

INTRIGUE . . .

3.74

Two-piece style in our best quality Celanese Taffeta . . . crisp and heavy, the kind that "swishes" as you walk! Knife pleating edges that smart new collar and the adorable pockets . . . a nosegay of field flowers for color accent. Covered ball buttons and loops. Skirt flared front and back. Exact copy of a $7.95 dress . . . same fine quality fabric, same careful finish. Shop at Sears and save!

MISSES' SIZES: 12 to 20, and JUNIOR SIZES: 13 to 19. *See size scale on Page 8. State bust measure and color.*

COLORS: Forest Green *313*, Navy Blue or Brown *623*.
31 F 4070 . . . . Shpg. wt., 1 lb., 10 oz.

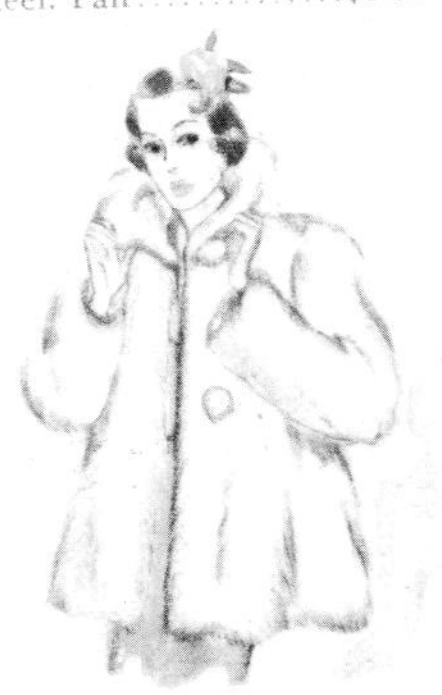

Genuine White Coney Fur Wrap . . . Smart with daytime or evening dresses. Rayon Taffeta lined and interlined. SIZES to fit bust 32, 34, 36, 38 in. Length, 24 in. *State bust.*
Shipping weight, 3 pounds.
17 F 2559—White . . . **$13.95**

The Dresses on this page shipped from New York City direct to you. You pay postage only from our nearest Mail Order House. Numbers after color names refer to Sears Color-Graph facing first index page in back of book.

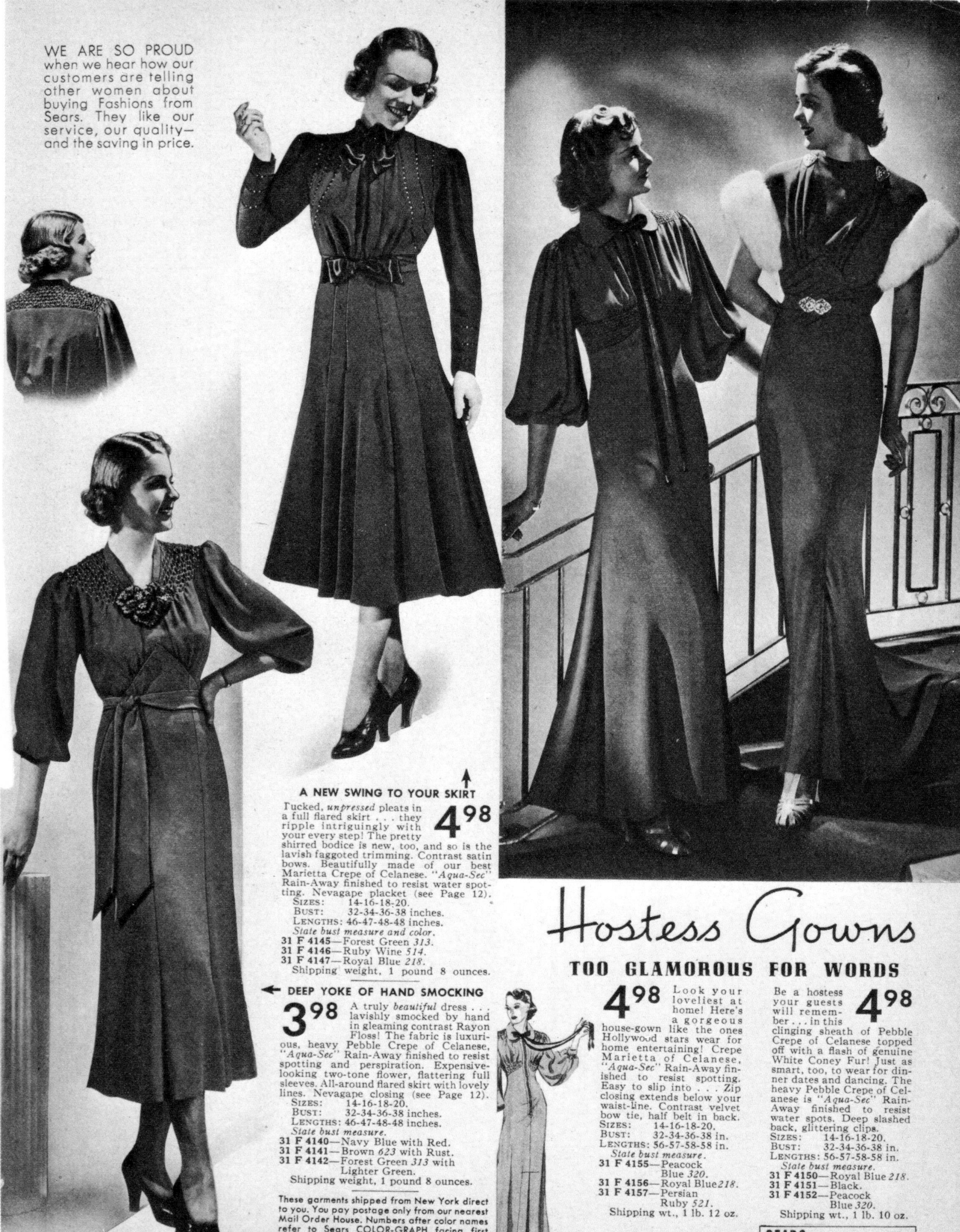

WE ARE SO PROUD when we hear how our customers are telling other women about buying Fashions from Sears. They like our service, our quality—and the saving in price.

A NEW SWING TO YOUR SKIRT

Tucked, *unpressed* pleats in a full flared skirt . . . they ripple intriguingly with your every step! The pretty shirred bodice is new, too, and so is the lavish faggoted trimming. Contrast satin bows. Beautifully made of our best Marietta Crepe of Celanese. "*Aqua-Sec*" Rain-Away finished to resist water spotting. Nevagape placket (see Page 12). **4.98**

SIZES: 14-16-18-20.
BUST: 32-34-36-38 inches.
LENGTHS: 46-47-48-48 inches.
State bust measure and color.
31 F 4145—Forest Green *313.*
31 F 4146—Ruby Wine *514.*
31 F 4147—Royal Blue *218.*
Shipping weight, 1 pound 8 ounces.

DEEP YOKE OF HAND SMOCKING

3.98 A truly *beautiful* dress . . . lavishly smocked by hand in gleaming contrast Rayon Floss! The fabric is luxurious, heavy Pebble Crepe of Celanese, "*Aqua-Sec*" Rain-Away finished to resist spotting and perspiration. Expensive-looking two-tone flower, flattering full sleeves. All-around flared skirt with lovely lines. Nevagape closing (see Page 12).

SIZES: 14-16-18-20.
BUST: 32-34-36-38 inches.
LENGTHS: 46-47-48-48 inches.
State bust measure.
31 F 4140—Navy Blue with Red.
31 F 4141—Brown *623* with Rust.
31 F 4142—Forest Green *313* with Lighter Green.
Shipping weight, 1 pound 8 ounces.

These garments shipped from New York direct to you. You pay postage only from our nearest Mail Order House. Numbers after color names refer to Sears COLOR-GRAPH facing first index page in back of book.

Hostess Gowns

TOO GLAMOROUS FOR WORDS

4.98 Look your loveliest at home! Here's a gorgeous house-gown like the ones Hollywood stars wear for home entertaining! Crepe Marietta of Celanese, "*Aqua-Sec*" Rain-Away finished to resist spotting. Easy to slip into . . . Zip closing extends below your waist-line. Contrast velvet bow tie, half belt in back.

SIZES: 14-16-18-20.
BUST: 32-34-36-38 in.
LENGTHS: 56-57-58-58 in.
State bust measure.
31 F 4155—Peacock Blue *320.*
31 F 4156—Royal Blue *218.*
31 F 4157—Persian Ruby *521.*
Shipping wt., 1 lb. 12 oz.

Be a hostess your guests will remember . . . in this clinging sheath of Pebble Crepe of Celanese topped off with a flash of genuine White Coney Fur! Just as smart, too, to wear for dinner dates and dancing. The heavy Pebble Crepe of Celanese is "*Aqua-Sec*" Rain-Away finished to resist water spots. Deep slashed back, glittering clips. **4.98**

SIZES: 14-16-18-20.
BUST: 32-34-36-38 in.
LENGTHS: 56-57-58-58 in.
State bust measure.
31 F 4150—Royal Blue *218.*
31 F 4151—Black.
31 F 4152—Peacock Blue *320.*
Shipping wt., 1 lb. 10 oz.

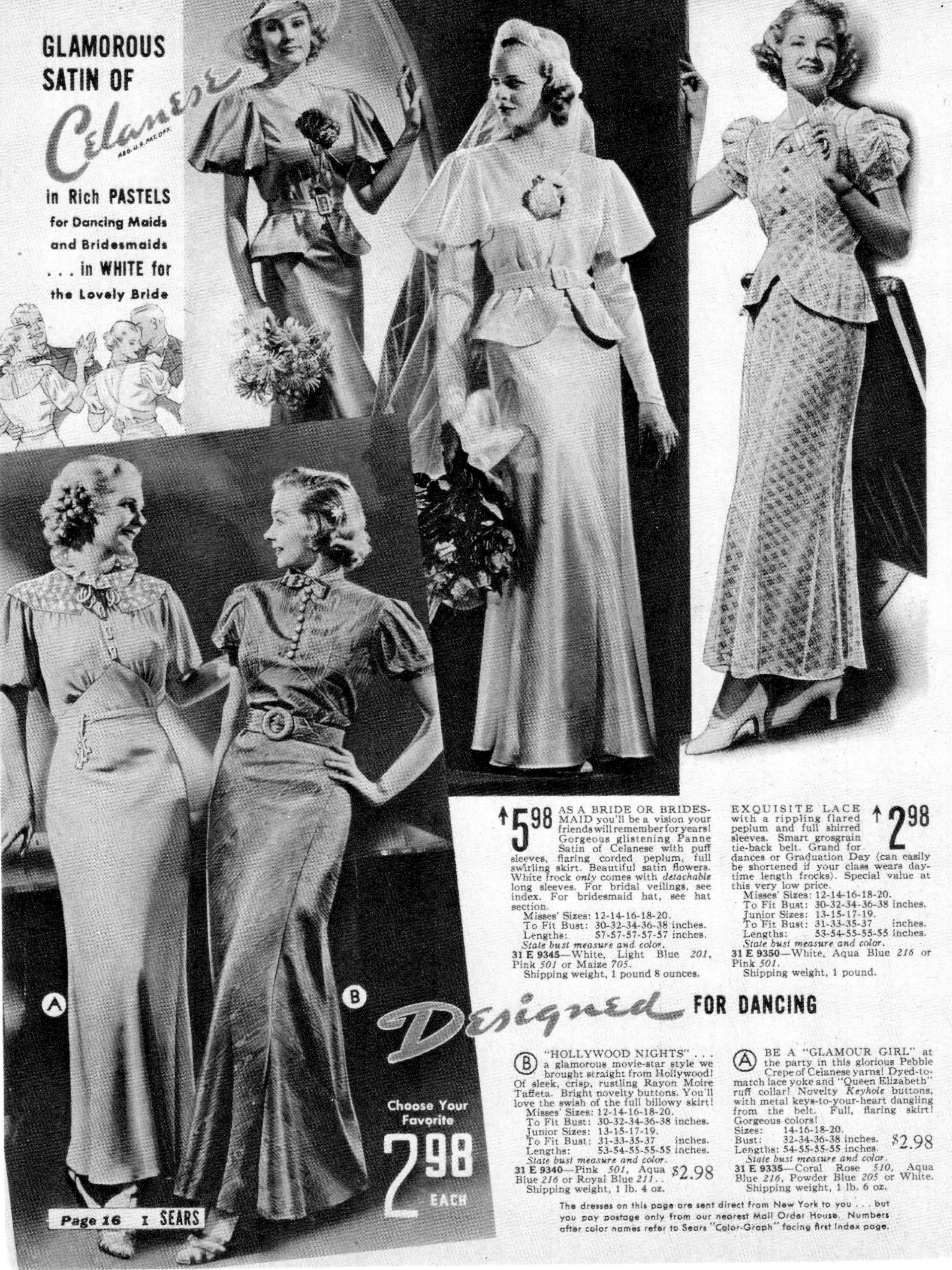
GLAMOROUS SATIN OF
Celanese
in Rich PASTELS
for Dancing Maids
and Bridesmaids
. . . in WHITE for
the Lovely Bride
5.98
AS A BRIDE OR BRIDESMAID you'll be a vision your friends will remember for years! Gorgeous glistening Panne Satin of Celanese with puff sleeves, flaring corded peplum, full swirling skirt. Beautiful satin flowers. White frock only comes with detachable long sleeves. For bridal veilings, see index. For bridesmaid hat, see hat section.
Misses' Sizes: 12-14-16-18-20.
To Fit Bust: 30-32-34-36-38 inches.
Lengths: 57-57-57-57-57 inches.
State bust measure and color.
31 E 9345—White, Light Blue 201, Pink 501 or Maize 705.
Shipping weight, 1 pound 8 ounces.
EXQUISITE LACE with a rippling flared peplum and full shirred sleeves. Smart grosgrain tie-back belt. Grand for dances or Graduation Day (can easily be shortened if your class wears daytime length frocks). Special value at this very low price.
Misses' Sizes: 12-14-16-18-20.
To Fit Bust: 30-32-34-36-38 inches.
Junior Sizes: 13-15-17-19.
To Fit Bust: 31-33-35-37 inches.
Lengths: 53-54-55-55-55 inches.
State bust measure and color.
31 E 9350—White, Aqua Blue 216 or Pink 501.
Shipping weight, 1 pound.
2.98
Designed FOR DANCING
(B) "HOLLYWOOD NIGHTS" . . . a glamorous movie-star style we brought straight from Hollywood! Of sleek, crisp, rustling Rayon Moire Taffeta. Bright novelty buttons. You'll love the swish of the full billowy skirt!
Misses' Sizes: 12-14-16-18-20.
To Fit Bust: 30-32-34-36-38 inches.
Junior Sizes: 13-15-17-19.
To Fit Bust: 31-33-35-37 inches.
Lengths: 53-54-55-55-55 inches.
State bust measure and color.
31 E 9340—Pink 501, Aqua Blue 216 or Royal Blue 211. . $2.98
Shipping weight, 1 lb. 4 oz.
(A) BE A "GLAMOUR GIRL" at the party in this glorious Pebble Crepe of Celanese yarns! Dyed-to-match lace yoke and "Queen Elizabeth" ruff collar! Novelty Keyhole buttons, with metal keys-to-your-heart dangling from the belt. Full, flaring skirt! Gorgeous colors!
Sizes: 14-16-18-20.
Bust: 32-34-36-38 inches.
Lengths: 54-55-55-55 inches. $2.98
State bust measure and color.
31 E 9335—Coral Rose 510, Aqua Blue 216, Powder Blue 205 or White.
Shipping weight, 1 lb. 6 oz.
Choose Your Favorite
2.98 EACH
Page 16 x SEARS
The dresses on this page are sent direct from New York to you . . . but you pay postage only from our nearest Mail Order House. Numbers after color names refer to Sears "Color-Graph" facing first Index page.

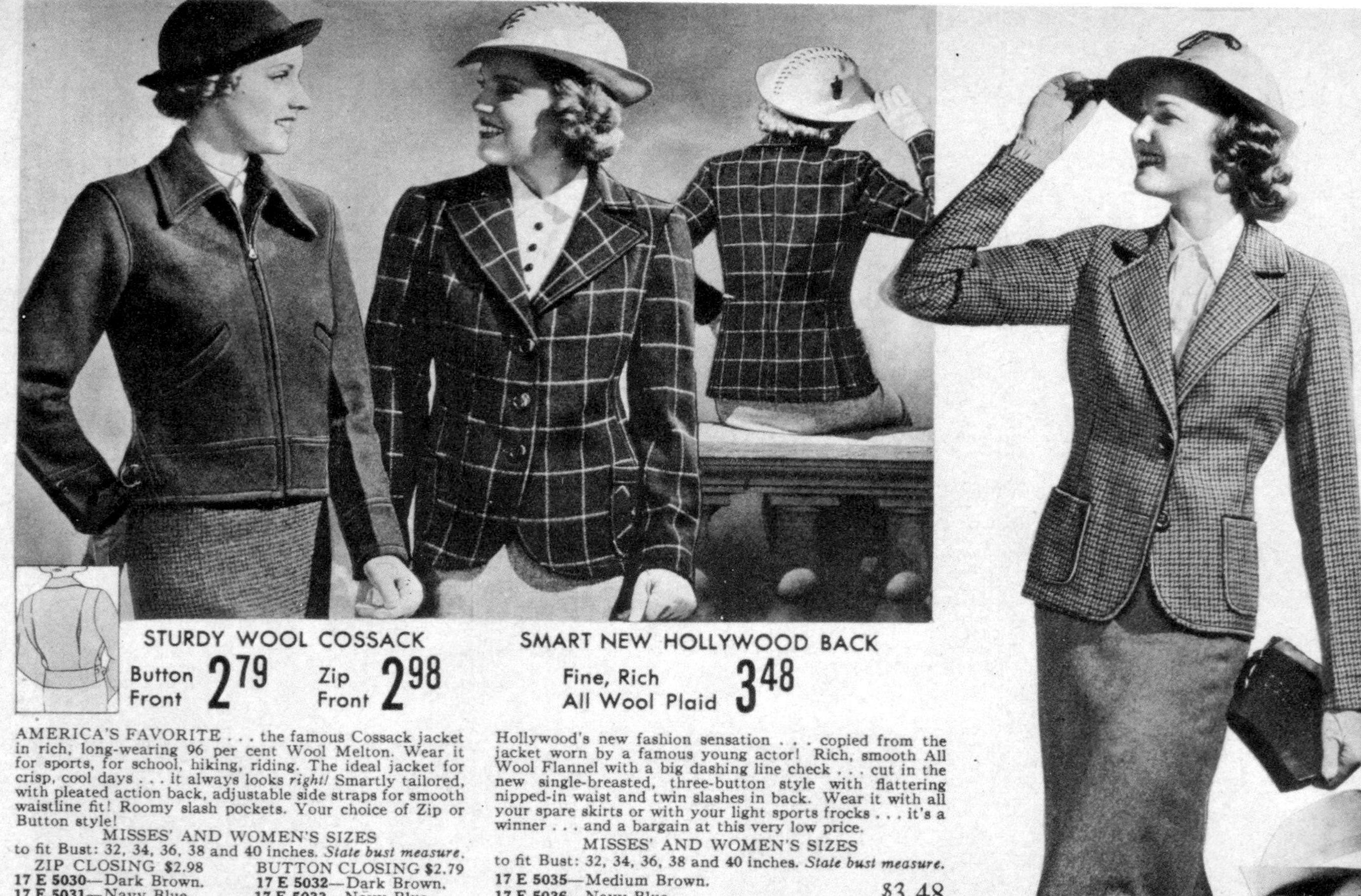

STURDY WOOL COSSACK

Button Front 2.79 Zip Front 2.98

AMERICA'S FAVORITE . . . the famous Cossack jacket in rich, long-wearing 96 per cent Wool Melton. Wear it for sports, for school, hiking, riding. The ideal jacket for crisp, cool days . . . it always looks *right!* Smartly tailored, with pleated action back, adjustable side straps for smooth waistline fit! Roomy slash pockets. Your choice of Zip or Button style!

MISSES' AND WOMEN'S SIZES to fit Bust: 32, 34, 36, 38 and 40 inches. *State bust measure.*

ZIP CLOSING $2.98
17 E 5030—Dark Brown.
17 E 5031—Navy Blue.

BUTTON CLOSING $2.79
17 E 5032—Dark Brown.
17 E 5033—Navy Blue.

Shipping weight, each, 2 pounds 4 ounces.

SMART NEW HOLLYWOOD BACK

Fine, Rich All Wool Plaid 3.48

Hollywood's new fashion sensation . . . copied from the jacket worn by a famous young actor! Rich, smooth All Wool Flannel with a big dashing line check . . . cut in the new single-breasted, three-button style with flattering nipped-in waist and twin slashes in back. Wear it with all your spare skirts or with your light sports frocks . . . it's a winner . . . and a bargain at this very low price.

MISSES' AND WOMEN'S SIZES to fit Bust: 32, 34, 36, 38 and 40 inches. *State bust measure.*

17 E 5035—Medium Brown.
17 E 5036—Navy Blue....................... $3.48

Shipping weight, 1 pound 6 ounces.

The garments on this and the opposite page are sent direct from New York to you . . . but you pay postage only from our nearest Mail Order House.

CLOSED
OPEN
LOCKING LEVER
Patented Slide Fastener Adjusts to Fit Every Waistline . . .
C
D
Fine All Wool Jersey 2.98

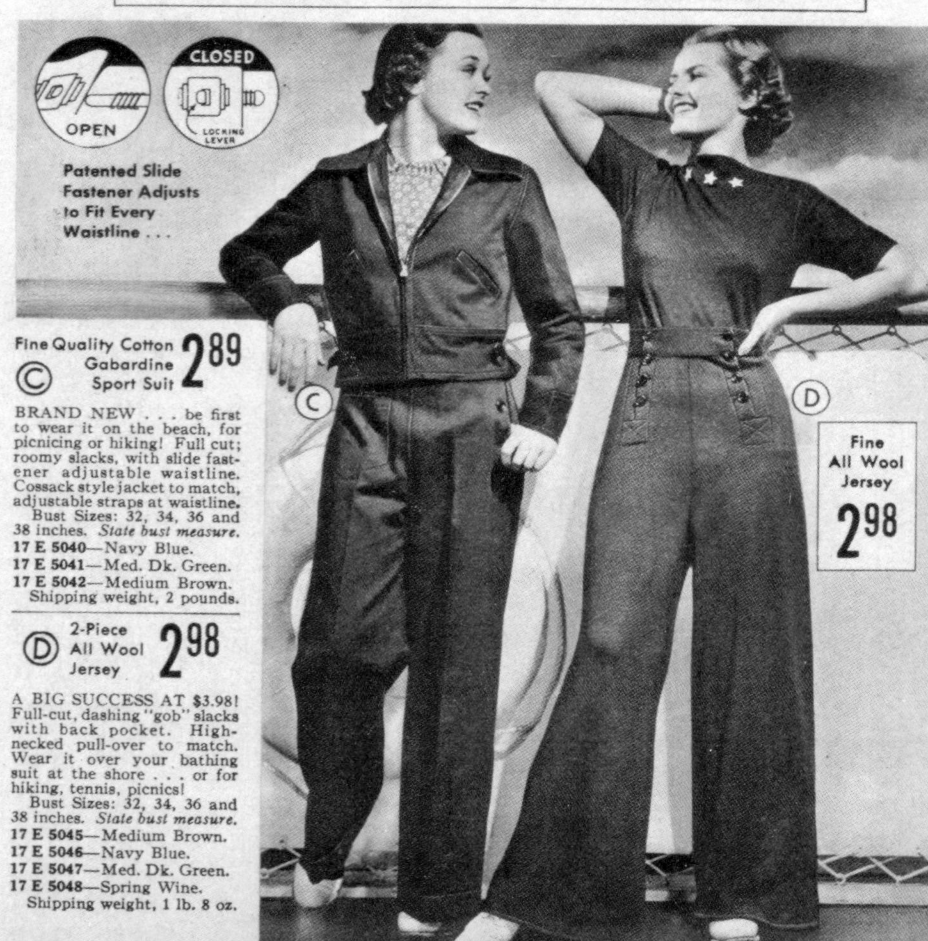

Fine Quality Cotton Gabardine Sport Suit Ⓒ 2.89

BRAND NEW . . . be first to wear it on the beach, for picnicing or hiking! Full cut; roomy slacks, with slide fastener adjustable waistline. Cossack style jacket to match, adjustable straps at waistline.

Bust Sizes: 32, 34, 36 and 38 inches. *State bust measure.*

17 E 5040—Navy Blue.
17 E 5041—Med. Dk. Green.
17 E 5042—Medium Brown.

Shipping weight, 2 pounds.

Ⓓ **2-Piece All Wool Jersey** 2.98

A BIG SUCCESS AT $3.98! Full-cut, dashing "gob" slacks with back pocket. High-necked pull-over to match. Wear it over your bathing suit at the shore . . . or for hiking, tennis, picnics!

Bust Sizes: 32, 34, 36 and 38 inches. *State bust measure.*

17 E 5045—Medium Brown.
17 E 5046—Navy Blue.
17 E 5047—Med. Dk. Green.
17 E 5048—Spring Wine.

Shipping weight, 1 lb. 8 oz.

3.98 Checked Coat with All Wool Flannel Skirt

WHAT A VALUE! This same style, quality and tailoring would cost much more in most shops! That dashing checked jacket, with its crisply tailored revers and slim nipped waistline, is about one-quarter fine Wool, balance Rayon for richness and longer wear. Don't you like that sporty action back? The smart kick-pleated skirt is of heavy All Wool Flannel, with Zip closing pocket and generous hem. Wear it three ways: as a suit, wear the jacket with dresses or other skirts, wear the skirt with all your sweaters and blouses. We predict you'll live in it all Spring . . . and love it!

MISSES' SIZES: 14-16-18-20.
TO FIT BUST: 32-34-36-38 inches.
State bust measure.

17 E 5050—Black and Gray Check Coat with Gray skirt.
17 E 5051—Brown and Tan Check Coat with Brown skirt.

Shipping weight, 2 pounds 12 ounces.

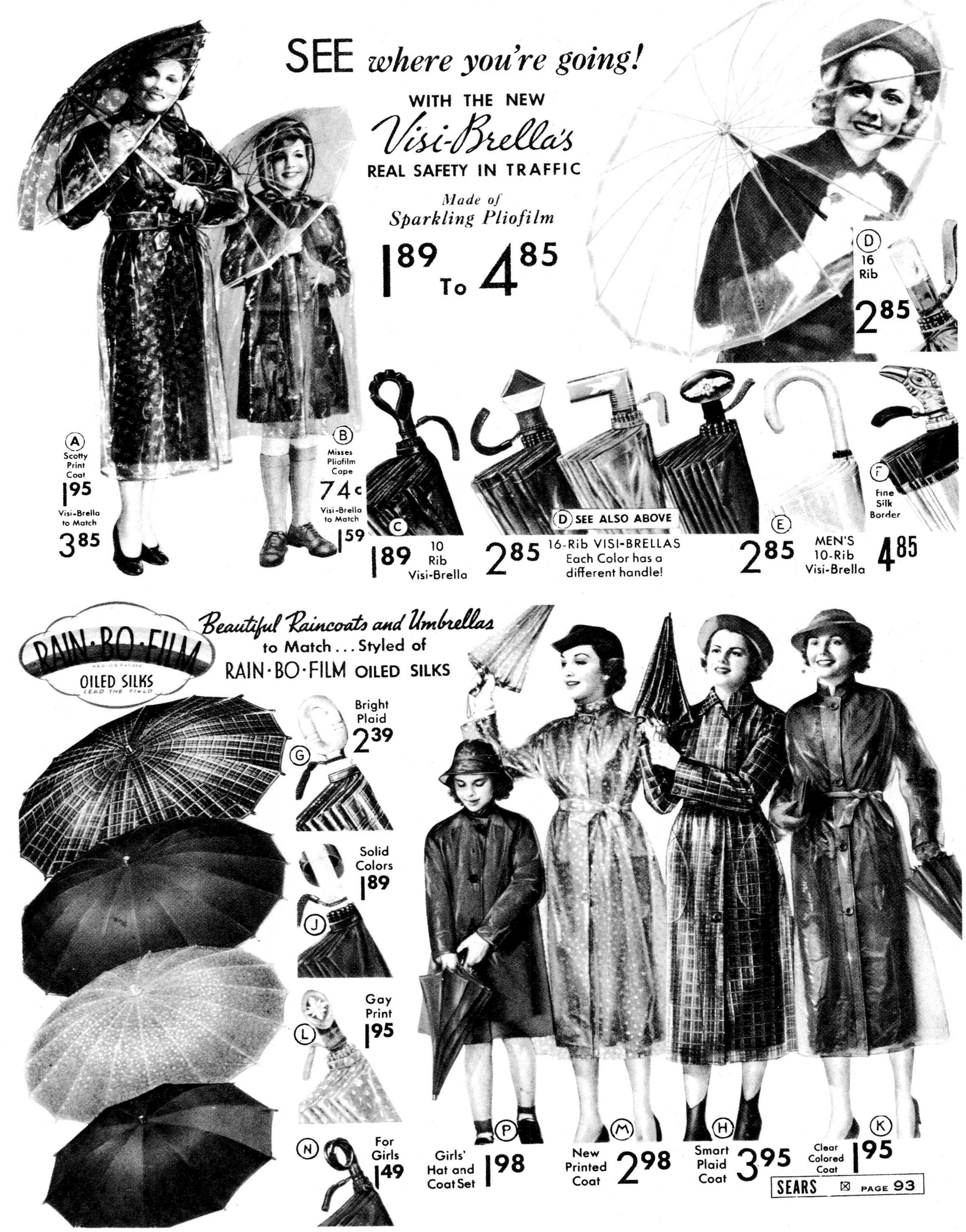

SEE *where you're going!*

WITH THE NEW

Visi-Brella's

REAL SAFETY IN TRAFFIC

Made of Sparkling Pliofilm

1.89 To 4.85

(A) Scotty Print Coat 1.95
Visi-Brella to Match 3.85

(B) Misses Pliofilm Cape 74c
Visi-Brella to Match 1.59

(D) 16 Rib 2.85

(C) 1.89 10 Rib Visi-Brella

(D) SEE ALSO ABOVE
2.85 16-Rib VISI-BRELLAS Each Color has a different handle!

(E) 2.85

(F) Fine Silk Border
MEN'S 10-Rib Visi-Brella 4.85

RAIN·BO·FILM REG. U.S. PAT. OFF. OILED SILKS LEAD THE FIELD

Beautiful Raincoats and Umbrellas to Match . . . Styled of RAIN·BO·FILM OILED SILKS

(G) Bright Plaid 2.39

(J) Solid Colors 1.89

(L) Gay Print 1.95

(N) For Girls 1.49

(P) Girls' Hat and Coat Set 1.98

(M) New Printed Coat 2.98

(H) Smart Plaid Coat 3.95

(K) Clear Colored Coat 1.95

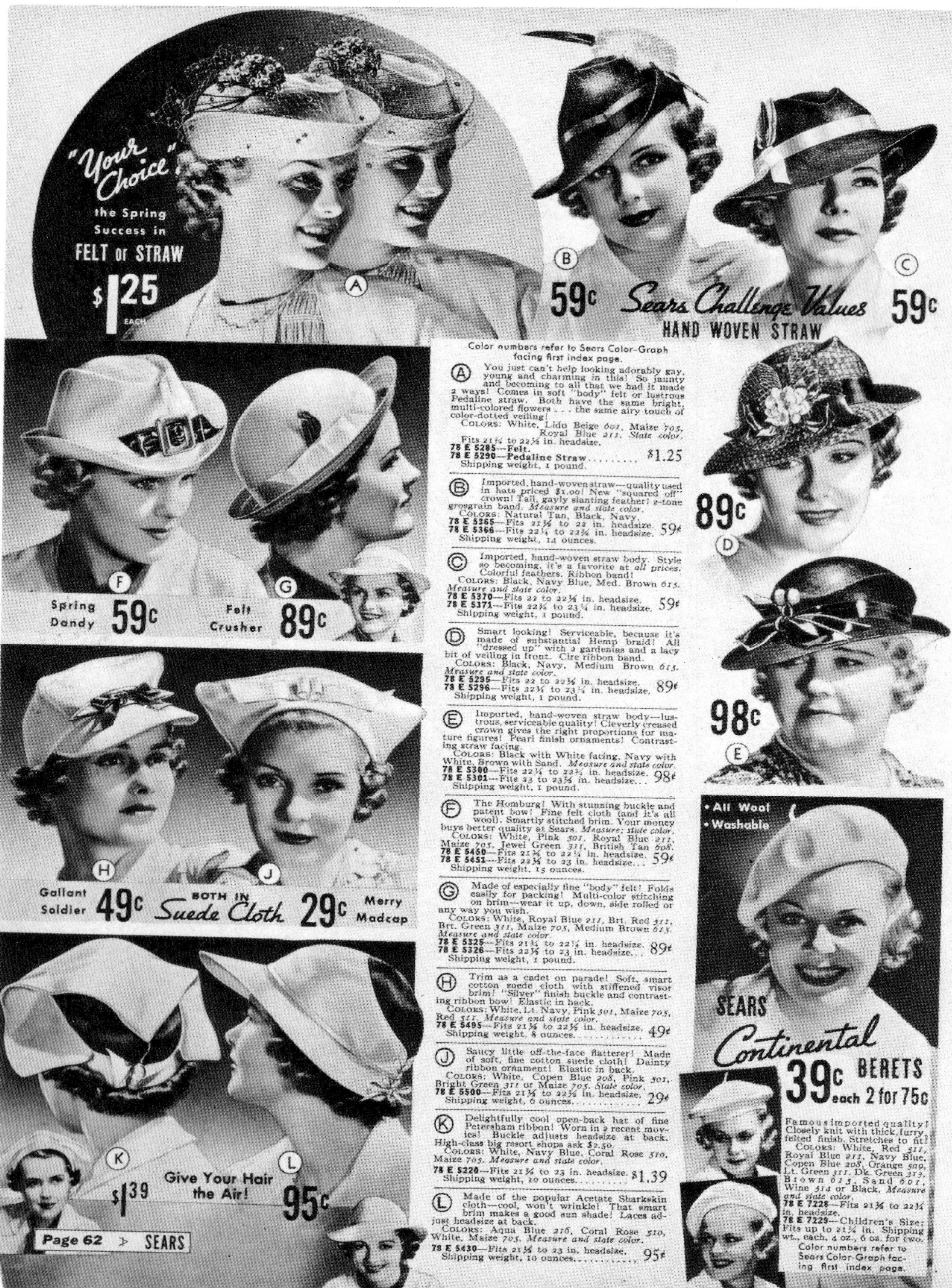

"Your Choice" the Spring Success in FELT or STRAW $1.25 EACH

A

B 59c Sears Challenge Values 59c C

HAND WOVEN STRAW

F Spring Dandy 59c

G Felt Crusher 89c

D 89c

E 98c

H Gallant Soldier 49c BOTH IN Suede Cloth 29c Merry Madcap J

K $1.39 Give Your Hair the Air! L 95c

Page 62 > SEARS

Color numbers refer to Sears Color-Graph facing first index page.

(A) You just can't help looking adorably gay, young and charming in this! So jaunty and becoming to all that we had it made 2 ways! Comes in soft "body" felt or lustrous Pedaline straw. Both have the same bright, multi-colored flowers . . . the same airy touch of color-dotted veiling!
COLORS: White, Lido Beige *601*, Maize *705*, Royal Blue *211*. *State color.*
Fits 21¾ to 22½ in. headsize.
78 E 5285—Felt.
78 E 5290—Pedaline Straw $1.25
Shipping weight, 1 pound.

(B) Imported, hand-woven straw—quality used in hats priced $1.00! New "squared off" crown! Tall, gayly slanting feather! 2-tone grosgrain band. *Measure and state color.*
COLORS: Natural Tan, Black, Navy.
78 E 5365—Fits 21⅞ to 22 in. headsize.
78 E 5366—Fits 22¼ to 22¾ in. headsize. 59¢
Shipping weight, 14 ounces.

(C) Imported, hand-woven straw body. Style so becoming, it's a favorite at *all* prices. Colorful feathers. Ribbon band!
COLORS: Black, Navy Blue, Med. Brown *615*. *Measure and state color.*
78 E 5370—Fits 22 to 22⅜ in. headsize.
78 E 5371—Fits 22¾ to 23¼ in. headsize. 59¢
Shipping weight, 1 pound.

(D) Smart looking! Serviceable, because it's made of substantial Hemp braid! All "dressed up" with 2 gardenias and a lacy bit of veiling in front. Cire ribbon band.
COLORS: Black, Navy, Medium Brown *615*. *Measure and state color.*
78 E 5295—Fits 22 to 22⅜ in. headsize.
78 E 5296—Fits 22¾ to 23¼ in. headsize. 89¢
Shipping weight, 1 pound.

(E) Imported, hand-woven straw body—lustrous, serviceable quality! Cleverly creased crown gives the right proportions for mature figures! Pearl finish ornaments! Contrasting straw facing.
COLORS: Black with White facing, Navy with White, Brown with Sand. *Measure and state color.*
78 E 5300—Fits 22¼ to 22¾ in. headsize.
78 E 5301—Fits 23 to 23⅜ in. headsize. . . 98¢
Shipping weight, 1 pound.

(F) The Homburg! With stunning buckle and patent bow! Fine felt cloth (and it's all wool). Smartly stitched brim. Your money buys better quality at Sears. *Measure; state color.*
COLORS: White, Pink *501*, Royal Blue *211*, Maize *705*, Jewel Green *311*, British Tan *608*.
78 E 5450—Fits 21¾ to 22¼ in. headsize.
78 E 5451—Fits 22⅜ to 23 in. headsize. . . 59¢
Shipping weight, 15 ounces.

(G) Made of especially fine "body" felt! Folds easily for packing! Multi-color stitching on brim—wear it up, down, side rolled or any way you wish.
COLORS: White, Royal Blue *211*, Brt. Red *511*, Brt. Green *311*, Maize *705*, Medium Brown *615*. *Measure and state color.*
78 E 5325—Fits 21¾ to 22¼ in. headsize.
78 E 5326—Fits 22⅜ to 23 in. headsize. . . 89¢
Shipping weight, 1 pound.

(H) Trim as a cadet on parade! Soft, smart cotton suede cloth with stiffened visor brim! "Silver" finish buckle and contrasting ribbon bow! Elastic in back.
COLORS: White, Lt. Navy, Pink *501*, Maize *705*, Red *511*. *Measure and state color.*
78 E 5495—Fits 21⅜ to 22⅜ in. headsize.
Shipping weight, 8 ounces. . . . . 49¢

(J) Saucy little off-the-face flatterer! Made of soft, fine cotton suede cloth! Dainty ribbon ornament! Elastic in back.
COLORS: White, Copen Blue *208*, Pink *501*, Bright Green *311* or Maize *705*. *State color.*
78 E 5500—Fits 21⅜ to 22⅛ in. headsize.
Shipping weight, 6 ounces. . . . . 29¢

(K) Delightfully cool open-back hat of fine Petersham ribbon! Worn in 2 recent movies! Buckle adjusts headsize at back. High-class big resort shops ask $2.50.
COLORS: White, Navy Blue, Coral Rose *510*, Maize *705*. *Measure and state color.*
78 E 5220—Fits 21⅜ to 23 in. headsize.
Shipping weight, 10 ounces. $1.39

(L) Made of the popular Acetate Sharkskin cloth—cool, won't wrinkle! That smart brim makes a good sun shade! Laces adjust headsize at back.
COLORS: Aqua Blue *216*, Coral Rose *510*, White, Maize *705*. *Measure and state color.*
78 E 5430—Fits 21⅜ to 23 in. headsize.
Shipping weight, 10 ounces. . . . . 95¢

• All Wool
• Washable

SEARS Continental BERETS 39c each 2 for 75c

Famous imported quality! Closely knit with thick, furry, felted finish. Stretches to fit!
COLORS: White, Red *511*, Royal Blue *211*, Navy Blue, Copen Blue *208*, Orange *509*, Lt. Green *311*, Dk. Green *313*, Brown *615*, Sand *601*, Wine *514* or Black. *Measure and state color.*
78 E 7228—Fits 21⅜ to 22¾ in. headsize.
78 E 7229—Children's Size: Fits up to 21¼ in. Shipping wt., each, 4 oz., 6 oz. for two.

Color numbers refer to Sears Color-Graph facing first index page.

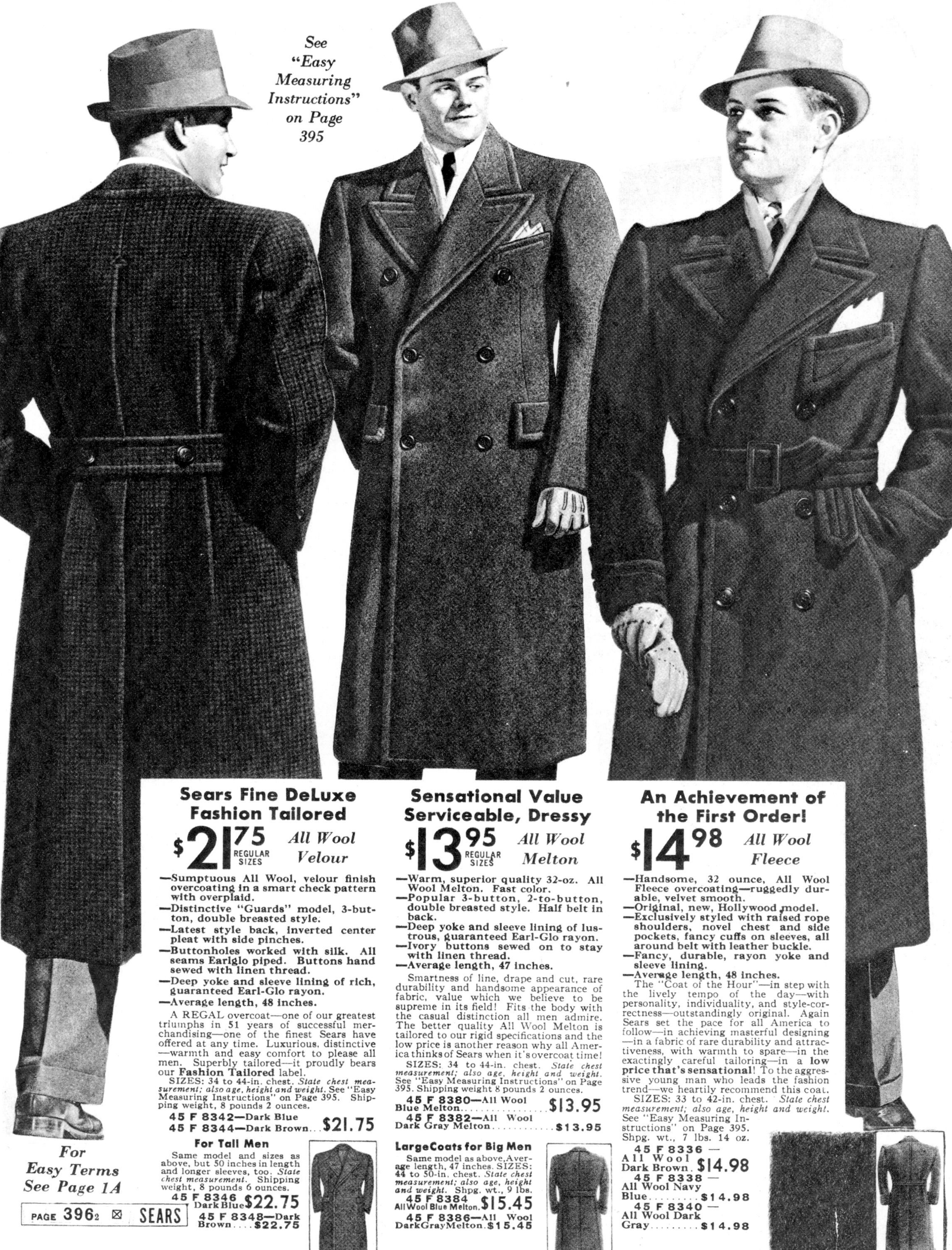

See "Easy Measuring Instructions" on Page 395

Sears Fine DeLuxe Fashion Tailored

$21.75 REGULAR SIZES *All Wool Velour*

—Sumptuous All Wool, velour finish overcoating in a smart check pattern with overplaid.
—Distinctive "Guards" model, 3-button, double breasted style.
—Latest style back, inverted center pleat with side pinches.
—Buttonholes worked with silk. All seams Earlglo piped. Buttons hand sewed with linen thread.
—Deep yoke and sleeve lining of rich, guaranteed Earl-Glo rayon.
—Average length, 48 inches.

A REGAL overcoat—one of our greatest triumphs in 51 years of successful merchandising—one of the finest Sears have offered at any time. Luxurious, distinctive—warmth and easy comfort to please all men. Superbly tailored—it proudly bears our **Fashion Tailored** label.

SIZES: 34 to 44-in. chest. *State chest measurement; also age, height and weight.* See "Easy Measuring Instructions" on Page 395. Shipping weight, 8 pounds 2 ounces.

45 F 8342—Dark Blue
45 F 8344—Dark Brown... $21.75

For Tall Men

Same model and sizes as above, but 50 inches in length and longer sleeves, too. *State chest measurement.* Shipping weight, 8 pounds 6 ounces.

45 F 8346 Dark Blue $22.75
45 F 8348—Dark Brown.... $22.75

Sensational Value Serviceable, Dressy

$13.95 REGULAR SIZES *All Wool Melton*

—Warm, superior quality 32-oz. All Wool Melton. Fast color.
—Popular 3-button, 2-to-button, double breasted style. Half belt in back.
—Deep yoke and sleeve lining of lustrous, guaranteed Earl-Glo rayon.
—Ivory buttons sewed on to stay with linen thread.
—Average length, 47 inches.

Smartness of line, drape and cut, rare durability and handsome appearance of fabric, value which we believe to be supreme in its field! Fits the body with the casual distinction all men admire. The better quality All Wool Melton is tailored to our rigid specifications and the low price is another reason why all America thinks of Sears when it's overcoat time!

SIZES: 34 to 44-in. chest. *State chest measurement; also age, height and weight.* See "Easy Measuring Instructions" on Page 395. Shipping weight 8 pounds 2 ounces.

45 F 8380—All Wool Blue Melton.............. $13.95
45 F 8382—All Wool Dark Gray Melton........... $13.95

LargeCoats for Big Men

Same model as above, Average length, 47 inches. SIZES: 44 to 50-in. chest. *State chest measurement; also age, height and weight.* Shpg. wt., 9 lbs.

45 F 8384 All Wool Blue Melton. $15.45
45 F 8386—All Wool DarkGrayMelton. $15.45

An Achievement of the First Order!

$14.98 *All Wool Fleece*

—Handsome, 32 ounce, All Wool Fleece overcoating—ruggedly durable, velvet smooth.
—Original, new, Hollywood model.
—Exclusively styled with raised rope shoulders, novel chest and side pockets, fancy cuffs on sleeves, all around belt with leather buckle.
—Fancy, durable, rayon yoke and sleeve lining.
—Average length, 48 inches.

The "Coat of the Hour"—in step with the lively tempo of the day—with personality, individuality, and style-correctness—outstandingly original. Again Sears set the pace for all America to follow—in achieving masterful designing—in a fabric of rare durability and attractiveness, with warmth to spare—in the exactingly careful tailoring—in a **low price that's sensational**! To the aggressive young man who leads the fashion trend—we heartily recommend this coat.

SIZES: 33 to 42-in. chest. *State chest measurement; also age, height and weight.* See "Easy Measuring Instructions" on Page 395. Shpg. wt., 7 lbs. 14 oz.

45 F 8336 — All Wool Dark Brown. $14.98
45 F 8338 — All Wool Navy Blue......... $14.98
45 F 8340 — All Wool Dark Gray......... $14.98

For Easy Terms See Page 1A

EASY TERMS
On Orders of $20.00 or More! See Easy Payment Page 951.

Gabardine
THE NATION'S FAVORITE

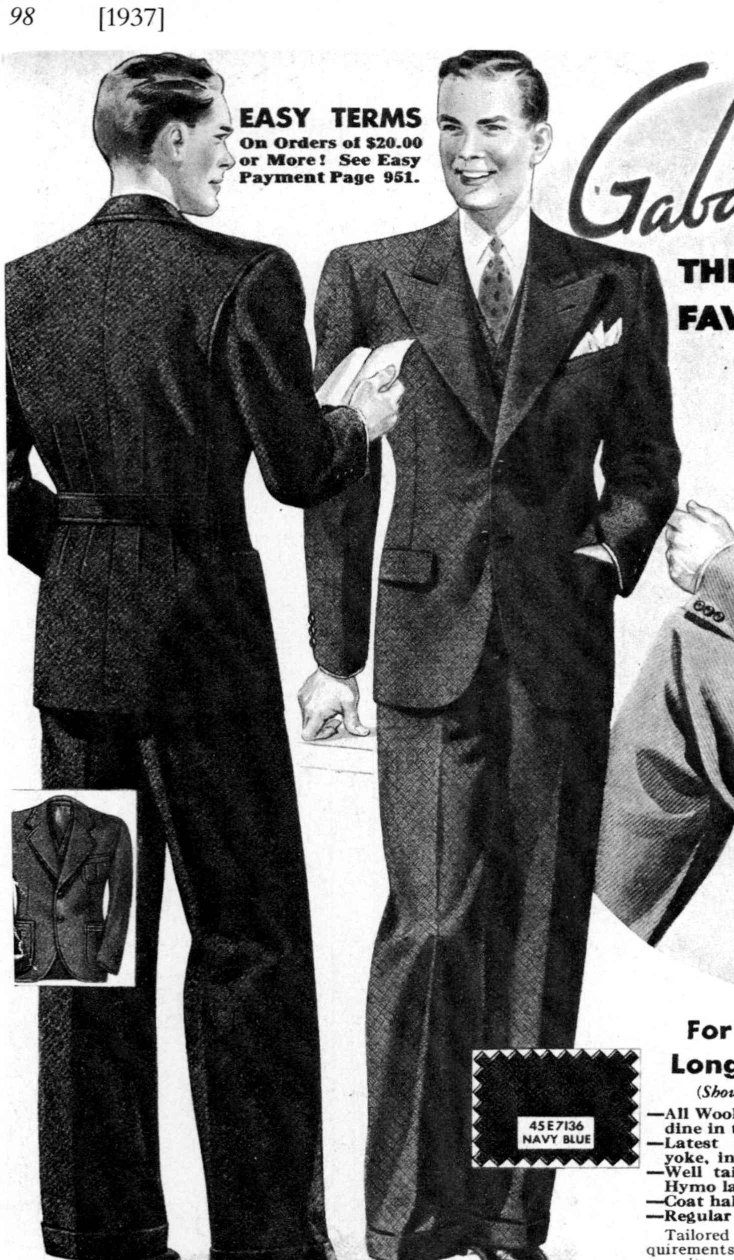

45E7165
NAVY BLUE

A Brand New Style Sensation! $13.50

—Smooth, firmly woven solid color All Wool Cassimere.

—Sporty, 2-button, notch lapel model with Bi-Swing back. Four tucks above the smart half belt.

—Inverted pleat patch pockets.

—Coat is half lined, sleeves fully lined with genuine, easy-slip Earl-Glo rayon.

—Pleated trousers have extension waistband, 21-in. cuffs.

Would you like to lead the style parade? Here is the very latest model in sports clothes and we predict that it will set a new record for popularity in 1937. Firmly woven, wear-resisting fabric . . . tailored to Sears exacting specifications . . . what more could you ask at such an extremely low price? Be one of the first to own this smart, beautifully styled new suit.

SIZES: 34 to 42 in. chest; 29 to 39 in. waist; 29 to 35 in. inseam. *State measurements; also age, height and weight.* See "How to Measure" on Page 293. Shipping weight, 5 pounds 7 ounces.

45 E 7180
Medium Dark Brown **$13.50**

45 E 7141
Medium Dark Blue. . . . **$13.50**

Snappy, DIAMOND-WEAVE Worsted! $15.45

—Pure, hard finished, Virgin Wool Worsted.

—Two-button, peak lapel model with athletic shoulders.

—Plain, form fitting back.

—Coat half lined, sleeves fully lined with Earl-Glo rayon.

—Wide 21-inch trouser cuffs.

This famous "Diamond Weave" fabric will give more honest-to-goodness wear and satisfaction than any we know of. It is firmly woven and will hold its shape even when given the roughest kind of hard wear. Splendid tailoring and smart, authoritative styling assure a well groomed appearance. And best of all, Sears offer you this rich-looking suit at a money-saving price that you can't afford to overlook. A small budget goes a long way in America's Largest Clothing Store! Look your best . . . and LET SEARS SAVE YOU MONEY!

SIZES: 34 to 42 in. chest; 28 to 39 in. waist; 29 to 35 in. inseam. *State measurements; also age, height and weight.* See "How to Measure" on Page 293. Shpg. wt. 5 lbs. 2 oz., with extra trousers, 6 lbs. 14 oz.

45 E 7136—Navy Blue. **$15.45**
45 E 7152—Navy Blue with Extra Trousers. **$19.45**
45 E 7137—Very Dark Oxford Gray. **$15.45**
45 E 7154—Very Dark Oxford Gray with Extra Trousers **$19.45**

For Extra Long Wear $17.85
(Shown Above)

—All Wool, 2-ply Worsted twill weave Gabardine in three popular Summer shades.

—Latest sports style, Action-Back, with yoke, inverted pleat and half belt.

—Well tailored. Coat has linen front and Hymo lapel interlining for lasting fit.

—Coat half lined, sleeves lined with Earl-Glo.

—Regular 20-inch trouser cuffs.

Tailored in the latest style to meet all the requirements of men who want the best. You can wear it as a complete suit or the coat may be worn correctly with contrasting trousers. The first day you wear this fine suit, you'll realize that it's a superior garment in every way and you'll see why other stores can sell it for as much as $25.00! Careful attention to minute tailoring details makes this a truly astonishing value!

SIZES: 34 to 42 in. chest; 29 to 39 in. waist; 29 to 35 in. inseam. *State measurements; also age, height and weight.* See "How to Measure" on Page 293. Shipping weight, 5 pounds 6 ounces.

45 E 7164—Medium Light Gray. . **$17.85**
45 E 7165—Navy Blue. **$17.85**
45 E 7166—Medium Brown. **17.85**

"Air Cooled" Wool Worsted $15.95
(Shown At Right)

—New, medium weight small check pattern Wool Worsted with rayon decorations. Sears famous "Poro-Twist" Worsted.

—Latest 2-button, notch lapel, sports model with inverted center pleat, and four tucks above the half belt. Patch pockets.

—Coat is ⅛ lined with Earl-Glo rayon. Sleeves fully lined.

—Six button vest is skeleton lined.

—Trousers have 21-inch cuffs.

Don't be hot and bothered this Summer. Wear one of these Poro-Twist "Air-Cooled" suits and you'll laugh at the hot weather. The new, porous, light weight fabric is specially woven to let the air get at you, and because it's wool worsted it is ideal for the cool days of Spring, too. Wears just like any regular suit. Beautifully and strongly tailored and will give lasting service at the very minimum of expense. We guarantee to fit you perfectly.

SIZES: 34 to 42 in. chest; 29 to 39 in. waist; 29 to 35 in. inseam. *State measurements; also age, height and weight.* See "How to Measure" on Page 293. Shipping weight, 5 pounds 6 ounces.

45 E 7123—Medium Light Tan "Poro" Tropical Twist. **$15.95**
45 E 7117—Light Gray "Poro" Tropical Twist. **$15.95**

GIRLS' OFFICIAL GYM SUITS

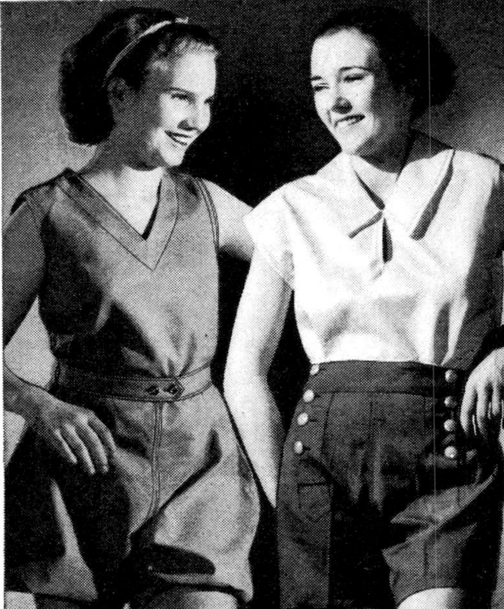

1-PIECE GYM SUITS 89c

- Good quality, cotton suiting material. Strong rugged weave. Inside pocket.
- Fast vat-dye colors.
- Button on one shoulder and lower down side; elastic at knee. Comfortable full fit.

EXTRA FULL CUT

Regular $1.25 value. Adopted as official by many girls' schools and colleges. Full cut patterns; V-shaped neck. Sleeveless to allow freedom of arms. Official size and specifications. Colors: Blue or Green. AGES: 10 to 22 years. State age-size and color. Shpg. wt., 12 oz.

6 F 1983..........89c

GYM BLOUSE 98c

- Slipover style with button combination.
- 1/4 length sleeves.
- "V" neck with square cut collar.

Made of medium weight, white jean cloth. SIZES: 30 to 36-in. bust. State size. Shipping weight, 12 oz.

6 F 1985........98c

GIRLS' GYM SHORTS

- Black Henrietta twill.
- Snappy pleated model.

Also ideal for soft ball, bicycle riding and other outdoor sports. Buttons as shown. SIZES: 24 to 30 in. waist. State size. Shpg. wt., 8 oz.

6 F 1984......95c

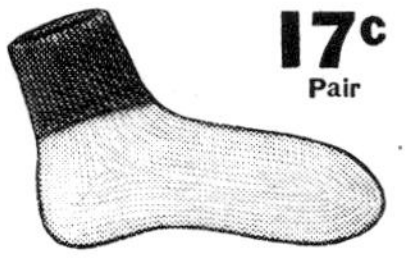

17c Pair GIRLS' COTTON SPORT SOCKS

Unusually low price for fine quality socks like these. Perfect match for girls' suits above. White body with blue, green, or black cuffs. SIZES: 9 and 10. State size and color trim. Shipping weight, 4 ounces.

6 F 2053—Pair..........17c

KEEP WARM FOR WINTER SPORTS

$1.00 $1.85

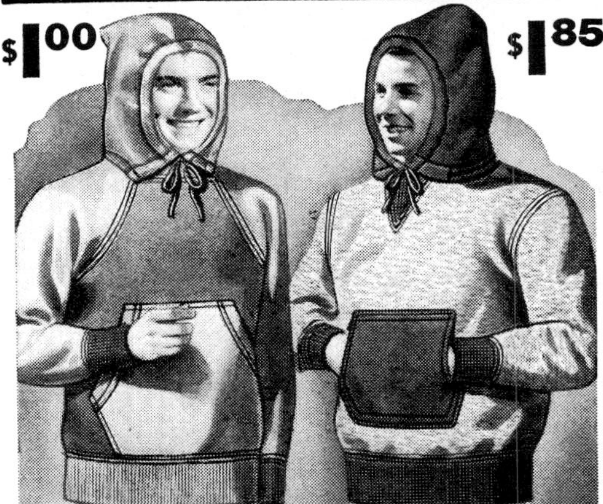

HOODED SWEATSHIRT GREAT FOR BOYS

- Medium weight cotton shirt with hood attached. Cotton fleece lined.
- Hood keeps ears and face warm, has drawstrings to pull tight around face.
- Raglan sleeve style.

"Muff" in front to warm hands or carry small things. Just the thing for school children who enjoy playing outdoors on chilly or cold winter days. Navy body with scarlet hood, muff and shoulders.

Boys' SIZES: 6 to 16 years. State age-size. Shpg. wt., 1 pound 4 ounces.

6 F 2009.......$1.00

HEAVYWEIGHT COTTON WINTER SPORT JACKET

- Double thickness sweatshirt cotton, fleeced backing turned toward inside; cannot touch or come off on clothes.
- "Muff" pocket on front.
- Hood with drawstrings for tight fit around face.

An ideal garment for skating, skiing and all other winter sports. Also, a good utility garment for those who work outdoors in cold weather. Silver gray body trimmed with Navy blue at cuffs, collar, bottom, hood and muff. SIZES: 32 to 46-in. chest. State size. Shpg. wt. 2 lbs. 2 oz.

6 F 2012......$1.85

Heavier, Roomier, More Finely Woven
THAN MOST SHIRTS AT THIS PRICE!

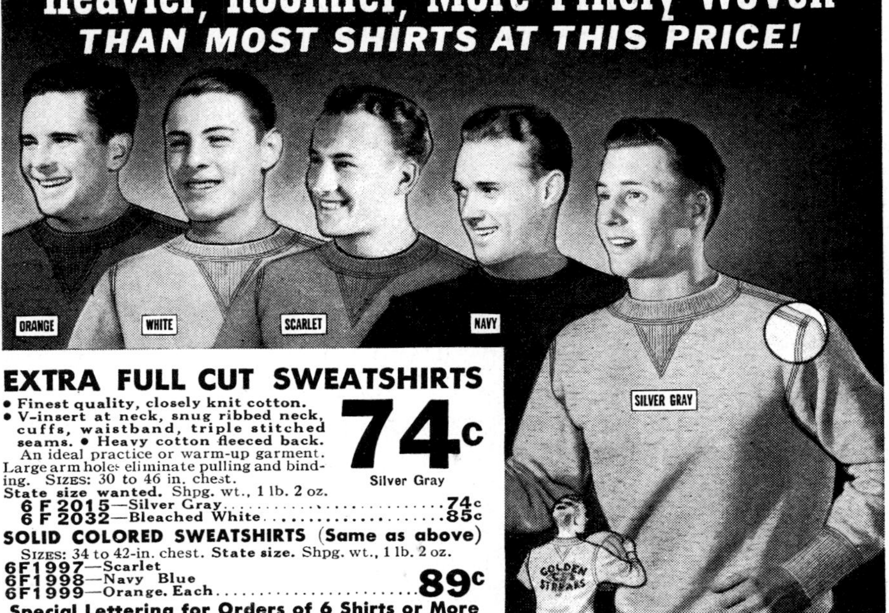

EXTRA FULL CUT SWEATSHIRTS 74c Silver Gray

- Finest quality, closely knit cotton.
- V-insert at neck, snug ribbed neck, cuffs, waistband, triple stitched seams. ● Heavy cotton fleeced back.

An ideal practice or warm-up garment. Large arm holes eliminate pulling and binding. SIZES: 30 to 46 in. chest. State size wanted. Shpg. wt., 1 lb. 2 oz.

6 F 2015—Silver Gray..........74c
6 F 2032—Bleached White..........85c

SOLID COLORED SWEATSHIRTS (Same as above)

SIZES: 34 to 42-in. chest. State size. Shpg. wt., 1 lb. 2 oz.

6F1997—Scarlet
6F1998—Navy Blue
6F1999—Orange. Each..........89c

Special Lettering for Orders of 6 Shirts or More

Now teams can have fabric letters or emblems or a combination of both in any athletic color ready attached to front or back of shirt only, (see how to order below). Lettering and design fused into shirt, cannot furnish separately. Fast colors. Will not shrink. We cannot fill orders for less than 6 shirts. Orders for at least six shirts must specify identical letters and design of same size and color on each shirt.

6 F 2097—Any amount of lettering, any size, including emblem (send sketch) on shirt front. Per Shirt 55c
6 F 2098—As above, except on back of shirt. Per Shirt 55c

How to Order Lettering on Sweatshirts

State size, color, and print plainly lettering wanted. Send pencil sketch of design wanted. Orders are shipped from factory within 5 days, but you pay postage only from our nearest mail order house.

Silver Gray Sweat Pants

Matches 6 F 2015 sweatshirt. Drawstrings at waist, ankles. Small, med. or large. State size. Shipping weight, 1 pound 4 ounces.

6 F 2044.......89c

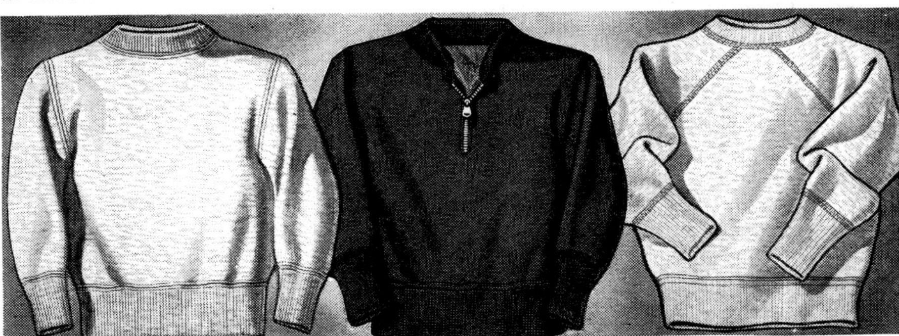

MEDIUM WEIGHT 67c

- Durable cotton silver gray sweatshirt.
- Ribbed for snug fit at neck, wrists and bottom.

Plenty of length and freedom in this serviceable garment. All seams triple stitched and flat locked. SIZES: 30 to 46-in. chest. State size. Shpg. wt., 15 oz.

6 F 2035—Silver Gray...67c

"ZIP" NECK STYLE 95c Silver Gray

- 7-inch Talon fastener.
- Medium weight cotton.
- Triple stitched seams.
- Cotton fleeced back.

Ribbed neck, cuffs and waistband. SIZES: 30 to 46-in. chest. State size. Shipping weight, 1 pound 3 ounces.

6 F 2018—Navy Blue.......99c
6 F 2017—Silver Gray......95c

RAGLAN SLEEVE STYLE 75c

- Long-wearing, medium weight cotton.
- Fleecing on inside.

Triple flat locked stitching throughout. Extra freedom in arms due to raglan sleeve. Silver Gray color. SIZES: 30 to 46-in. chest. State size. Shpg. wt., 1 lb.

6 F 2011—Silver Gray....75c

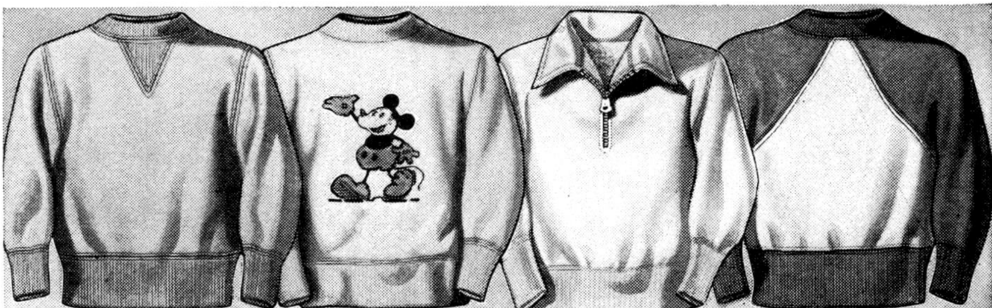

DOUBLE WT. COTTON $1.69

- Flat locked triple stitching throughout.
- Full cut for freedom.

An extra warm garment of double thickness sweatshirt cloth. Both layers fleeced, but fleecing is faced in to keep from touching or coming off on the clothes. Excellent for winter sports and general winter wear. Gun metal color.

SIZES: 30 to 46-in. chest. State size. Shipping wt., 1 lb. 12 oz.

6 F 2008......$1.69

"MICKEY MOUSE" 55c White

- Extra full cut.
- Cotton fleeced back. ● Ribbed neck, cuffs and waistband.

Good quality cotton sweatshirt with Walt Disney's famous "Mickey Mouse" emblem. Popular "knock-about" for youngsters. AGES: 6 to 16 yrs. State age-size. Shipping weight, 10 ounces.

6 F 2014—White..55c
6 F 2043—Yellow, Cadet Blue, or Jockey Red. State color..............65c

PULLOVER JACKET $1.09

- Expertly cut and tailored.
- Snappy rolled collar.
- Talon opener at neck.

Sears best! Made of fine quality cotton with cotton fleece backing. Makes an ideal sport garment for beach wear, tennis, golf and around camp. White. SIZES: 34 to 42-in. chest. State size. Shipping wt., 1 lb. 10 oz.

6 F 2013
$1.09

TWO-TONE SHIRT 99c

- Heavy-weight cotton.
- Shoulder insert.
- Cotton fleece back.

Ideal sweatshirt for football. Orange insert, navy blue body; or navy insert with cardinal red body. SIZES: 32 to 42-in. chest. State size, color. Shpg. wt., 1 lb.

6 F 2467........99c

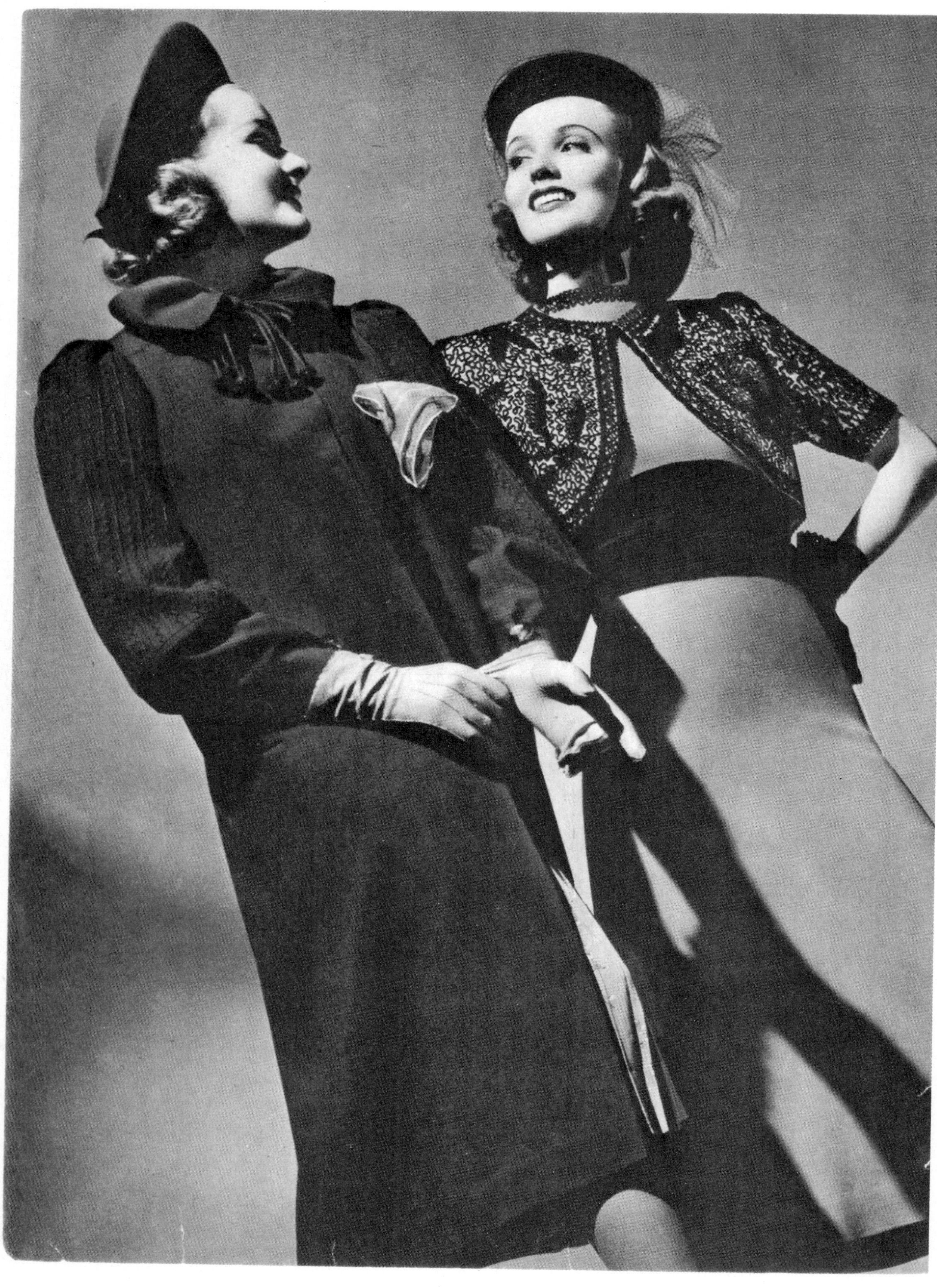

FOR QUALITY FASHIONS

1. Soft Chamois-like Leather Interlinings for Fur Coat Warmth
2. Superior Styling for Wear Through Many Seasons
3. Expert Tailoring in Fine Fabrics of Enduring Beauty
4. Rich, Durable Linings Guaranteed for 2 Years

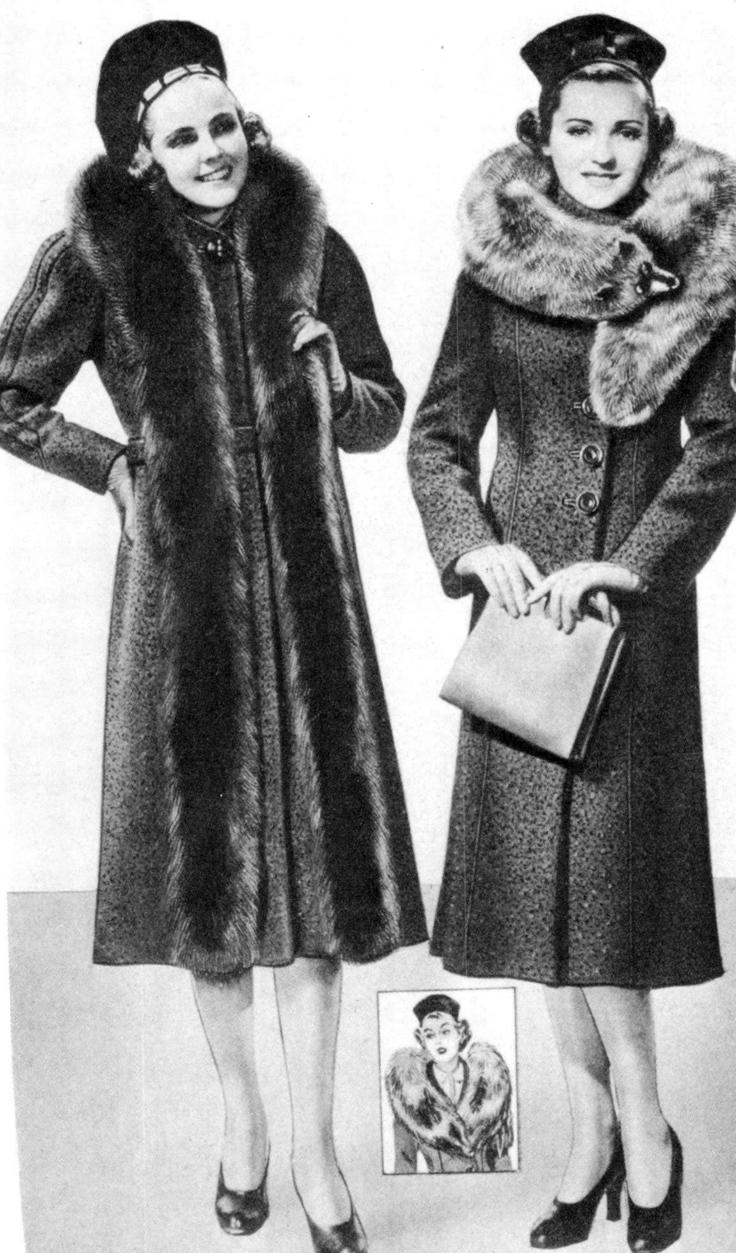

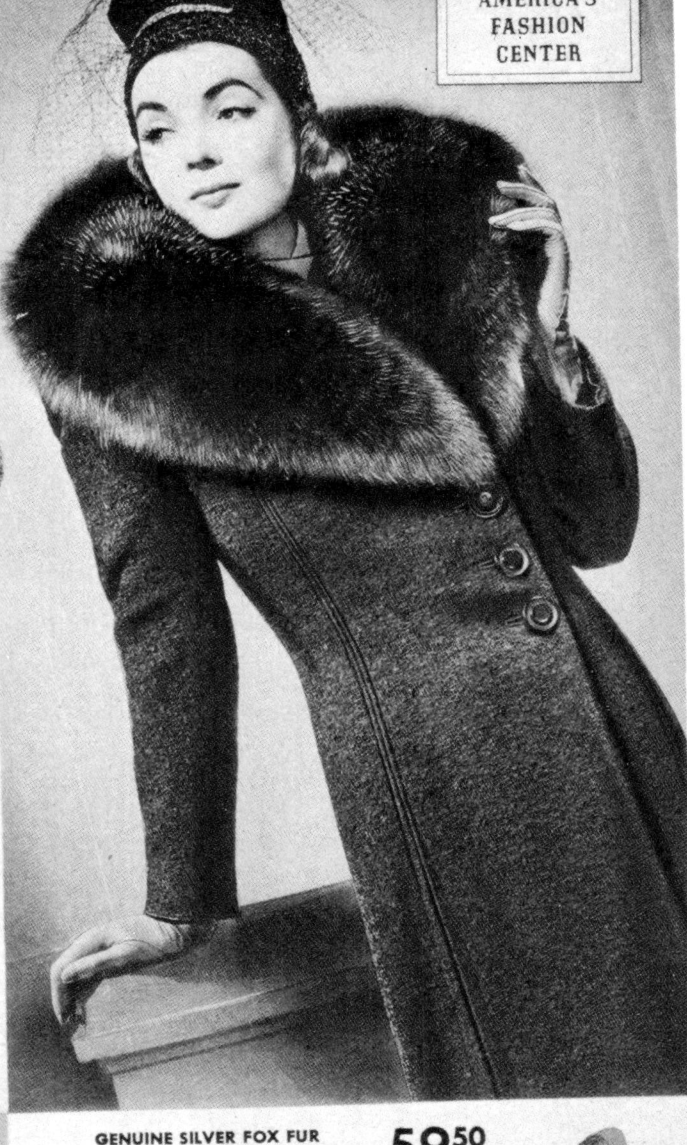

27.50 GENUINE MANCHURIAN WOLF-DYED DOG FUR

Swirls in fluffy black elegance 'round your shoulders clear down to the hem! Tailored of handsome ALL WOOL Nubbed Boucle . . . the rich, soft-textured quality usually found only in far higher-priced coats. Slim princess lines with a softly flared skirt—so beautifully cut you can wear it with or without the matching belt. Rayon Panné Satin lining, guaranteed for two years; warm interlining. Extra interlining of soft Chamois-like leather to the waist.

SIZES: 14-16-18-20-22.
BUST: 32-34-36-38-40 in.
LENGTH: 44-45-45-46-46 in. **State bust.**
17 K 8610—Grape Wine *908*.
17 K 8611—Rich Black.
Shipping weight, 6 pounds 6 ounces.

MANY-WAY COLLAR OF GENUINE AMUR RACCOON 24.98

Amur Raccoons are the finer-quality, longer-haired pelts that look like fluffy fox. Full-skin collar with head and paws . . . you can wear it four or five flattering ways! Handsome, new, ALL WOOL Nubbed Boucle Coating, the quality you see in expensive coats. Lined with weighted Silk Crepe-Back Satin . . . interlined. Extra interlining of soft Chamois-like leather to the waist.

SIZES: 14-16-18-20-22-42-44-46.
BUST: 32-34-36-38-40-42-44-46 in.
LENGTH: 46-47-47-48-48-48-48-48 in.
State bust measure.
17 K 8620—Brown *623* with Natural Brownish Tan Fur.
17 K 8621—Black with Silvery Black Fur.
Shipping weight, 5 pounds 6 ounces.

GENUINE SILVER FOX FUR
Our Finest "BOTANY" ALL WOOL Boucle 59.50

SILVER-DYED RUSSIAN FOX
FINE ALL WOOL BOUCLE 39.50

TWO GREAT SEARS TRIUMPHS . . . supreme in style and value! Coats of distinguished beauty such as you would find in big-city specialty shops! Glamorously furred, tailored by skilled craftsmen of our finest ALL WOOL Boucle coatings . . . extra-warm, rich, heavily nubbed. Long, slender, perfect-fitting princess lines do the utmost for your figure. Stitched-down pleats give the all-important new skirt detail. Silk weighted Crepe-Back Satin linings are guaranteed for two years; warm interlinings. Extra interlining in the back of soft Chamois-like leather to the waist. Collar can be buttoned high on cold days.

SIZES: 14-16-18-20-22-42-44-46.
BUST: 32-34-36-38-40-42-44-46 in.
LENGTH: 46-47-47-48-48-48-48-48 in. **State bust measure.**

WITH GENUINE SILVER FOX COLLAR

Queen of all luxury furs . . . so flattering, so rare and costly it's the choice of America's wealthiest women! Hand-picked pelts only, rich with shining "silver" . . . a huge rippling collar that swathes your shoulders in a wealth of black-and-silver glory. $59.50
17 K 8615—Rich Black only . . . .

WITH GENUINE SILVER-DYED RUSSIAN FOX COLLAR

Gloriously fluffy, hand-picked pelts, skillfully dyed to give the silver-tipped beauty of Silver Fox.
17 K 8618—Black with Silver-dyed Russian Fox.
17 K 8619—Seal Brown *623*; Brown-dyed Fox. $39.50
Shipping weight, each, 6 pounds.

These coats are sent direct from New York to you . . . you pay postage only from our nearest Mail Order House.

Numbers after Color names refer to Sears COLOR-GRAPH following index pages in back of book.

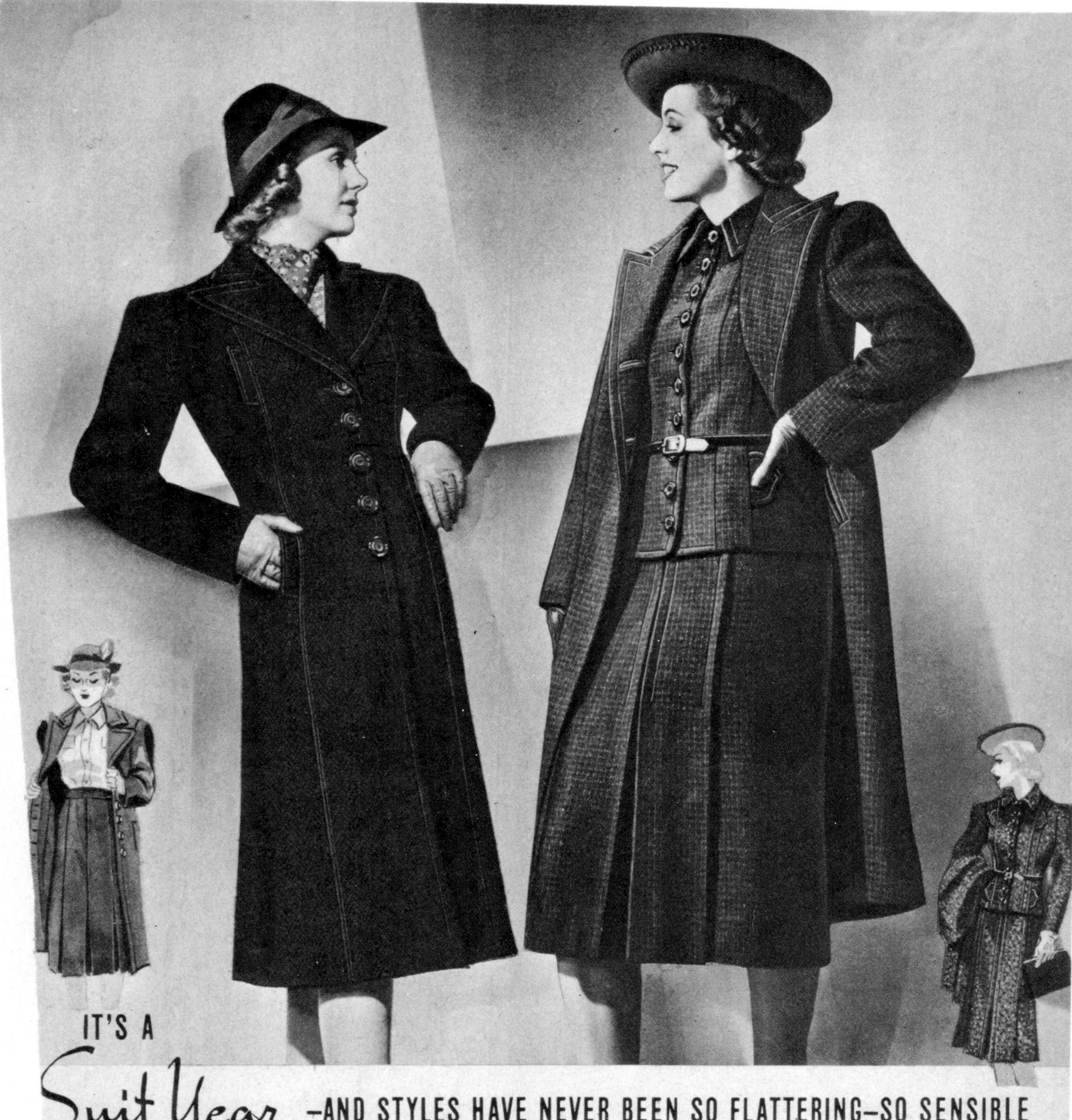

IT'S A Suit Year —AND STYLES HAVE NEVER BEEN SO FLATTERING—SO SENSIBLE

2-Piece Reefer Suit . . . All Wool Shetland

Now's the time to invest your capital in a Suit , . . a good suit that you can wear right through until Spring! And remember that fine fabric, and painstaking workmanship mean long wear and satisfaction!

This Two-piece ALL WOOL Shetland Suit qualifies 100% as the perfect all year 'round outfit—correct any place . . . any time! It's flawlessly tailored on simple classic lines that will never go out of style. The ALL WOOL fabric is soft and warm and durable . . . the finer quality that you would expect to find in a much higher priced suit! The full length coat can be worn all winter long as a topcoat over all your dresses, for it's lined with sturdy Rayon Taffeta and warmly interlined. Its fitted Princess lines are pencil slim . . . its shoulders padded just enough to square them off! Tucks and gores give the back a graceful flare. There are four slash pockets. The skirt fits beautifully. It has a smooth-closing Zip placket, and three kick pleats in front to give you plenty of walking room. The skirt and coat are not sold separately!

17 K 8920—Rich Black.
17 K 8921—Navy Blue.
17 K 8922—Rust Brown *615*.

SIZES: 14-16-18-20.
TO FIT BUST: 32-34-36-38 in.
LENGTHS: 44-44-45-45 in.

State bust measure. Shipping weight, 4 lbs. 8 oz.

10.98

3-Piece Suit in Your Choice of 2 Fabrics

This winter, no wardrobe will be complete without a suit . . . and when the suit can be as useful and as smart as this, it's big news!

It's three-piece: Topcoat, Jacket and Skirt, in your choice of the two fabrics shown. The stunning Checked Suiting (large view) is 80% Wool, balance Rayon and Cotton. The fabric shown in the small sketch is fine ALL WOOL Nubbed Suiting.

The top coat is lined with two year guaranteed Rayon and warmly interlined. The shoulders are squared, the coat hangs slim and straight. The fitted jacket is lined with lustrous Rayon. Has four pockets, and an imitation leather belt. The skirt placket is Zip-closed and has two box pleats in the front. (Coat or Skirt not sold separately).

SIZES: 14-16-18-20-22.
TO FIT BUST: 32-34-36-38-40 in.

LENGTH Topcoat 44 inches.
State bust measure. Shpg. wt., ea., 8 lbs.

CHECKED SUITING (Large View)
Rayon Taffeta Lining

17 K 8910—Navy Blue.
17 K 8911—Oxford Gray.
17 K 8912—Dark Brown

13.98

ALL WOOL Nubbed Suiting
(Small View)
Earl-glo Rayon Satin Lining

17 K 8915—Copper Wine *536*.
17 K 8916—Navy Blue. . . . .

19.98

These suits are sent direct from New York to you . . . you pay postage only from our nearest Mail Order House.

Numbers after Color names refer to Sears COLOR-GRAPH following index pages in back of book.

SEARS * PAGE 21

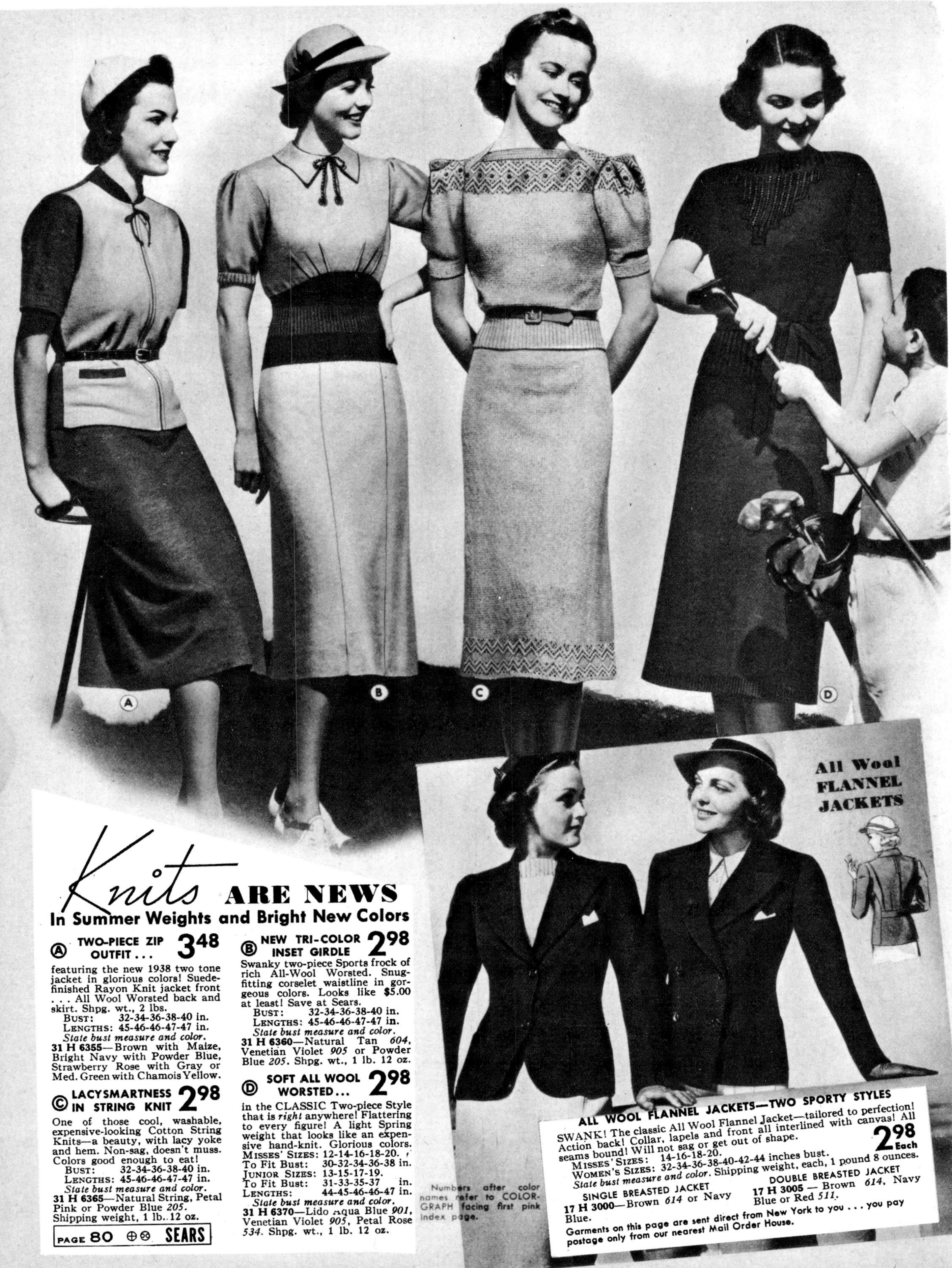
A
B
C
D
All Wool
FLANNEL
JACKETS
Knits ARE NEWS
In Summer Weights and Bright New Colors
(A) TWO-PIECE ZIP OUTFIT . . . 3.48
featuring the new 1938 two tone jacket in glorious colors! Suede-finished Rayon Knit jacket front . . . All Wool Worsted back and skirt. Shpg. wt., 2 lbs.
BUST: 32-34-36-38-40 in.
LENGTHS: 45-46-46-47-47 in.
State bust measure and color.
31 H 6355—Brown with Maize, Bright Navy with Powder Blue, Strawberry Rose with Gray or Med. Green with Chamois Yellow.
(C) LACYSMARTNESS IN STRING KNIT 2.98
One of those cool, washable, expensive-looking Cotton String Knits—a beauty, with lacy yoke and hem. Non-sag, doesn't muss. Colors good enough to eat!
BUST: 32-34-36-38-40 in.
LENGTHS: 45-46-46-47-47 in.
State bust measure and color.
31 H 6365—Natural String, Petal Pink or Powder Blue 205.
Shipping weight, 1 lb. 12 oz.
PAGE 80 SEARS
(B) NEW TRI-COLOR INSET GIRDLE 2.98
Swanky two-piece Sports frock of rich All-Wool Worsted. Snug-fitting corselet waistline in gorgeous colors. Looks like $5.00 at least! Save at Sears.
BUST: 32-34-36-38-40 in.
LENGTHS: 45-46-46-47-47 in.
State bust measure and color.
31 H 6360—Natural Tan 604, Venetian Violet 905 or Powder Blue 205. Shpg. wt., 1 lb. 12 oz.
(D) SOFT ALL WOOL WORSTED . . . 2.98
in the CLASSIC Two-piece Style that is right anywhere! Flattering to every figure! A light Spring weight that looks like an expensive hand-knit. Glorious colors.
MISSES' SIZES: 12-14-16-18-20.
To Fit Bust: 30-32-34-36-38 in.
JUNIOR SIZES: 13-15-17-19.
To Fit Bust: 31-33-35-37 in.
LENGTHS: 44-45-46-46-47 in.
State bust measure and color.
31 H 6370—Lido Aqua Blue 901, Venetian Violet 905, Petal Rose 534. Shpg. wt., 1 lb. 12 oz.
Numbers after color names refer to COLOR-GRAPH facing first pink index page.
ALL WOOL FLANNEL JACKETS—TWO SPORTY STYLES
SWANK! The classic All Wool Flannel Jacket—tailored to perfection! Action back! Collar, lapels and front all interlined with canvas! All seams bound! Will not sag or get out of shape.
2.98 Each
MISSES' SIZES: 14-16-18-20.
WOMEN'S SIZES: 32-34-36-38-40-42-44 inches bust.
State bust measure and color. Shipping weight, each, 1 pound 8 ounces.
SINGLE BREASTED JACKET
17 H 3000—Brown 614 or Navy Blue.
DOUBLE BREASTED JACKET
17 H 3005 — Brown 614, Navy Blue or Red 511.
Garments on this page are sent direct from New York to you . . . you pay postage only from our nearest Mail Order House.

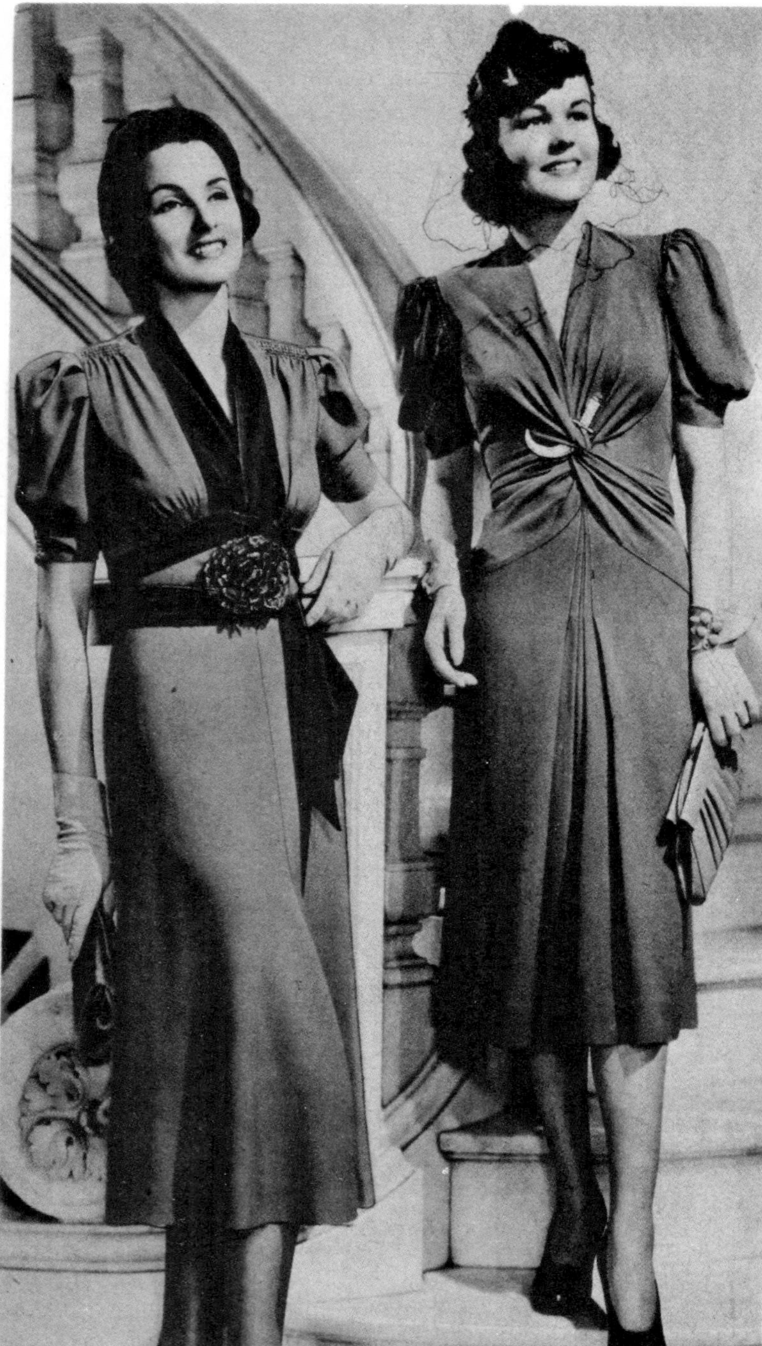

Fashion's Highest Honors Go to These Adaptations of

THE VIONNET DRAPE

3.98 Featuring two of the season's "top" fashions: the lovely Vionnet draped bust line—and glorious two-tone color contrast! Inspired by a famous French designer, especially famous for her deftness in draping materials to the body! In this—the darker color sash flows down from the neck—crosses under bosom to back—and ties at side in a superb cascade of color! Beautiful . . . in keeping with the fine DeLuxe Celanese Rayon Pebble Crepe! Deep-toned double flower! An unusual value at this economy price!
SIZES: 14-16-18-20-22.
BUST: 32-34-36-38-40 inches.
LENGTHS: 45-46-46-47-47 inches.
State bust measure and color.
31 H 6270—Venetian Violet *905* with Purple, Powder Blue *205* with Navy or Navy with Powder Blue.
Shipping weight, 1 lb. 4 oz.

4.98 One of the most important dresses of this season! The Vionnet draped line does simply grand things to your figure: gives you that slim look about the waist and hips, with a delicately up-curving line about the bosom! Notice how the cloth is twisted and draped at the "midriff"—with one enormous glittering scimitar pin for dramatic contrast. All of it—including the half-sash that buckles in the back and self covered buttons—is DeLuxe Celanese Rayon Pebble Crepe. Looks every cent of twice its low price!
SIZES: 14-16-18-20-22.
BUST: 32-34-36-38-40 inches.
LENGTHS: 45-46-46-47-47 inches.
State bust measure and color.
31 H 6265—Venetian Violet *905*, Adriatic Green *906*, Chinese Peacock *228* or Cliquot Beige *637*.
Shipping weight, 1 lb. 4 oz.

These dresses sent direct from New York . . . you pay postage only from our nearest Mail Order House.

Numbers after color names refer to COLOR-GRAPH facing first pink index page.

DARK WITH LIGHT
is Fashion Right

3.98

CHIC AND COOL!

Ultra-Smart Embroidered Rayon Marquisette . . . in the new *dark* background that is so popular for summer! Embroidered with white threads for contrast! Made crisp and full, with *double* organdy collar (white underneath) and puff sleeves trimmed with organdy. Rustling Rayon Taffeta slip included—*dark*, of course, to match the dress! All this glory for the low price of only $3.98!
SIZES: 14-16-18-20-22.
BUST: 32-34-36-38-40 inches.
LENGTHS: 45-46-46-47-47 inches.
State bust measure and color.
31 H 6275—Wine, Black or Navy.
Shipping weight, 1 lb. 6 oz.

3.98

RIC RAC TRIM IS NEW!

Look twice at this dress—for it's well on its way to being a big summer success! It features a *dark* color fabric "striped" with *white* Ric Rac braid from top to bottom! *Very* new and *very* slenderizing! Fabric is the big summer hit, SUN-SHAN . . . the stunning spun rayon in shantung effect that washes so beautifully! Detachable cuffs, collar-and-bib of white Cotton Pique. Real value!
SIZES: 14-16-18-20-22.
BUST: 32-34-36-38-40 inches.
LENGTHS: 45-46-46-47-47 inches.
State bust measure and color.
31 H 6280—Black or Navy.
Shipping weight, 1 lb. 4 oz.

TAKE A SEARS BASIC "Many-Way" DRESS

CHANGE ACCESSORIES!

..You have a different dress for every day in the week!

"SEARS FOR THE RIGHT ACCESSORY"
You always get the Most For Your Money
MOST VALUE . . . MOST STYLE

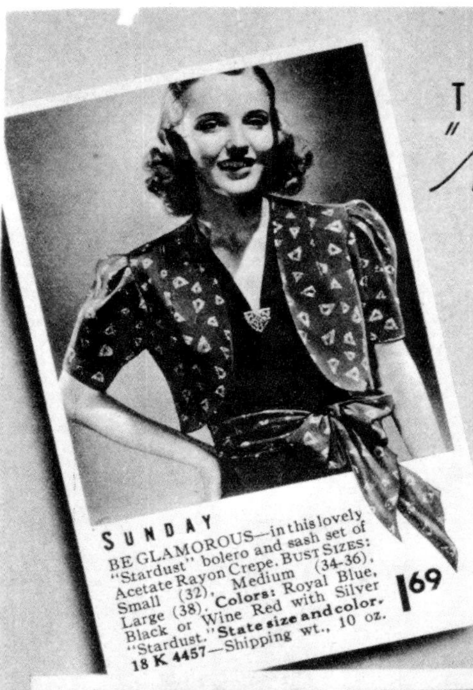

SUNDAY
BE GLAMOROUS—in this lovely "Stardust" bolero and sash set of Acetate Rayon Crepe. BUST SIZES: Small (32), Medium (34-36), Large (38). **Colors:** Royal Blue, Black or Wine Red with Silver "Stardust." **State size and color.**
18 K 4457—Shipping wt., 10 oz. 1.69

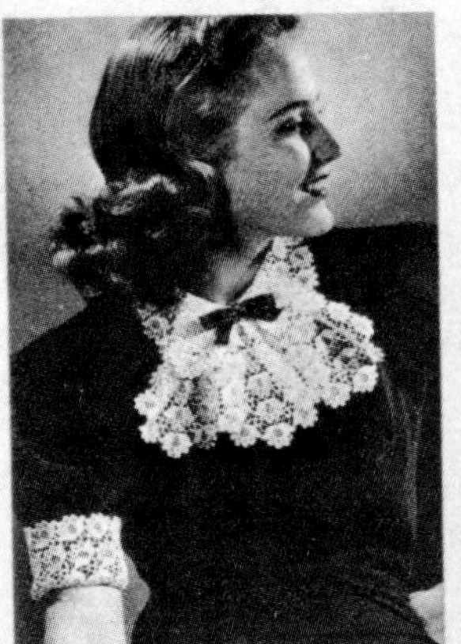

MONDAY
BE PERT AND GAY in this young-looking collar and cuff set of embroidered Venise type lace. Frilly jabot at the front caught by a small black ribbon bow. Bewitching on a simple dress! Easy to launder. **Colors:** White or Ecru.
State color.
18 K 4458—Shipping weight, 5 ounces. 59c

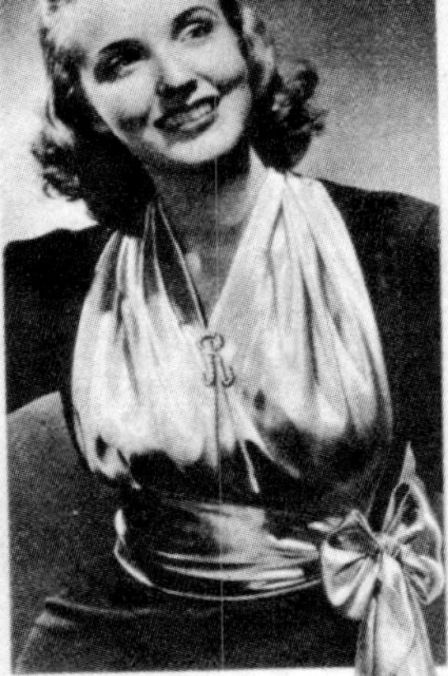

TUESDAY
BE STRIKING—genuine "Topette". State rhinestone initial wanted.
18 K 4459—In Celanese Rayon Satin. **Colors:** Gold or White.
18 K 4490—In Rayon Crepe. **Colors:** Rust *617*, Green *321* or Norse Blue *911*. Shpg. wt., ea., 8 oz. EACH 94c

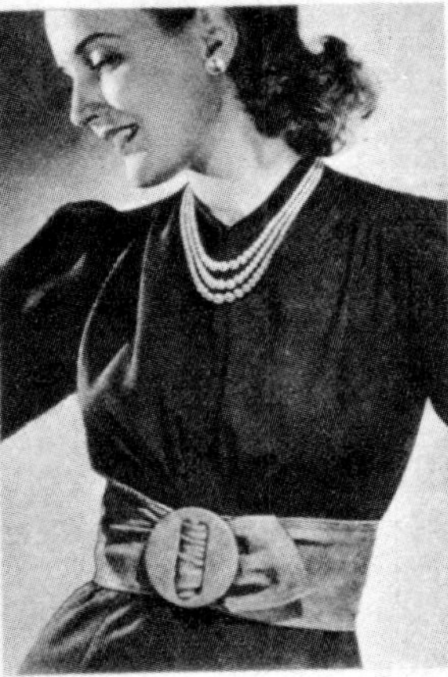

WEDNESDAY
BE SOPHISTICATED—
18 K 2103—Belt. Genuine Suede; 4-in. wide. WAIST SIZES: 26 to 36. **Colors:** Black or Copper Brown *913*. Shpg. wt., 5 oz. 94c
4 K 3809—Pearl Necklace (Simulated). 3-strand. **Color:** White. Shipping wt., 5 oz. 59c
4 K 3810—Pearl Earrings (Simulated). Screw style. **Color:** White. Shpg. wt., 3 oz.... 59c

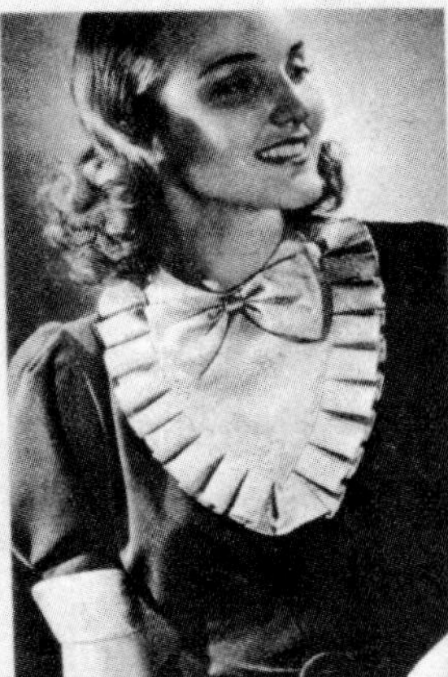

THURSDAY
BE THRILLINGLY FEMININE—in this collar and cuff set of embossed Rayon Satin. Gorgeous metal brocade effect. **Colors:** Gold or Silver.
18 K 4460—State color. Shipping weight, 6 oz. 59c SET

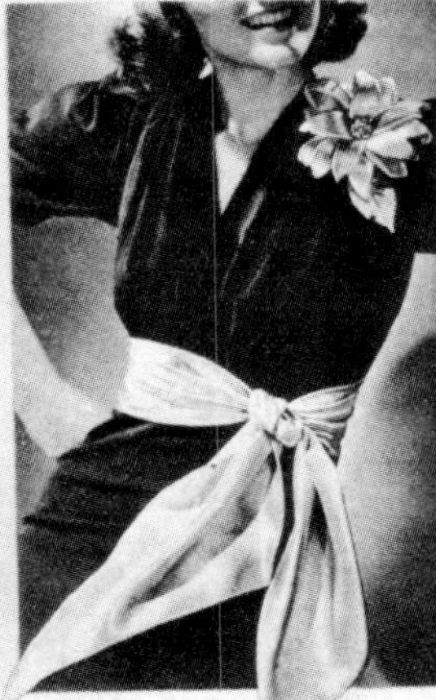

FRIDAY
BE STUNNING—in a flower and sash set of lustrous Celanese Panné Satin (Rayon). Sash measures 8 x 56 in. **Colors:** Gold, Red *530* or Green *321*.
18 K 4461—State color. Shipping weight 6 oz. 79c

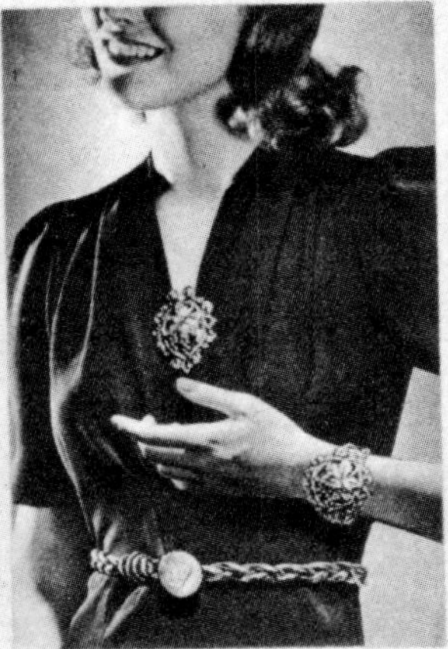

SATURDAY
BE A GOLDEN GIRL in gold colored belt, metal bracelet and clip.
18 K 2104 — Belt. Braided belt material. SIZES: 26 to 36 in. waist.
4 K 3504—Bracelet.
4 K 3503—Clip to match. Shipping wt., each, 4 oz. 59c EACH

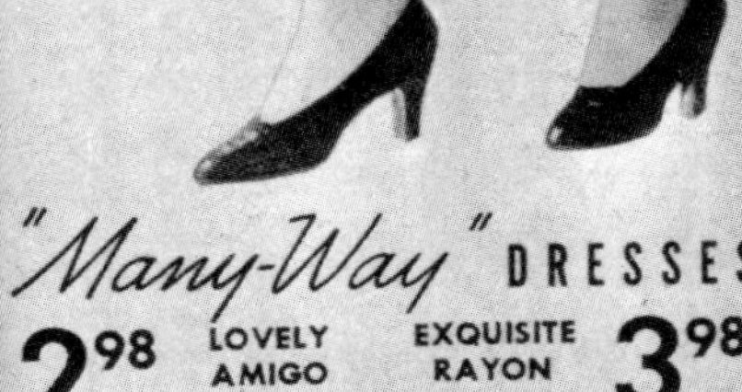

"Many-Way" DRESSES

2.98 LOVELY AMIGO CREPE

Ⓐ A beautifully styled "Many-Way" basic dress of superior quality Satin-back CREPE AMIGO in Celanese Rayon. Notice the rich-looking shirring at the shoulders—the tucks that drape the waistline so gracefully—the five gore skirt front—the puffed, short sleeves—and Crown Zip placket! All go to make this an exceptional basic dress. Convertible high-low neckline. SIZES: 14 to 22 (see table below). **Colors:** Black or Navy Blue. **State size and color.**
18 K 4455—Shipping weight, 1 lb. 2 oz.

EXQUISITE RAYON ALPACA 3.98

Ⓑ An unusually fine material, plus expert workmanship! Of Celanese Rayon Alpaca, a flat, basket-weave that falls softly, wears splendidly. Lastex cuffs fit snugly above or below the elbow. Skirt flares with 5 gores in back as well as in front. Graceful shirring at the shoulder and sleeve-tops. Crown Zip placket. Convertible high or low neckline. SIZES: 14 to 44 (see table below). **Colors:** Black or Navy Blue. **State size and color.**
18 K 4456—Shipping weight, 1 lb. 5 oz.

SIZE:	14	16	18	20	22	42	44	
BUST:	32	34	36	38	40	42	44	inches
LENGTHS:	45	46	46	47	47	48	48	inches

Numbers after Color names refer to Sears COLORGRAPH following index pages in back of book.

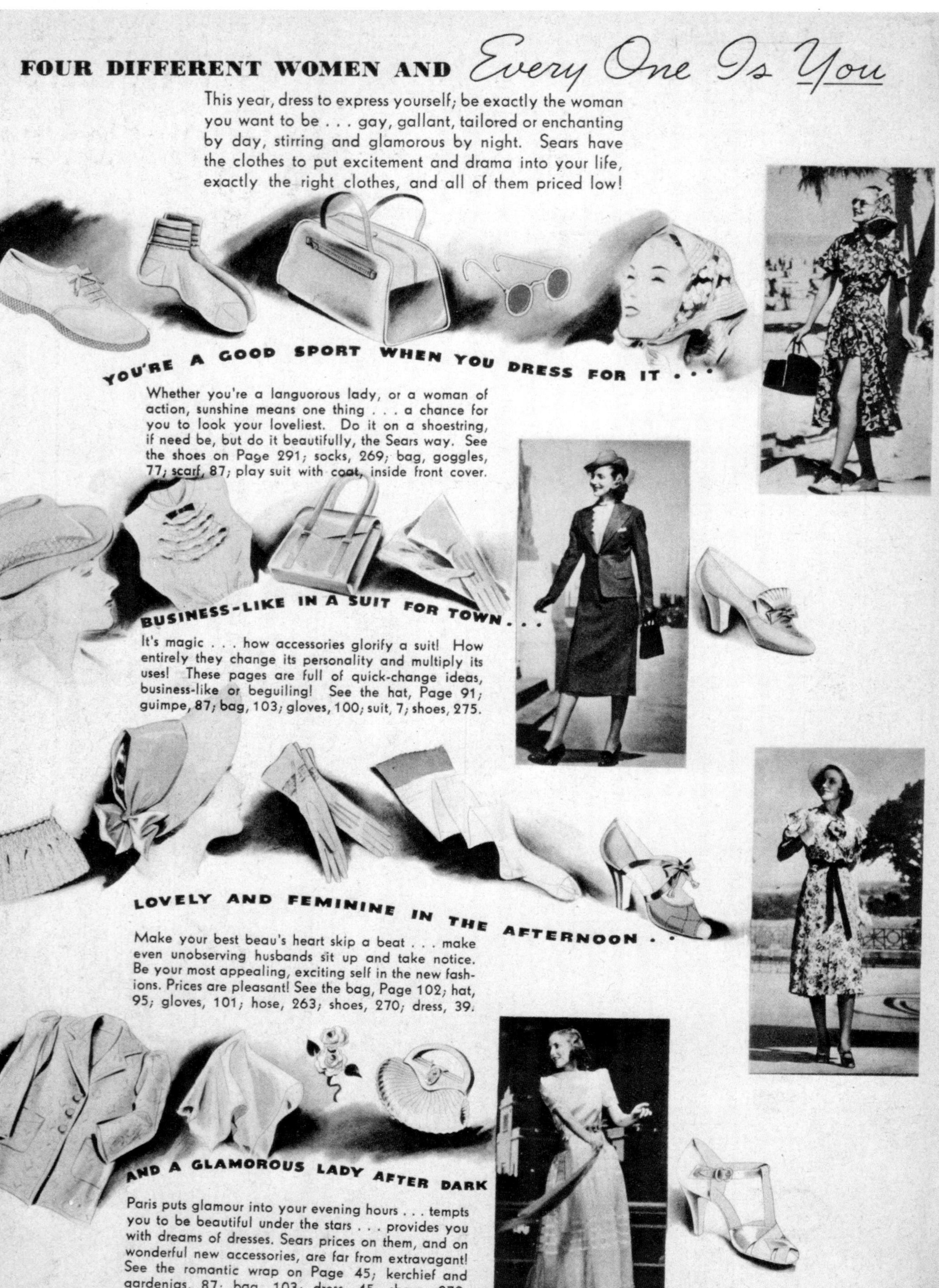
FOUR DIFFERENT WOMEN AND Every One Is You
This year, dress to express yourself; be exactly the woman you want to be . . . gay, gallant, tailored or enchanting by day, stirring and glamorous by night. Sears have the clothes to put excitement and drama into your life, exactly the right clothes, and all of them priced low!
YOU'RE A GOOD SPORT WHEN YOU DRESS FOR IT . . .
Whether you're a languorous lady, or a woman of action, sunshine means one thing . . . a chance for you to look your loveliest. Do it on a shoestring, if need be, but do it beautifully, the Sears way. See the shoes on Page 291; socks, 269; bag, goggles, 77; scarf, 87; play suit with coat, inside front cover.
BUSINESS-LIKE IN A SUIT FOR TOWN . . .
It's magic . . . how accessories glorify a suit! How entirely they change its personality and multiply its uses! These pages are full of quick-change ideas, business-like or beguiling! See the hat, Page 91; guimpe, 87; bag, 103; gloves, 100; suit, 7; shoes, 275.
LOVELY AND FEMININE IN THE AFTERNOON . .
Make your best beau's heart skip a beat . . . make even unobserving husbands sit up and take notice. Be your most appealing, exciting self in the new fashions. Prices are pleasant! See the bag, Page 102; hat, 95; gloves, 101; hose, 263; shoes, 270; dress, 39.
AND A GLAMOROUS LADY AFTER DARK
Paris puts glamour into your evening hours . . . tempts you to be beautiful under the stars . . . provides you with dreams of dresses. Sears prices on them, and on wonderful new accessories, are far from extravagant! See the romantic wrap on Page 45; kerchief and gardenias, 87; bag, 103; dress, 45; shoes, 270.
SEARS PAGE 21

WEAR OR GIVE A "Personal" SCARF

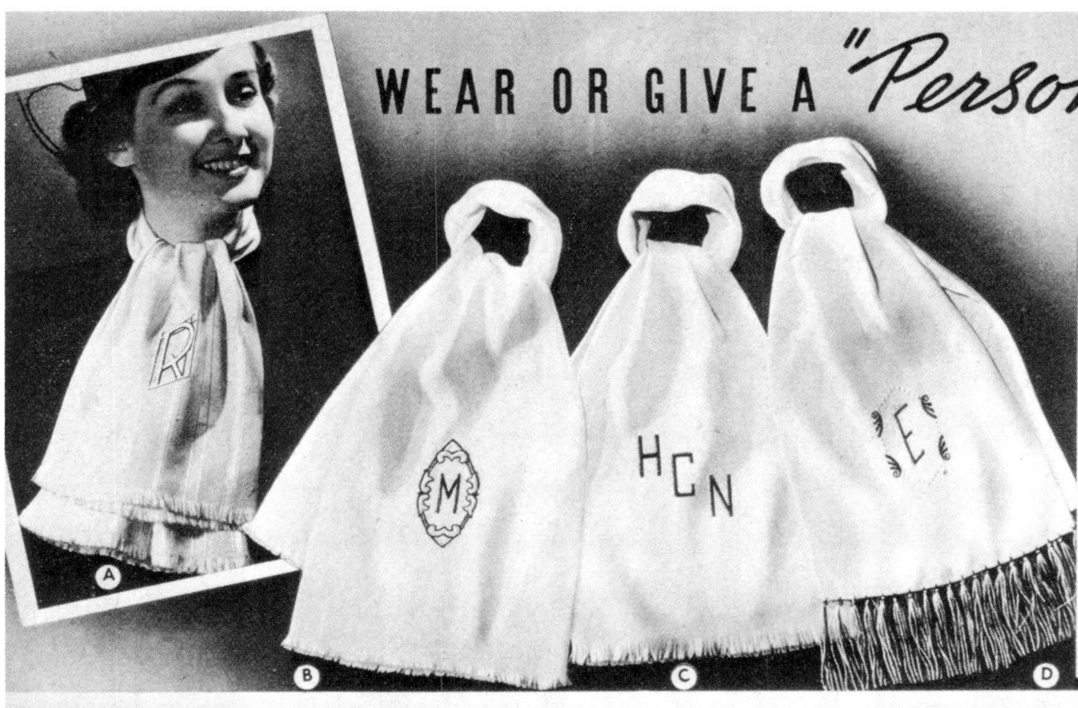

SMARTLY INITIALED! CORRECT FOR EVERY AGE AND COSTUME!

All scarfs in white only with black embroidered initials. Scarfs A, B and D come with all initials except I, O, Q, U, V, X, Y and Z. **Print initial.**

OUR FINEST SILK CREPE SCARF
(A) Exquisite, satin-striped double Silk, weighted. Size, 9 x 42 in. **Print initial.** 1.00
18 K 4384—Shipping wt., 9 oz.

SILK CREPE (weighted)
(B) Special value. Doubled. Size, 9 x 42 in. **Print initial.** 47c
18 K 4385—Shpg. wt., 7 oz.

WITH EVERY INITIAL
(C) Fine quality weighted silk crepe. Tubular. Initialed to your order in one, two or three letters. Allow 5 days for initialing. Size, 9 x 42 in. 85c
18 K 4386—Shipping wt., 7 oz.

KNOTTED FRINGE EDGE
(D) Silk crepe (weighted). Hand-knotted fringe. Tubular. Size, 9x47 in. **Print initial.** 59c
18 K 4345—Shipping wt., 7 oz.

Numbers after Color names refer to Sears COLOR-GRAPH following index pages in back of book.

SAVE ON SQUARES!

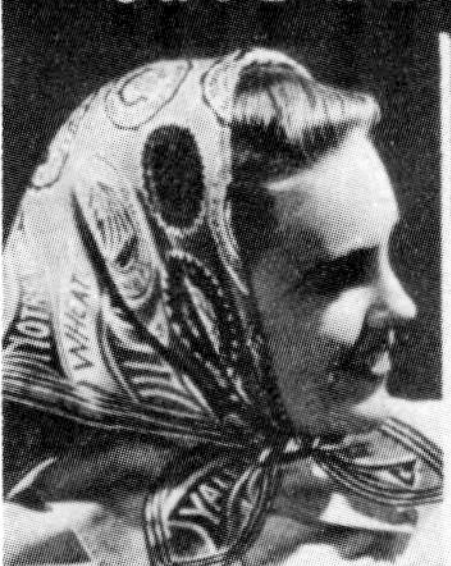

49c CAMPUS SQUARE

Many college pennants on this gorgeous Silk Satin (weighted) square! Rolled edges. Wear it on your head or as a neckerchief. 23 inches square.
Background Colors: Red, Brown or Green. **State color.**
18 K 4388—Shipping weight, 4 ounces.

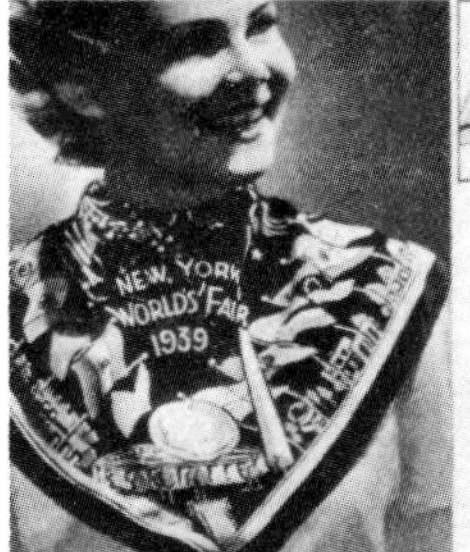

25c WORLD'S FAIR

1938 fashion with a 1939 pattern! Flags of the coming New York World's Fair printed on this lovely Rayon square. Gay and colorful! Picot edges. 19 inches square.
Background Colors: Red, Brown or Navy Blue. **State color.**
18 K 4389—Shpg. wt., 4 ounces.

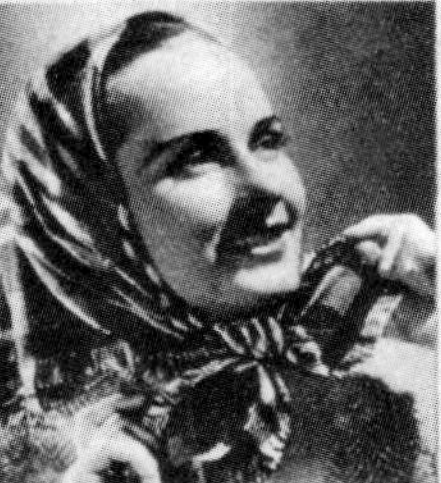

45c SHEER WOOL

Sheer, all wool square that can be worn as a scarf or a head-kerchief. Scotch-type plaid check design. Self-fringed edges. 24 inches square.
Colors: Brown with Orange or Red with Navy Blue. **State color.**
18 K 4390—Shpg. wt., 6 ounces.

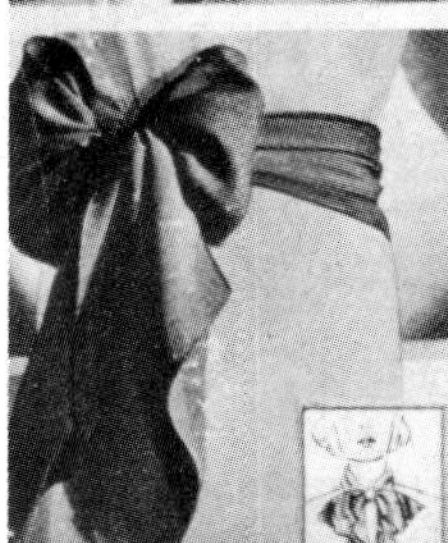

SCARF OR SASH
25c Roman Striped or Solid Color. In lovely rayon. Measures 62 x 6½ inches.
18 K 4391—Multi-color Roman Stripes only.
18 K 4392—Solid color.
Colors: Green *321*, Red *508* or Royal Blue *218*. **State color.**
Shpg. wt., ea., 5 oz.

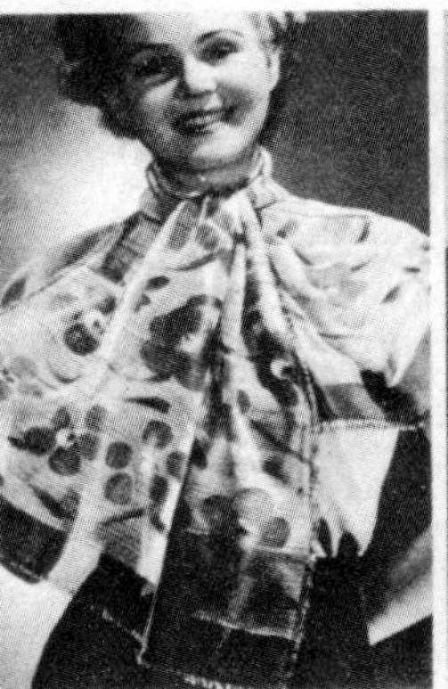

STUNNING PRINT OR SOLID COLORS
Long silk Chiffon Scarfs.

FLORAL PRINT
18 K 4393—**Border Colors:** Navy Blue, Brown or Wine. Size: 19 x 46½ inches. **State color.** 98c

SOLID COLOR
18 K 4318—**Colors:** Royal Blue *212*, Green *311*, Red *511* or White... 49c
Size: 15½ x 53 in.
Shipping wt., each, 6 oz.

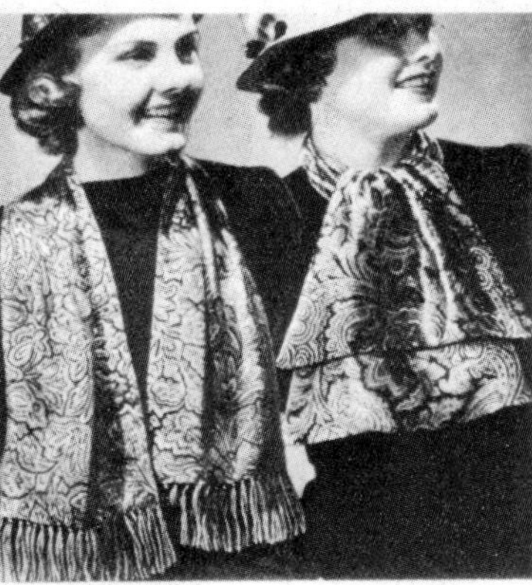

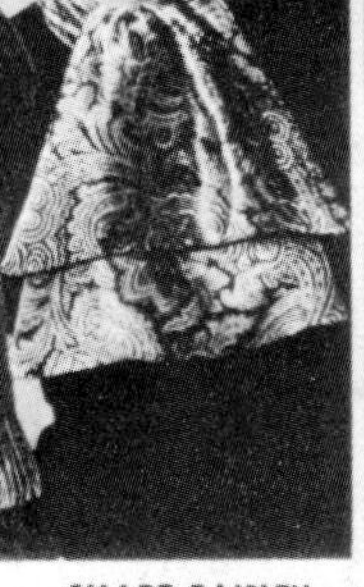

FRINGED PAISLEY TUBULAR
98c All silk weighted satin. Rich jewel-like colors in Oriental pattern. Knotted fringed edges. Tubular style—wear it tied also!
Background Colors: Brown, Wine or Royal Blue. **State color.** Size: 46 x 9 in.
18 K 4394—Shipping weight, 9 oz.

SMART PAISLEY ASCOT
89c Richly colored Paisley scarf, in popular ascot style, gorgeous Rayon Satin, lined with weighted silk crepe.
Size: 37½ x 10½.
Background Colors: Brown, Royal Blue or Lustrous Black. **State color.**
18 K 4395—Shipping weight, 7 ounces.

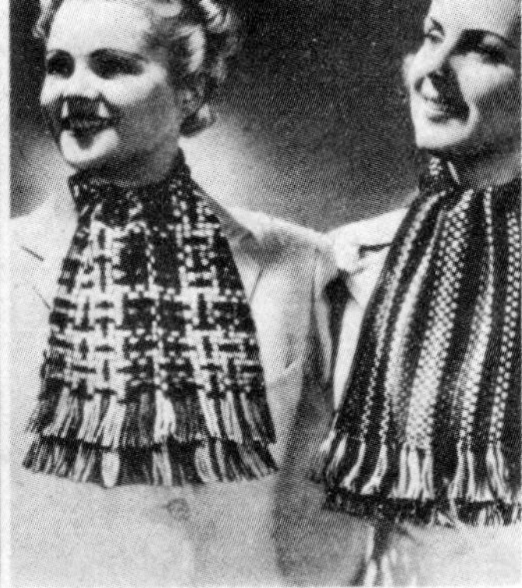

ALL WOOL GAY PLAID
29c Brightly colored all wool worsted scarf. Self-fringed edge. A thrilling value, a grand gift!
Size: 10 x 45 in.
Plaid Colors: Navy Blue, Red, Brown or Green. **State color.**
18 K 4396—Shpg. wt., 7 oz.

KNOTTED WOOL FRINGE
59c Soft all Zephyr wool. Hand-knotted fringe. Multi-colored.
Size: 10 x 45 in.
Background Colors: Royal Blue, Red, Brown or Solid White. **State color.**
18 K 4397—Shpg. weight, 7 oz.

WEAR THE V-scarf
REG. U.S. PAT. OFF.

Many Different Ways

95c It's the cleverest scarf in years! No end to the number of ways you'll wear it! Pictures below show a few ideas, you'll discover more. Brightens the whole dress front. Smart print design in weighted silk satin. Hemmed edges. "V" length, 62 in. x 8 in.
Colors: Brilliant stripes with background of Navy Blue, Bright Green, or Red. **State color.**
18 K 4398—Shpg. wt., 6 oz.

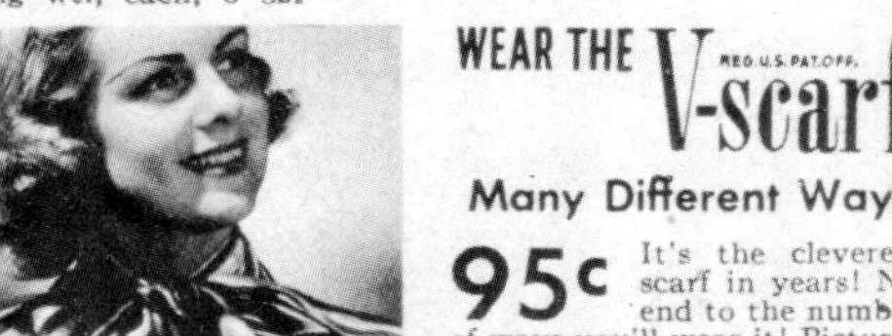

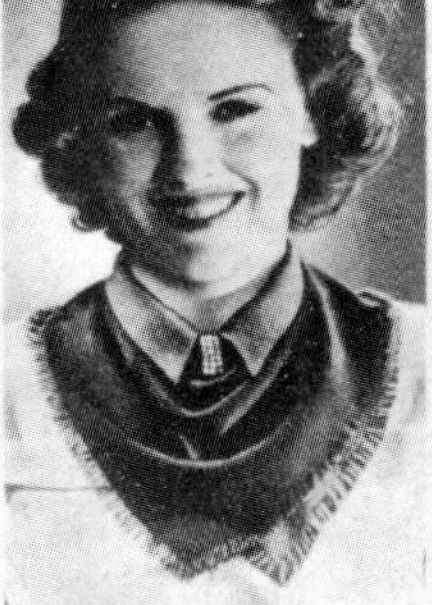

25c Reversible two tone scarf of Rayon Crepe.
Size: 24 x 16¾ in.
Colors: Red with Navy or Brown with Rust. **State color.**
18 K 4399—Shipping weight, 5 ounces.

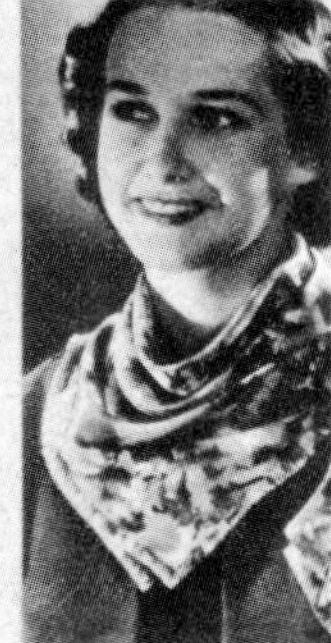

39c Scarf and Hanky Set of Rayon. Batik pattern.
Scarf Size: 19 in. square.
Backgrounds of Red or Brown.
18 K 4383—Shpg. weight, 5 ounces.

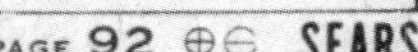

SEARS

Finest Styles

THESE TWO HAVE HAND BAGS IN COLORS TO MATCH

- NEWEST FASHIONS
- QUALITY MATERIALS
- FINE WORKMANSHIP
- CHOICE OF A, B, C, D WIDTHS

HANDBAGS $1.95 EACH

SHOES ON THIS PAGE $2.98 PAIR

Ⓛ *Flattering Shoe*

Slenderizing, for it's low cut on one side. Fine materials, and fine fit. Peek toes. Leather soles. 2-inch Cuban heel.

Women's Sizes 5, 5½, 6, 6½, 7, 7½, 8, 8½, 9 in A width (very narrow) and B width (narrow). **Sizes** 3½, 4, 4½, 5, 5½, 6, 6½, 7, 7½, 8, 8½, 9 in C width (medium) and D width (medium wide). **State size and width.** Shipping weight, 1 pound 4 ounces.

15K2833–Brown Copper Calfskin.
15K2834–Canberry Red Calfskin.
15K2835–Black Patent. Pr. **$2.98**

Ⓜ **THE BAG:** Stunning top handle style. **Colors:** Brown Copper or Cranberry Red in Calf leather or Black in Patent leather. **Size:** 11x 7¼ inches. Shipping weight, 1 pound 6 ounces.

18 K 3480—**State color**.... **$1.95**

Ⓝ *Sides Swing Low*

Shows all the exquisite workmanship that went into it. Leather sole. 2-inch Cuban heel.

Women's Sizes 5, 5½, 6, 6½, 7, 7½, 8, 8½, 9 in A width (very narrow) and B width (narrow). **Sizes** 3½, 4, 4½, 5, 5½, 6, 6½, 7, 7½, 8, 8½, 9 in C width (medium) and D width (medium wide). **State size and width.** Shpg. wt., 1 lb. 4 oz.

15 K 2905—Black Suede.
15 K 2903—Brown Copper Calf.
15 K 2904—Navy Blue Calf.
Pair.......................... **$2.98**

Ⓟ **THE BAG:** Beautiful stitched quilted effect. Top zip style. **Colors:** Brown Copper or Navy Blue in Calf leather, or Black in Suede leather. **Size:** 9½x8¼ inches. Shpg. wt., 1 lb. 3 oz.

18 K 3481—**State color**... **$1.95**

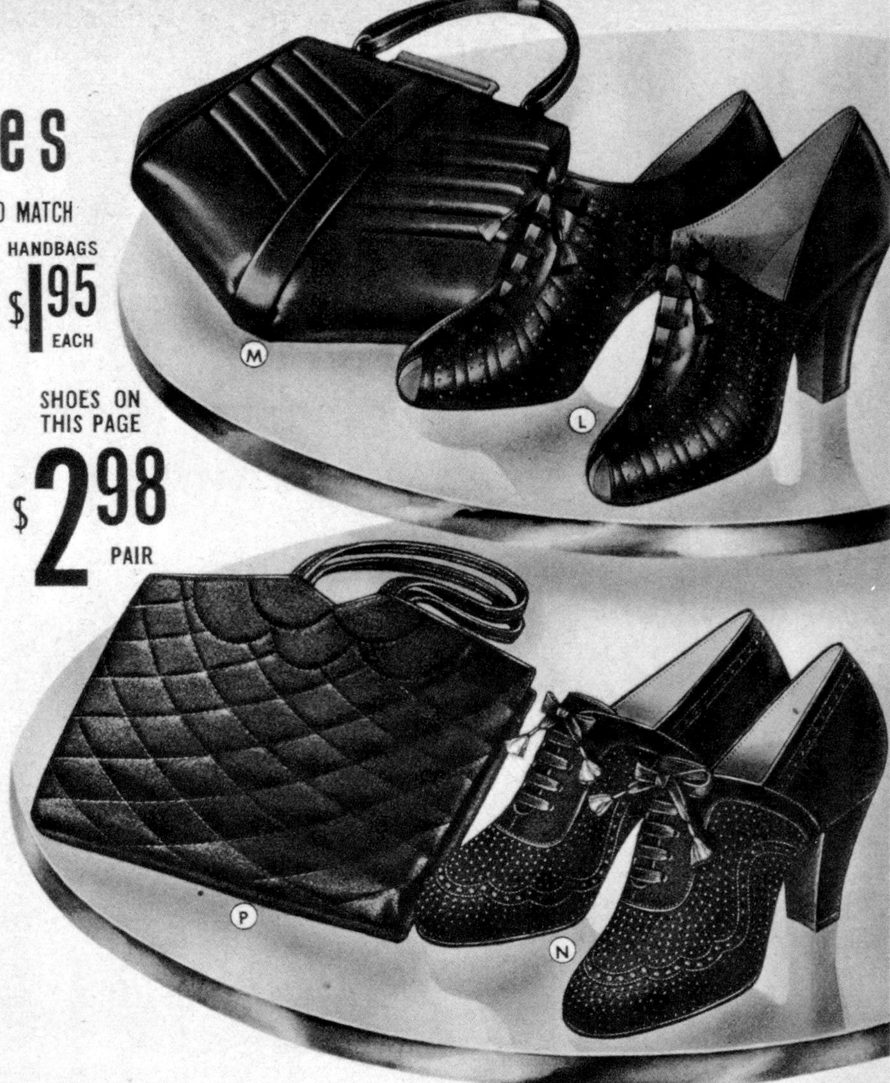

..And These Three "Step Out" Alone

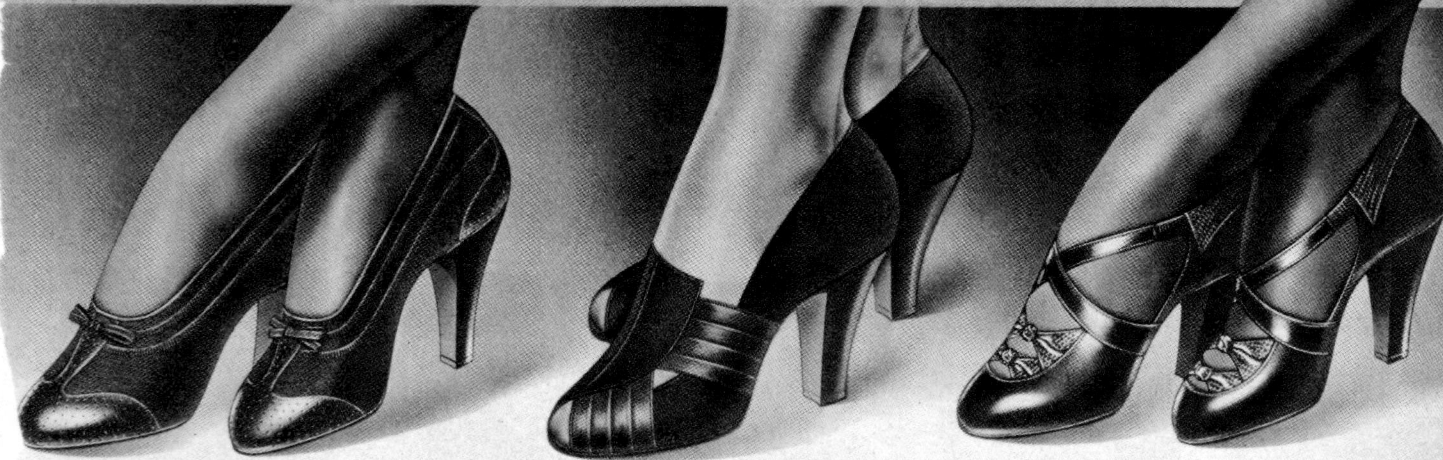

Shoes Have Braid and Fancy Bows

Braided and finished off with little bows . . . this is perfect. A perfect fit, too. Excellent quality gabardine and calf, tricked out with perforations. Blue or black, both are pretty and well made. Leather sole. 2½-inch Spike heel.

Women's Sizes 5, 5½, 6, 6½, 7, 7½, 8, 8½, 9 in A width (very narrow) and B width (narrow). **Sizes** 3½, 4, 4½, 5, 5½, 6, 6½, 7, 7½, 8, 8½, 9 in C width (medium) and D width (medium wide). **State size and width.** Shipping weight, 1 pound 4 ounces.

15 K 2909—Black. 15 K 2908—Blue. Pr..... **$2.98**

Smart! New Softly Draped Side

For all its soft look (the mark of lovely material), this step-in fits splendidly. Snug side gores, open toes. Suede, fine leather trim. Leather sole. 2½-inch Spike heel.

Women's Sizes 5, 5½, 6, 6½, 7, 7½, 8, 8½, 9 in A width (very narrow) and B width (narrow). **Sizes** 3½, 4, 4½, 5, 5½, 6, 6½, 7, 7½, 8, 8½, 9 in C width (medium) and D width (medium wide). **State size and width.** Shipping weight, 1 lb. 4 oz.

15 K 2919—Desert Rust.
15 K 2920—Black. Pr................ **$2.98**

Wear a Smart Lizard Collar on Your Heel

Lizard grained leather for collar and vamp. Cross-straps give a high-arch effect like very expensive shoes. That's Sears beautiful workmanship for you! Glove-fit. Leather sole. 2¼-inch Continental heel.

Women's Sizes 5, 5½, 6, 6½, 7, 7½, 8, 8½, 9 in A width (very narrow) and B width (narrow). **Sizes** 3½, 4, 4½, 5, 5½, 6, 6½, 7, 7½, 8, 8½, 9 in C width (medium) and D width (medium wide). **State size and width.** Shpg. wt., 1 lb. 4 oz.

15 K 2911—Black Kidskin.
15 K 2910—Blue Kidskin.
15 K 2912—Black Patent. Pair...... **$2.98**

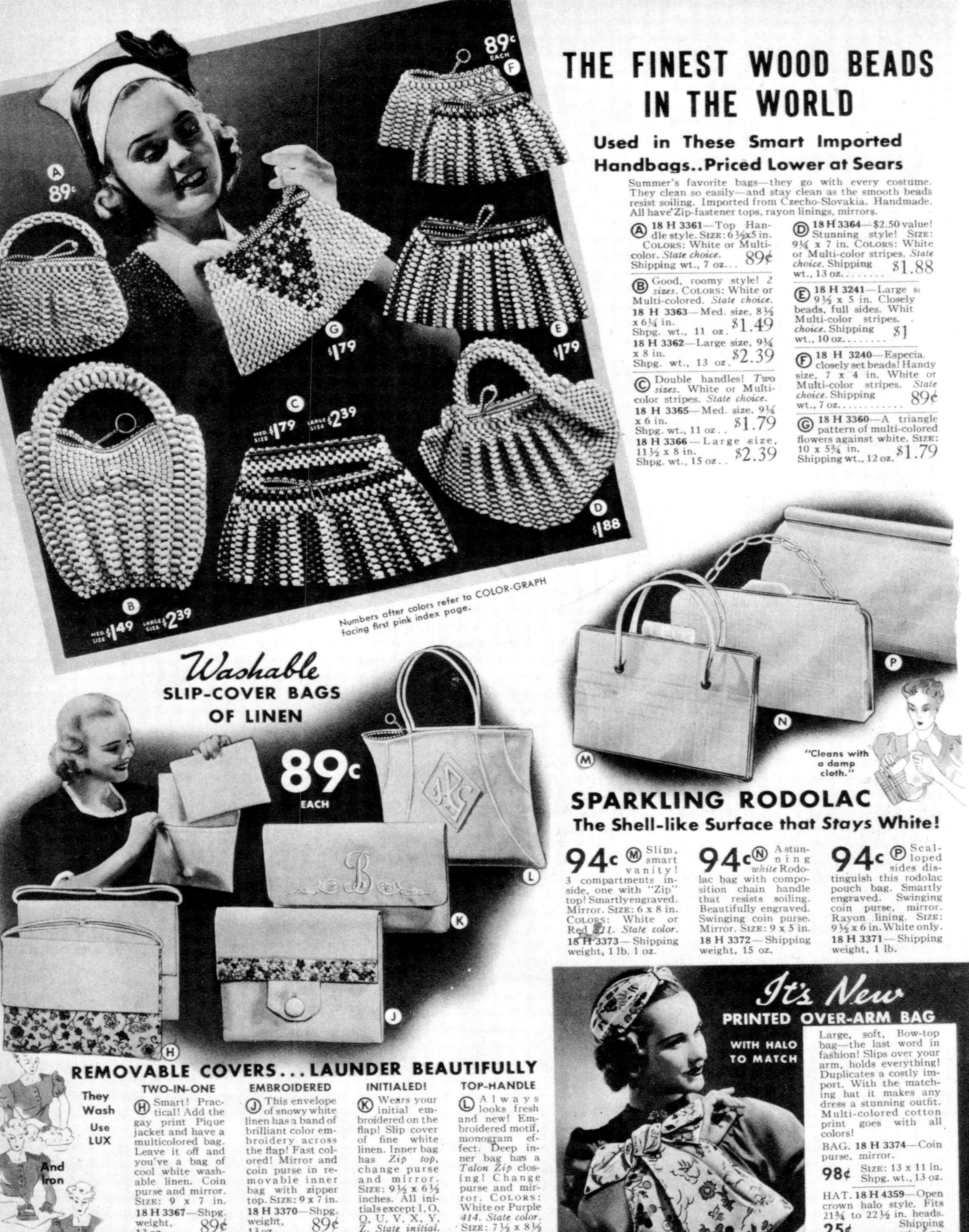
THE FINEST WOOD BEADS IN THE WORLD
Used in These Smart Imported Handbags..Priced Lower at Sears
Summer's favorite bags—they go with every costume. They clean so easily—and stay clean as the smooth beads resist soiling. Imported from Czecho-Slovakia. Handmade. All have Zip-fastener tops, rayon linings, mirrors.
(A) 18 H 3361—Top Handle style. SIZE: 6½x5 in. COLORS: White or Multi-color. State choice. Shipping wt., 7 oz... 89¢
(B) Good, roomy style! 2 sizes. COLORS: White or Multi-colored. State choice. 18 H 3363—Med. size, 8½ x 6¼ in. Shpg. wt., 11 oz. $1.49 18 H 3362—Large size, 9¼ x 8 in. Shpg. wt., 13 oz. $2.39
(C) Double handles! Two sizes. White or Multi-color stripes. State choice. 18 H 3365—Med. size, 9¼ x 6 in. Shpg. wt., 11 oz.. $1.79 18 H 3366—Large size, 11½ x 8 in. Shpg. wt., 15 oz.. $2.39
(D) 18 H 3364—$2.50 value! Stunning style! SIZE: 9¼ x 7 in. COLORS: White or Multi-color stripes. State choice. Shipping wt., 13 oz....... $1.88
(E) 18 H 3241—Large si 9½ x 5 in. Closely beads, full sides. Whit Multi-color stripes. choice. Shipping wt., 10 oz........ $1
(F) 18 H 3240—Especia. closely set beads! Handy size, 7 x 4 in. White or Multi-color stripes. State choice. Shipping wt., 7 oz........... 89¢
(G) 18 H 3360—A triangle pattern of multi-colored flowers against white. SIZE: 10 x 5¾ in. Shipping wt., 12 oz. $1.79
A 89c
B MED. SIZE $1.49 LARGE SIZE $2.39
C MED. SIZE $1.79 LARGE SIZE $2.39
D $1.88
E $1.79
F 89c EACH
G $1.79
Numbers after colors refer to COLOR-GRAPH facing first pink index page.
Washable SLIP-COVER BAGS OF LINEN
89c EACH
REMOVABLE COVERS...LAUNDER BEAUTIFULLY
They Wash Use LUX And Iron Like New
TWO-IN-ONE
(H) Smart! Practical! Add the gay print Pique jacket and have a multicolored bag. Leave it off and you've a bag of cool white washable linen. Coin purse and mirror. SIZE: 9 x 7 in. 18 H 3367—Shpg. weight, 13 oz...... 89¢
EMBROIDERED
(J) This envelope of snowy white linen has a band of brilliant color embroidery across the flap! Fast colored! Mirror and coin purse in removable inner bag with zipper top. SIZE: 9 x 7 in. 18 H 3370—Shpg. weight, 13 oz...... 89¢
INITIALED!
(K) Wears your initial embroidered on the flap! Slip cover of fine white linen. Inner bag has Zip top, change purse and mirror. SIZE: 9½ x 6½ inches. All initials except I, O, Q, U, V, X, Y, Z. State initial. 18 H 3369—Shpg. wt., 12 oz.... 89¢
TOP-HANDLE
(L) Always looks fresh and new! Embroidered motif, monogram effect. Deep inner bag has a Talon Zip closing! Change purse and mirror. COLORS: White or Purple 414. State color. SIZE: 7½ x 8½ inches. 18 H 3368—Shpg. wt., 12 oz.... 89¢
PAGE 102 SEARS
"Cleans with a damp cloth."
SPARKLING RODOLAC
The Shell-like Surface that Stays White!
94c (M) Slim, smart vanity! 3 compartments inside, one with "Zip" top! Smartly engraved. Mirror. SIZE: 6 x 8 in. COLORS: White or Red 211. State color. 18 H 3373—Shipping weight, 1 lb. 1 oz.
94c (N) A stunning white Rodolac bag with composition chain handle that resists soiling. Beautifully engraved. Swinging coin purse. Mirror. SIZE: 9 x 5 in. 18 H 3372—Shipping weight, 15 oz.
94c (P) Scalloped sides distinguish this rodolac pouch bag. Smartly engraved. Swinging coin purse, mirror. Rayon lining. SIZE: 9½ x 6 in. White only. 18 H 3371—Shipping weight, 1 lb.
It's New
PRINTED OVER-ARM BAG
WITH HALO TO MATCH
Large, soft, Bow-top bag—the last word in fashion! Slips over your arm, holds everything! Duplicates a costly import. With the matching hat it makes any dress a stunning outfit. Multi-colored cotton print goes with all colors!
BAG. 18 H 3374—Coin purse, mirror.
98¢ SIZE: 13 x 11 in. Shpg. wt., 13 oz.
HAT. 18 H 4359—Open crown halo style. Fits 21¾ to 22½ in. heads.
25¢ Shipping wt., 5 oz.

SAVE! SMARTER SWIM STYLES FOR LESS!

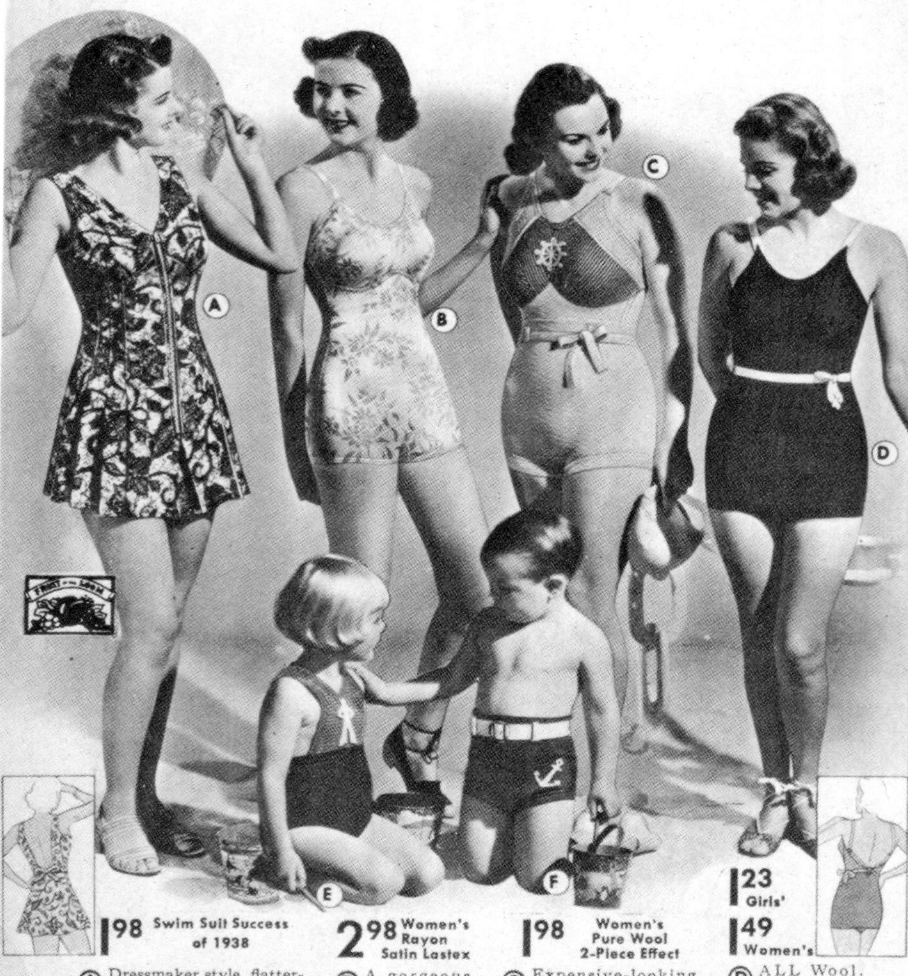

Worth ~~$5.00~~

Catalina LASTEX TRUNKS A Smash Hit!

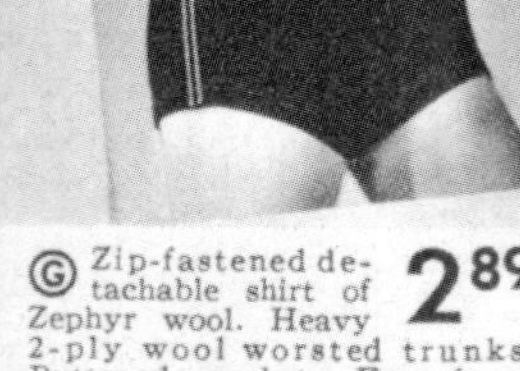

1.98 Swim Suit Success of 1938

(A) Dressmaker style, flattering to all figures. Quick-fastening, rustless Talon-Zip in front. Famous Fruit-of-the-Loom cotton in gorgeous, colorfast batik print. Skillfully made over a skin-snug, pantie lining of wool Jersey in protective matching dark color. Graceful pleated skirt. Sash ties. Same quality usually sells for $3.00 in exclusive shops. Women's Even Sizes: 32 to 42 in. bust.

PREDOMINATING COLORS: Wine or Dark Blue. *State size and color.*

18 H 5670 — Shpg. wt., 1 lb. 3 oz. $1.98

2.98 Women's Rayon Satin Lastex

(B) A gorgeous suit! Usually priced at $5.00 in smart shops! Shimmering Satin Lastex stretches crosswise for figure control. Woven of rayon, lastex and cotton. Skirtless style, with cotton lined front, deep sun back.

COLORS White ground with Royal Blue, Red or Black print. WOMEN'S EVEN SIZES: 32 to 40 in. bust. *State size and color.*

18 H 5641—Shipping weight, 1 lb. 1 oz. $2.98

1.98 Women's Pure Wool 2-Piece Effect

(C) Expensive-looking fancy stitch. Cotton lined from waist down.

18 H 1603 — Women's EVEN SIZES: 32 to 40 in. bust. COLORS: Jockey Red and White, Ocean Green and White, Navy Blue and White or Pink with Brown stripes. *State size and color.*

Shipping wt., 12 oz. $1.98

18 H 1703—Girls' EVEN AGE-SIZES: 8 to 16 years (26 to 34 in. bust). COLORS: Brown and Orange, Maroon and Gray or Royal Blue and White. *State size; color.*

$1.74 Shipping wt., 12 oz.

1.23 Girls' **1.49** Women's

(D) ALL Wool. Our famous classic "skirted" suit! Knit of all wool worsted. Shaped, lined bust. Moderate sun back.

State size; color.

18 H 1643—Women's Even Sizes: 34 to 42 in. bust. COLORS: Royal Blue, Jockey Red, Ocean Green or Black.

Shpg. wt. 12 oz.... $1.49

18 H 1713—Girls' Skirtless Suit. SIZES: 8 to 16 yrs. COLORS: French Blue, Jockey Red or Dark Green.

Shpg. wt. 8 oz..... $1.23

(E) Boys' or Girls' All Wool sun back suit. AGE-SIZES: 2, 4, 6 or 8 yrs. COLORS: Maroon with Red top, Royal with French Blue or Myrtle with Ocean Green. *State size and color.* **69c**

18 H 1554—Shipping wt., 4 oz.

(F) Warm, All Wool trunks permit healthful suntan. Colorful felt applique. AGE-SIZES: 2, 4, 6 or 8 yrs. COLORS: Navy Blue, Orange or dark Green. *State age size and color.* **54c**

18 H 1575—Shipping wt., 4 oz.

At Last!
STRAPLESS SWIM FOUNDATION
Easily Attached ← to Suit
GIRDLE 47c

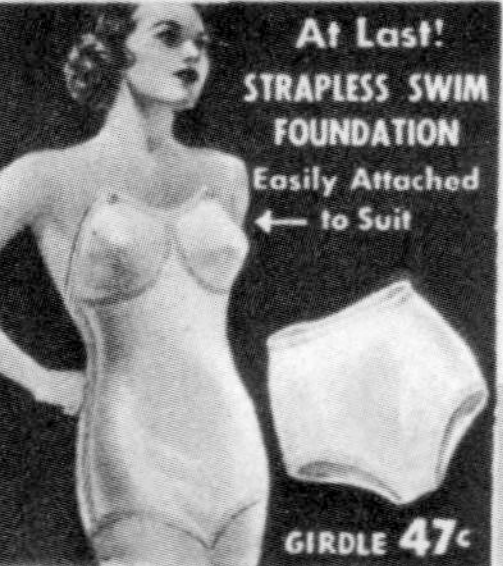

Wear a sheer suit with ease and confidence! Both in flesh color rubber. SIZES: Petite (26-28); SMALL (29-31); Medium (32-34); Regular (35-36 in. waist).

18 H 5654—Foundation. Shpg., wt., 10 oz. .... 89¢

18 H 1653 — Pantie Girdle. Shpg. wt., 7 oz. .... 47¢

PAGE 78 2 ⊕ ⊗

BEACH NECESSITIES

18 H 1679—Gay cotton mesh sandals with rubber soles and heels. COLORS: Multi-color or White. SIZES: 4 to 8; no half sizes. Shpg. wt. 17 oz. **49c** a pair

18 H 5681—All rubber with crepe effect rubber soles. COLORS: White, Red or Blue with multi-color toe trim. SIZES: 4 to 8; no half sizes. Shipping wt., 1 lb. **25c** a pair

18 H 1648—Patented Howland rubber cap. Keeps hair dry. COLORS: White or Turquoise Blue. SIZES: Small, Medium or Large. Shipping wt., 5 oz. **49c**

For Sun Glasses See Page 77

"Marcel" rubber caps. *State color.* **25c** each

18 H 1646—Women's size. COLORS: White, Black or Blonde.

18 H 1579 Child's size. White only. Shpg. wt., 4 oz.

(G) Zip-fastened detachable shirt of Zephyr wool. Heavy 2-ply wool worsted trunks. Buttoned pocket. Extra-brace elastic supporter. Lastex belt. **2.89**

MEN'S EVEN SIZES: 34 to 44 in. chest. COLORS: Navy Blue trunks with White top or Navy with Med. Blue. *State size; color.*

18 H 1811—Shipping wt., 1 lb. 4 oz. $2.89

(H) Famous CATALINA quality! Stretchable lastex makes them fit better, look better. Light weight, satin finish rayon, woven with lastex and cotton. Fine wool supporter. Belt. **2.95**

MEN'S EVEN SIZES: 28 to 38 in. waist. COLORS: Royal Blue, Maroon or Black. *State size and color.*

18 H 5806 — Shpg. wt., 1 lb. 2 oz.

(J) Athletic cut White Zephyr wool shirt, zip fastened to trunk. All wool worsted Navy Blue trunks with elastic supporter. Belt. **1.98** Men's

18 H 1310—Men's EVEN SIZES: 34 to 44 in. chest. *State size.* Shipping weight 11 oz..... $1.98

18 H 1405—Boys' Sizes: 28 to 34 in. chest. No supporter. *State size.* Shipping wt., 8 oz. Boys' $1.78

(K) Worth much more! Good all wool worsted; bar welt stitch! Simulated fly-front. Fine belt. COLORS: Navy Blue, Royal Blue or Maroon. *State size and color.* **1.00** Men's

18 H 1800—Men's EVEN SIZES: 28 to 40 in. waist. Has supporter. Shipping weight, 8 oz.

18 H 1901—Boys' Sizes: 22 to 30 in. waist. Shipping wt., 7 oz. Boys' 94c

(L) Stretchable Lastex! Woven with quick drying rayon and cotton—most perfect fitting fabric we've seen! In corded rib of enduring elasticity. Simulated fly front. Built-in supporter. **1.98**

MEN'S EVEN SIZES: 28 to 40 in. waist. COLORS: Royal Blue, Black or Gray. *State size; color.*

18 H 5804—Shipping wt., 1 lb. 1 oz.

STURDY 2-PLY WOOL
MEN'S AND BOYS' SIZES
$2.49 value! Worsted wool. Pocket. Elastic supporter.
1.69 Men's
COLORS: Navy Blue, Royal Blue or Gray. State size, color.
18 H 1801 — Men's Even Sizes: 28 to 40 in. waist. Shpg. wt., 11 oz.
18 H 1903 — Boys' Sizes: 24 to 30 in. waist. Shipping wt., 9 oz. $1.49

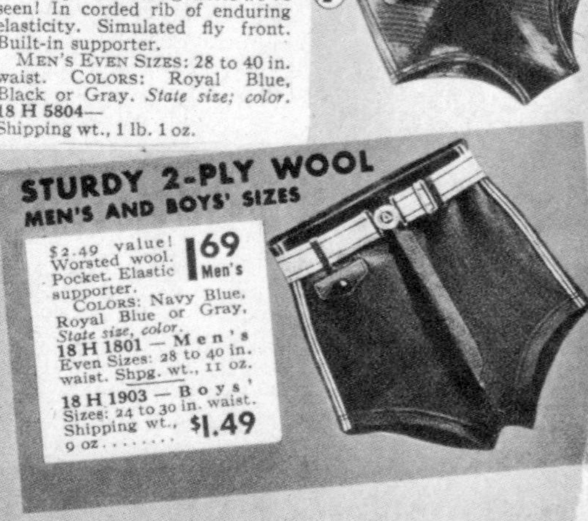

Vee Line SHIRTS AND SHORTS GIVE THAT STREAMLINE FIT

• They Hug Your Body Lines . . . S-T-R-E-T-C-H For Action . . . Snap Back and Stay in Shape

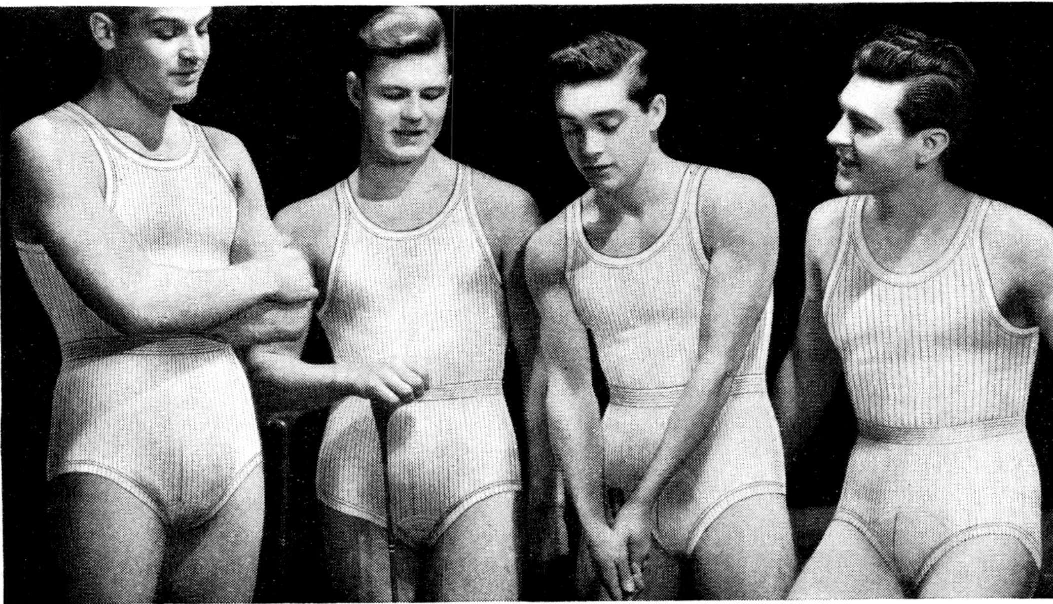

Wide lastex band in Top takes down stomach bulge..Gives you a new feeling of fitness and a real athlete's figure.

"Sta-Trim" SHORTS

47c EACH

The famous Swiss ribbed shorts with the deep Lastex top that keeps your waistline trim . . . supports abdominal muscles, makes you *look* fit and *feel* fit. Sta-Trims are supremely comfortable, yet give just enough restraint to promote better posture, and improved muscle tone. Fast becoming a favorite for sports and everyday wear. They're *combed* cotton—that's why they wear so long, feel so soft. Brief leg bottom bound with Lastex. Elastic binding at waist to keep it from curling down, to give extra comfort. Fly front.

COLOR: White. SIZES: Small (30–32); Medium (34–36); Large (38–40); Extra Large (42–44) inch waist. *State size.* Shipping weight, 5 ounces.

16 H 5202—Each.......... **47c**

REAL BARGAIN

15c EACH GARMENT

Lowest price for Swiss ribbed Vee Lines, the favorite shirts and shorts of men of action! Finely knit of good sturdy cotton yarns. Elastic waistband; ribbed hem on leg openings. Fly front.

16 H 5198—Shirts
16 H 5199—Shorts
Each. **15c** 4 for....... **57c**

COMBED COTTON

19c EACH GARMENT

For just a few pennies more you get combed cotton Vee Lines, which means only long fibered yarns are used. Swiss ribbed. Lastex waistband; ribbed hem on leg openings. Fly front.

16 H 5150—Shirts
16 H 5151—Shorts
Each. **19c** 4 for....... **72c**

EXTRA FINE

33c EACH GARMENT

Soft! Unusually smooth and comfortable against your body because it's *extra fine* combed cotton. Close rib knit. Finely tailored. Lastex waistband. Fly front. Double crotch.

16 H 5164—Shirts
16 H 5165—Shorts
Each. **33c** 3 for........ **95c**

FINE LISLE

39c EACH GARMENT

Say "lisle" and you're saying "a wonder for wear." Very finely ribbed knit of extra fine cotton lisle yarns, tailored to perfection. Extra soft, rich, smooth. Lastex waistband. Fly front. Double crotch.

16 H 5174—Shirts
16 H 5175—Shorts
Each garment........... **39c**

All above **SHORTS**—COLOR: White. SIZES: Small (30–32); Medium (34–36); Large (38–40) inch waist. *State size.*
All the above **SHIRTS**—COLOR: White. SIZES: Small (34–36); Medium (38–40); Large (42–44) inch chest. *State size.* All have tubular neck and armholes; bottoms shaped to go with brief-leg shorts. Shipping weight, each 3 ounces; 4 garments, 9 ounces.

"GOB" STYLE ALL PURPOSE SHIRT

IT'S AN UNDERSHIRT
IT'S AN OUTERSHIRT

FOR CAMPING – SPORTS – WORK

Here's the latest—the Gob-style shirt! It looks like a very smart sports shirt. Wear it as an outer-shirt for sports and for lounging, or as an undershirt—it's practical, correct, either way. Flat knit, so it's cool, doesn't cling. Loose fitting—good summer weight . . . with round neck and short sleeves. Choice of good quality cotton or better looking, long wearing *combed* cotton. For all around comfort, try Gob-style shirts.

COLOR: White. EVEN SIZES: 34 to 46-inch chest. *State size.* Shipping weight, each, 4 ounces.

Good Quality Cotton 24c Each
16 H 5204—Sturdy dependable cotton.

Combed Cotton 33c Each
16 H 5206—Softer; longer wearing.

BALBRIGGAN SHIRTS AND DRAWERS

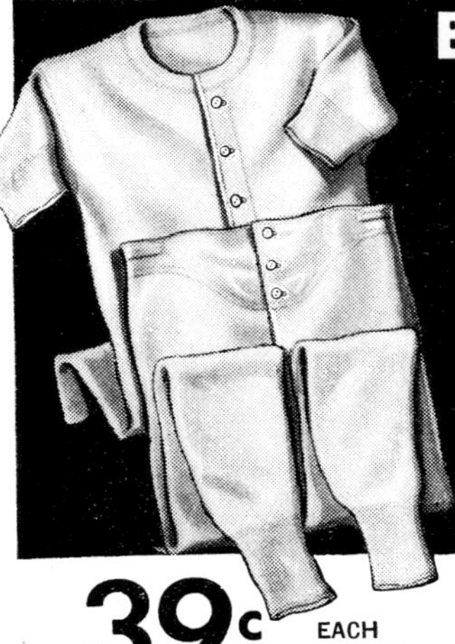

39c EACH GARMENT

Dependable quality at a low price! Flat knit fine gauge cotton Balbriggans. *State size.* COLOR: Cream. Shpg. wt., ea., 7 oz.; 3 garments, 18 oz.

Undershirts

EVEN SIZES 34 to 46-inch chest. Collarette neck; short sleeves.
16 H 5044—Short sleeves
16 H 5046—Long sleeves
Each.. **39c** 3 for...... **$1.15**

Drawers

EVEN SIZES: 30 to 44-inch waist.
16 H 5045—Ankle length. Adjustable strap back. Reinforced crotch. Each **39c** 3 for **$1.15**

Our Finest COMBED COTTON

Now Only 58c EACH GARMENT

Our finest Balbriggans give you biggest value. They wear longer, they're softer, they fit better. Flat knit of fine *combed* cotton.

COLOR: Cream. Shipping weight, each, 8 ounces.

Undershirts

EVEN SIZES: 36 to 56-inch chest. *State size.*
16 H 5062—Short sleeves
16 H 5032—Long sleeves
Each.................. **58c**

Drawers

EVEN SIZES: 32 to 56-inch waist. *State size.*
16 H 5033—Ankle length. Double seat. Reinforced crotch. Sateen waistband. Each.. **58c**

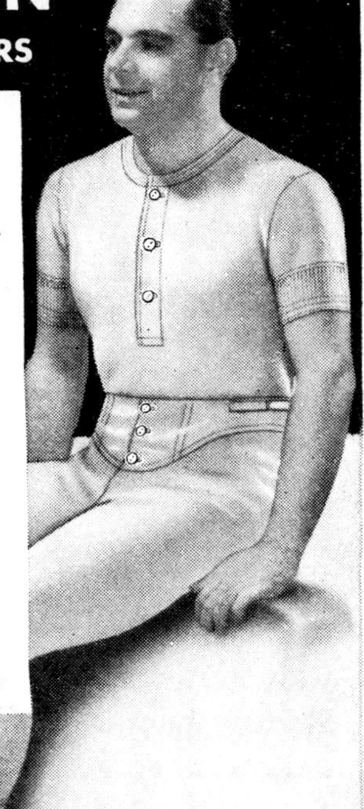

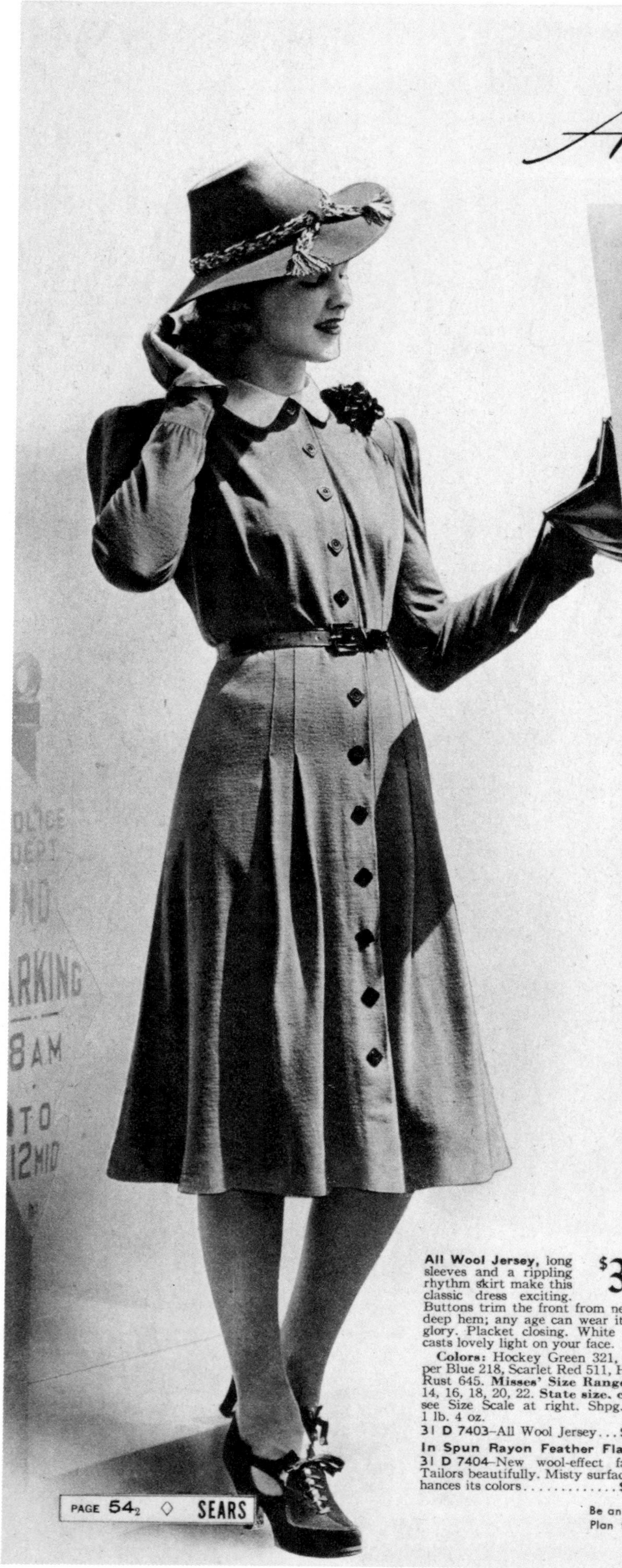

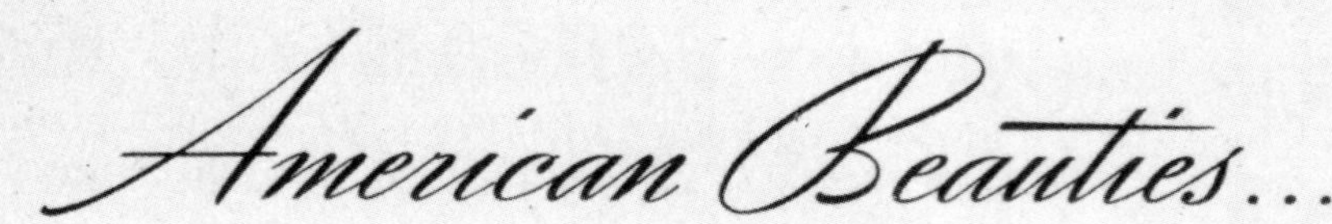

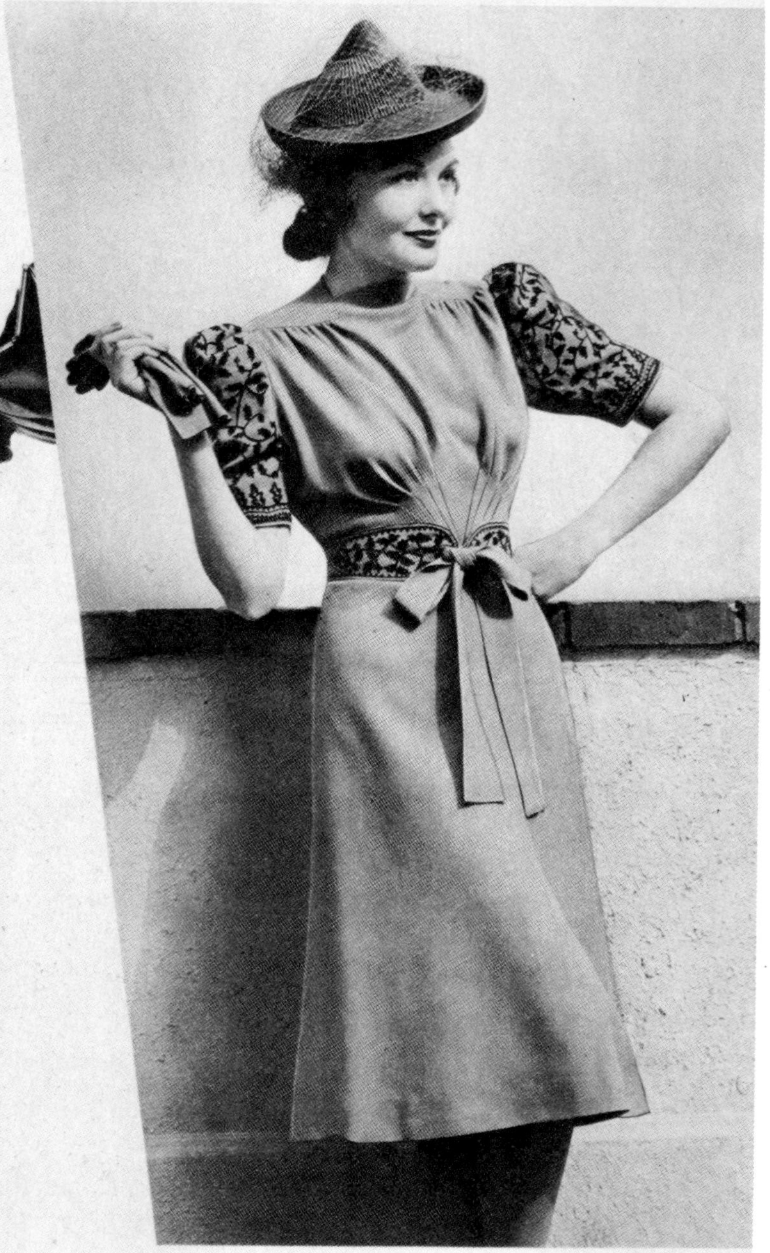

All Wool Jersey, long sleeves and a rippling rhythm skirt make this classic dress exciting. Buttons trim the front from neck to deep hem; any age can wear it with glory. Placket closing. White collar casts lovely light on your face.

$3.98 UP

Colors: Hockey Green 321, Skipper Blue 218, Scarlet Red 511, Henna Rust 645. **Misses' Size Range:** 12, 14, 16, 18, 20, 22. **State size, color;** see Size Scale at right. Shpg. wt., 1 lb. 4 oz.

31 D 7403–All Wool Jersey... **$3.98**

In Spun Rayon Feather Flannel

31 D 7404–New wool-effect fabric. Tailors beautifully. Misty surface enhances its colors............. **$4.98**

Fashion says: "Wear a dressy wool-type frock this winter". We echo the cry and give you this pretty winner in Sears wonderful new wool-like Crown Tested Spun Rayon *Duo-Spun*. Luscious light-hearted colors are enriched by contrasting embroidery on both sleeves and belt.

$3.98

Your waist is softly emphasized, hips neatly minimized, by fan-stitched tucks at the waist. Crown zip placket. A parade of style points at a low Sears price!

Colors: Henna Rust 645, Rancho Rose 527, Limegreen 339 or Gold 720. **Misses' Size Range:** 12, 14, 16, 18, 20, 22. **State size and color;** see Size Scale at right.

31 D 7406—Shpg. wt., 1 lb. 2 oz. **$3.98**

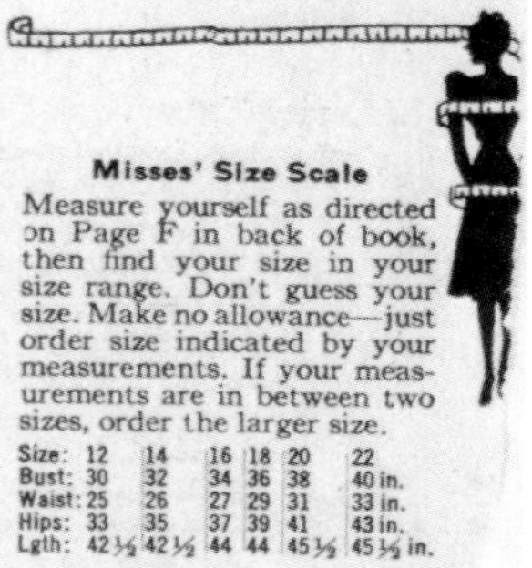

Misses' Size Scale

Measure yourself as directed on Page F in back of book, then find your size in your size range. Don't guess your size. Make no allowance—just order size indicated by your measurements. If your measurements are in between two sizes, order the larger size.

Size:	12	14	16	18	20	22
Bust:	30	32	34	36	38	40 in.
Waist:	25	26	27	29	31	33 in.
Hips:	33	35	37	39	41	43 in.
Lgth:	42½	42½	44	44	45½	45½ in.

Be an American Beauty, the American way. Use Sears Easy Payment Plan to buy lovely dresses like these. Full details on Page 11.

Select your Charmette BACKGROUND DRESS complete with accessory

Your choice of any ONE of these accessory changes included in price of dress . . .

When you have given us the correct catalog number, size and color of the dress you desire, then also indicate the accessory desired. Indicate accessory choice by Letter, A, B, or C, as shown below. **State color** desired if you choose B or C.

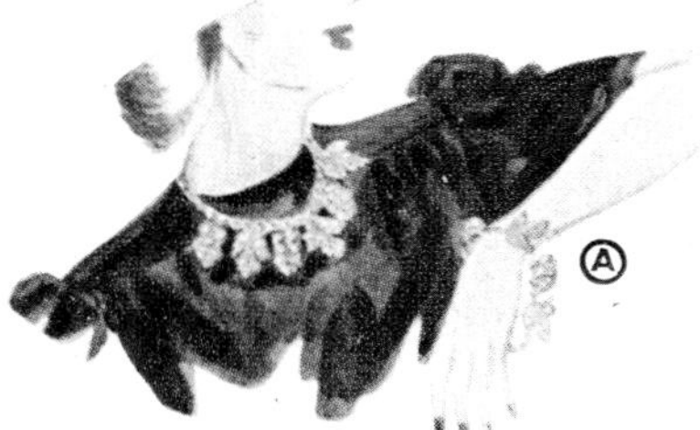

Ⓐ **Bangle** bracelet and necklace of tinkling grapes and leaves in gold colored metal. Both pieces yours if you choose A!

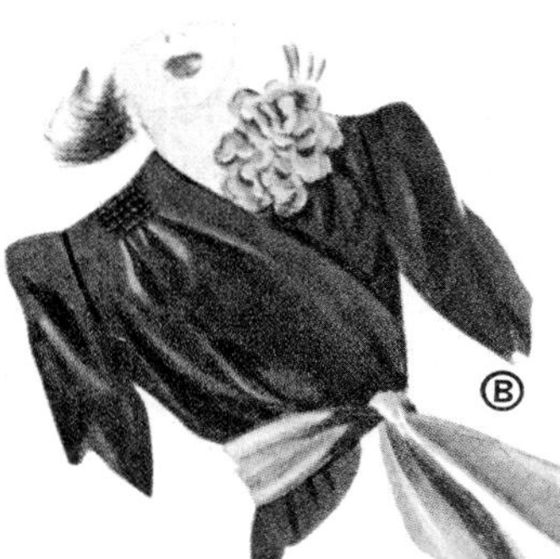

Ⓑ **Corsage** and **Sash** 2 yds. long in Rayon and Cotton Bengaline! **Colors:** American Beauty, Skipper Blue or Aster Pink. **State color.**

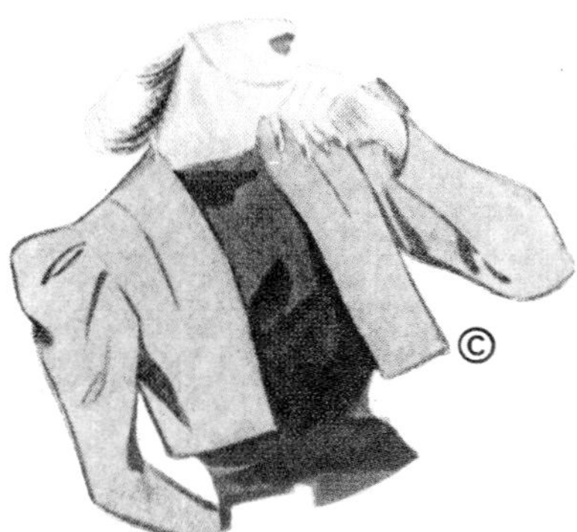

Ⓒ **Bolero** of Rayon and Cotton Bengaline, same sizes as dresses. **Colors:** Limegreen, Skipper Blue or Aster Pink. **State color.**

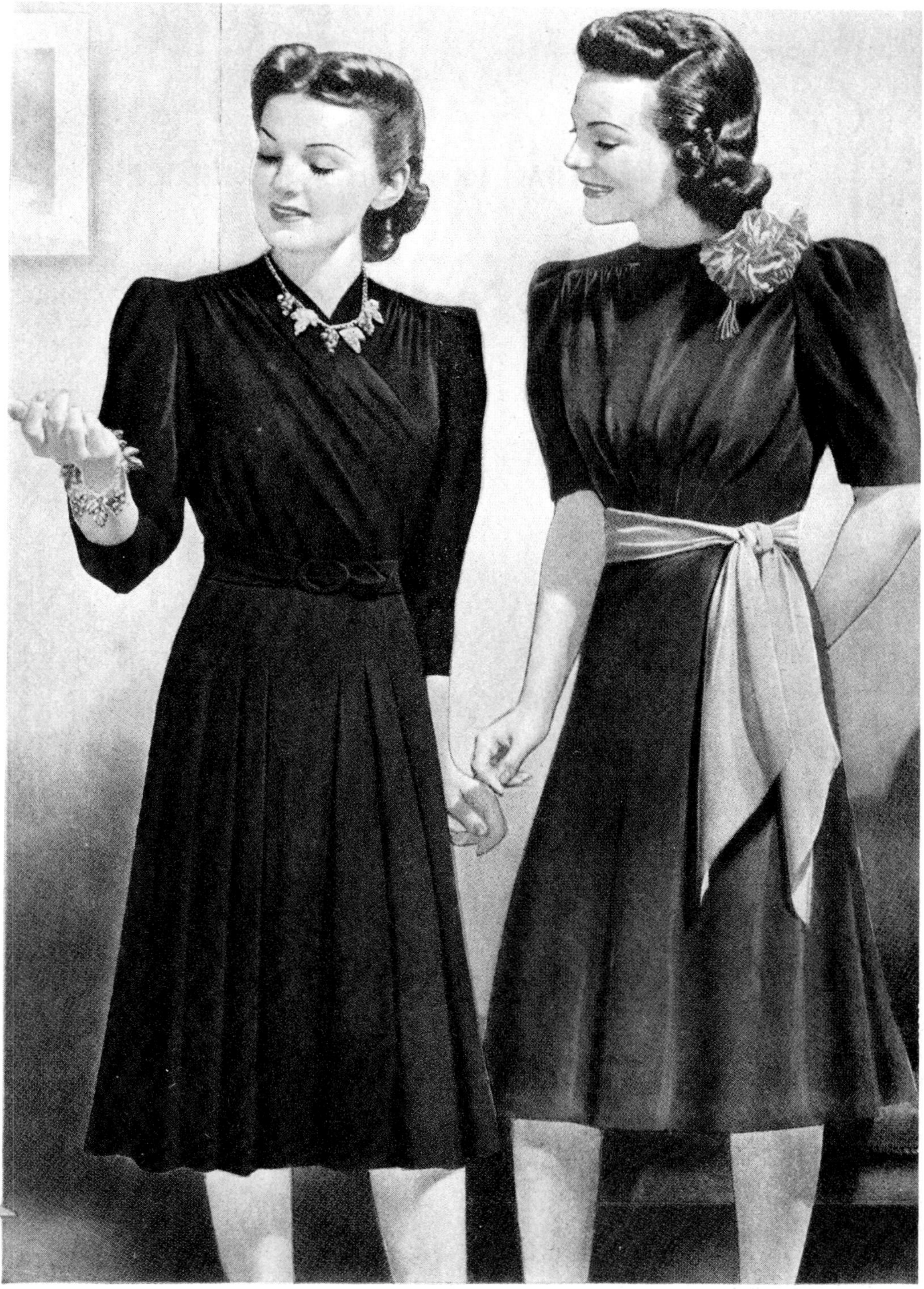

CHARMETTE DRESS

$5.98

What every woman wants! A really good dress with exquisite line and perfect fit. Smart enough to be lovely just as it is . . . or adaptable to accessory changes. Well-named, the *background* dress. Softly draped surplice bodice. Gently flared skirt has the very new unpressed pleats across the front. Self-belt and buckle. Crown zip placket. In our best quality Celanese Rayon Crepe Ariel, a fine Alpaca-type fabric (shown with accessory A).

Colors: Navy, Black or Nuberry Wine. **State size and color and accessory preferred.**

31 D 7464—**Women's Size Range:** 34, 36, 38, 40, 42 and 44. Size Scale, Page 64.
31 D 7465—**Sears New Shorter Women's Size Range:** 16½, 18½, 20½, 22½, 24½, 26½. Size Scale, Page 64.
Shipping weight, 1 lb. 10 oz. $5.98

MISS CHARMETTE

$4.98

Superbly simple background dress that's perfect when worn unadorned . . . and takes accessories with the greatest of ease! Wins you fame as the Girl who has Lots of Clothes, without costing you lots of money!

The lovely style is essentially young . . . with its envelope shoulder, high straight neckline and slightly fulled bodice. Sleeves come just to the elbow. Self-fabric buckled belt; Crown zip placket and zip neck closing at back.

Our best quality Celanese Rayon Crepe Ariel, a fine Alpaca-type fabric . . . perfect for fall and winter (Shown with accessory B.)

Colors: Nuberry Wine, Navy or Black.
Misses' Size Range: 12, 14, 16, 18 only. **State size and color and accessory preferred.** See Size Scale on Page 54.

31 D 7426 Shipping weight, 1 lb. 10 oz. **$4.98**

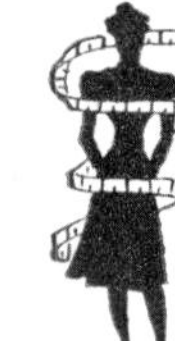

How to tell if you should wear Sears new Shorter Women's Sizes

If you are shorter than average—5 feet 3 inches or less—if you need a dress that is not so long in the sleeves, not so far between waistline and shoulders, somewhat shorter in the skirt—then you wear shorter women's sizes. You'll be delighted to know that the Charmette dress shown above comes in these new shorter sizes, as well as other dresses on pages 44, 45, 64, 65, 66, 67 and 69. See them all, and for a perfect fit follow the measurement directions on page F.

Buy these new Color-Rich dresses on Sears Easy Payment Plan. See details on Page II.

To check the colors listed in these dresses see swatches on opposite page or illustrated garments.

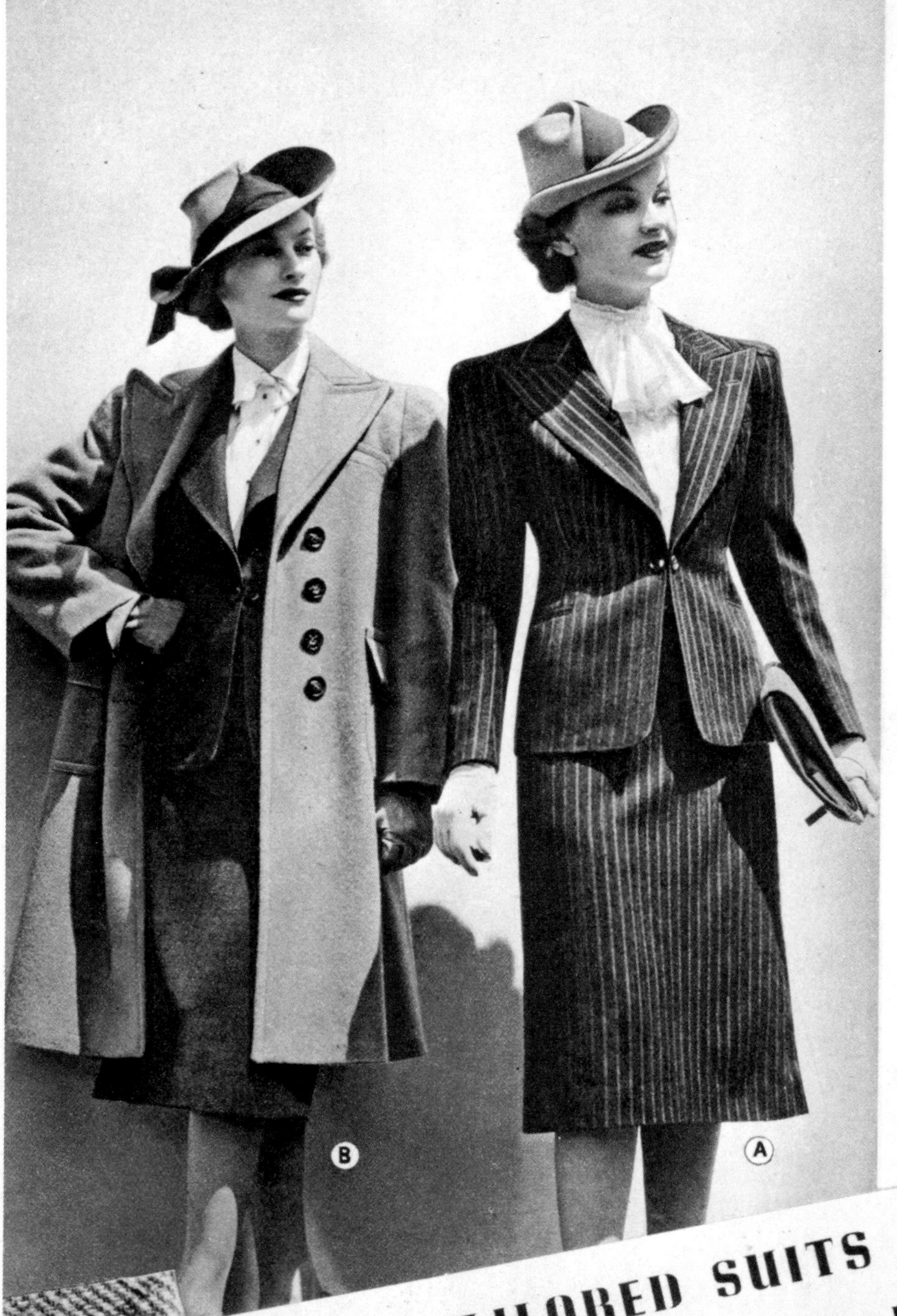

Ⓐ Two-Piece Suit in Three Fabrics

$9.98

THE classic man-tailored suit of the year—carefully designed, cleverly styled so it's becoming to all, with the masterly touches for which Sears suits have long been famous! Lots of fashion news about it this year . . . we've adapted some of England's bright ideas to this crisp young link-button jacket. Its sleek, figure-moulding lines are done with smart tucks at the waist giving it the newest English drape. A Crown zip makes the skirt fit smoothly, and kick pleats on each side flare with every step.

Misses' Size Range: 12, 14, 16, 18, 20, 22. **State size, color;** See Size Scale, Page 37. Shpg. wt., each, 2 lbs. 8 oz.

In Our Best All Wool Worsted

Tailored flawlessly and finished beautifully in our finest quality All Wool Worsted Twill, a closely woven, high-twist fabric that holds its press and wears marvelously. Neva-Moth processed, thoroughly Mothproof! Earl-Glo Rayon Serge lining is guaranteed for the life of the suit.

In Chalk Stripes
17 D 5820—Navy Blue or Black $9.98

In Plain Colors
17 D 5810—Navy, Black, or Banker's (Med.) Gray . $9.98

In Our Better Quality All Wool Suiting

$7.98

Same smart link-button style but in our better quality All Wool Menswear Suiting—closely woven, holds its shape! Rayon Serge lining guaranteed to wear 2 years. **State size, color.**

In Chalk Stripes
17 D 5823—Navy Blue or Oxford Gray $7.98

In Plain Colors
17 D 5813—Navy, Dark Oxford Gray, or Banker's (Med.) Gray $7.98

In Our Good Quality Mannish Suiting

$5.98

Same good-looking link-button style. Well-tailored in a good quality, durable mannish-type Suiting, 50% Wool, balance Rayon and Silk. Rayon Serge lining. **State size, color.**

In Chalk Stripes
17 D 5825—Navy Blue or Oxford Gray $5.98

In Plain Colors
17 D 5815—Banker's (Med.) Gray, or Navy Blue . . . $5.98

Ⓑ Classic Swagger Coat in Three Fabrics

$6.98 UP

The most wearable coat ever to appear on the American fashion scene! You see it in fashion photos, newsreels, on all smart women in everyday life! Wear it over a suit and you have a style-right, three-piece outfit for all year 'round. It's a coat designed by experts, with a swing that spells comfort, grace and youth! Wide, clean-cut revers have been specially tailored to hold their crisp outlines. Straight-cut, slot seamed back. Deep, comfortable pockets.

Misses' Size Range: 12, 14, 16, 18, 20, 22. **State size, color;** Size Scale, Page 20. Shpg. wt., ea., 4 lbs. 2 oz.

Our Best—Half Camel's Hair, Half Wool

Earl-Glo Rayon Serge lining, guaranteed for the life of the coat. Winter-weight interlining.
17 D 5600—Camel Tan 604, Black or Henna Rust 645. $10.98

Our Better Quality All Wool Tweed (See swatch)

Ultra-smart two-tone diagonal weave. Rayon Satin lining, guaranteed to wear two years. Winter-warm interlining.
17 D 5603—Gray Mixture, or Wine Mixture $8.98

Our Good Quality All Wool Fleece

Closely woven. Rayon Taffeta lined, warmly interlined.
17 D 5605—Nuberry (Grape) Wine 514, Navy Blue, or Henna Rust 645 . . . . $6.98

MAN-TAILORED SUITS

To Make a Woman Look Her Feminine Best

They're newer, smarter, more flattering than ever
THANKS to the new English drape
THANKS to the trimly squared, padded shoulders
THANKS to the easy-fitting slim skirt
THANKS to the new classic topcoat by which you make a winter-warm three-piece suit

Want To Buy Your Suit On Easy Terms? See Page 11

What Man-Tailored Really Means At Sears:

1. Collars felled and shrunk to fit.
2. Shoulders squared, padded.
3. Lapels interlined with genuine Menswear Canvas.
4. Jacket fronts interlined with crisp Menswear Canvas.
5. Non-sag pockets.
6. Non-fray buttonholes.
7. Reinforced armholes.
8. Open vent cuffs.
9. Crown zip closed skirts.

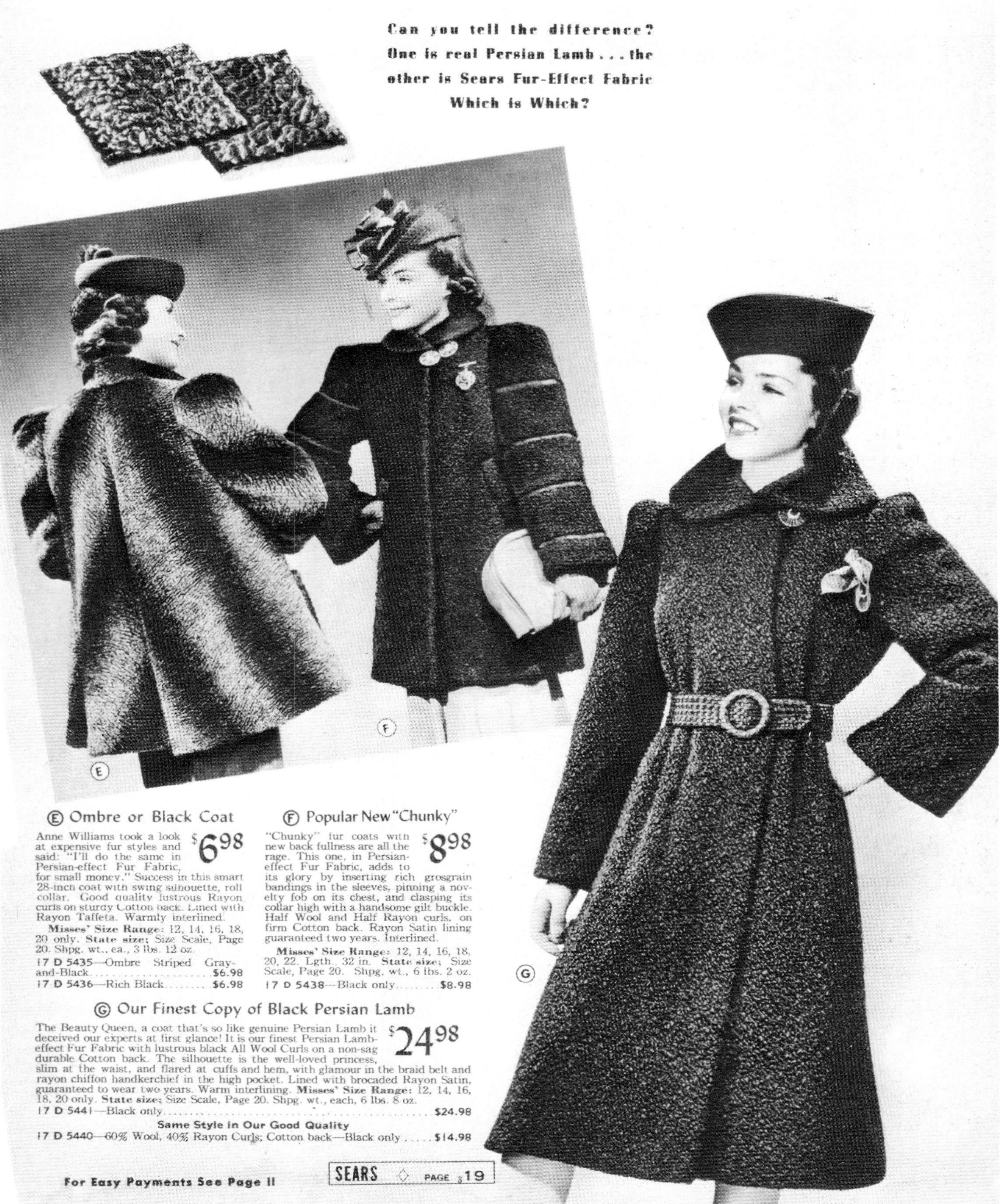

FASHION COPIES OF REAL PERSIAN FUR

Can you tell the difference? One is real Persian Lamb . . . the other is Sears Fur-Effect Fabric Which is Which?

(E) Ombre or Black Coat

$6^{98}

Anne Williams took a look at expensive fur styles and said: "I'll do the same in Persian-effect Fur Fabric, for small money." Success in this smart 28-inch coat with swing silhouette, roll collar. Good quality lustrous Rayon curls on sturdy Cotton back. Lined with Rayon Taffeta. Warmly interlined.

Misses' Size Range: 12, 14, 16, 18, 20 only. **State size;** Size Scale, Page 20. Shpg. wt., ea., 3 lbs. 12 oz.

17 D 5435—Ombre Striped Gray-and-Black.......... $6.98
17 D 5436—Rich Black.......... $6.98

(F) Popular New "Chunky"

$8^{98}

"Chunky" fur coats with new back fullness are all the rage. This one, in Persian-effect Fur Fabric, adds to its glory by inserting rich grosgrain bandings in the sleeves, pinning a novelty fob on its chest, and clasping its collar high with a handsome gilt buckle. Half Wool and Half Rayon curls, on firm Cotton back. Rayon Satin lining guaranteed two years. Interlined.

Misses' Size Range: 12, 14, 16, 18, 20, 22. Lgth., 32 in. **State size;** Size Scale, Page 20. Shpg. wt., 6 lbs. 2 oz.

17 D 5438—Black only.......... $8.98

(G) Our Finest Copy of Black Persian Lamb

$24^{98}

The Beauty Queen, a coat that's so like genuine Persian Lamb it deceived our experts at first glance! It is our finest Persian Lamb-effect Fur Fabric with lustrous black All Wool Curls on a non-sag durable Cotton back. The silhouette is the well-loved princess, slim at the waist, and flared at cuffs and hem, with glamour in the braid belt and rayon chiffon handkerchief in the high pocket. Lined with brocaded Rayon Satin, guaranteed to wear two years. Warm interlining. **Misses' Size Range:** 12, 14, 16, 18, 20 only. **State size;** Size Scale, Page 20. Shpg. wt., each, 6 lbs. 8 oz.

17 D 5441—Black only.......... $24.98

Same Style in Our Good Quality

17 D 5440—60% Wool, 40% Rayon Curls; Cotton back—Black only..... $14.98

For Easy Payments See Page 11

SEARS ◇ PAGE 319

FOR YOUR MOST GLAMOROUS EVENINGS

...in This Romantic Era

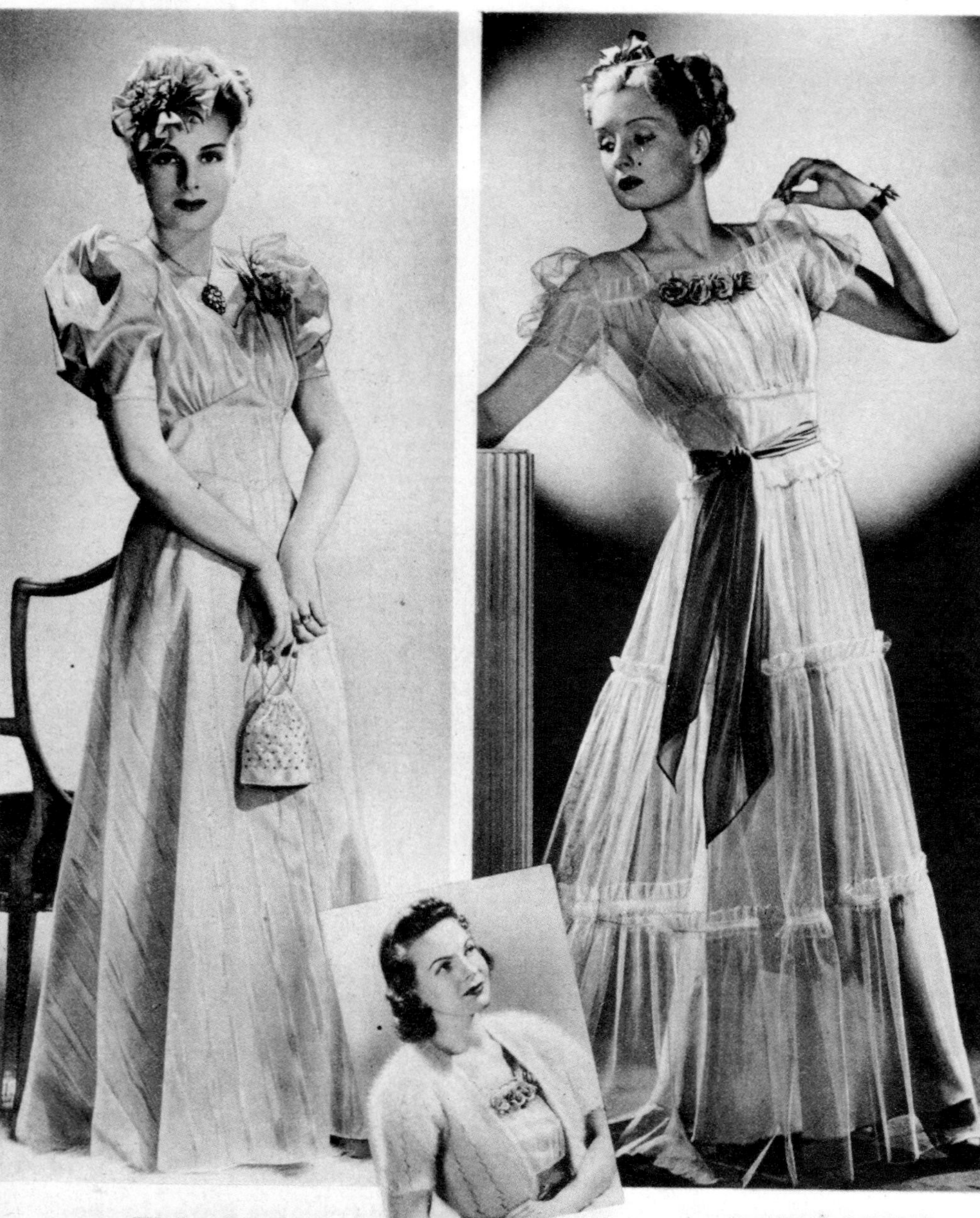

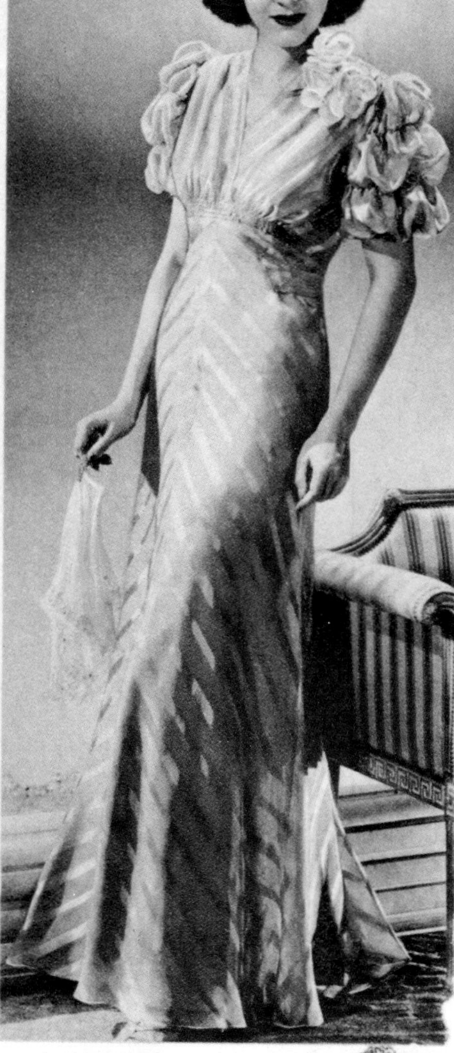

Waltz Song

YOU—a dream of romance in a gown of rustling Moire Rayon Taffeta! A frilly little Rayon Taffeta evening hat included! A most becoming heart-shaped neckline and crisp flower. Gay Nineties puffed sleeves and a sweeping skirt to float you through any dance! Length, 59 inches. For long, evening slip see Slip pages. **$2.98**

Sizes: 12-14-16-18-20.
To Fit Bust: 30-32-34-36-38 in.
State size and color.
Shipping weight, 1 pound 6 ounces.
31 L 2046—Petal Rose 534, Romance Aqua 918, White or Orchid 416.

CUDDLE-PUFF BOLERO

Thrill of the moment! Cuddly bolero, softly knitted of fine Zephyr Wool and 15% fluffy Angora rabbit hair. You can dress-up anything with it! Wear it on big evenings when glamour reigns, or with any of your daytime clothes.
Sizes: 12-14-16-18-20.
To Fit Bust: 30-32-34-36-38 in.
State size and color.
Shipping weight, 1 pound.
31 L 2055—White, Sky Blue 202, Petal Pink 501. **$2.98**

Moonlight Sonata

YOU—winsome and desirable in clouds of Rayon Net, your tiny waist sashed with whispering Rayon Taffeta! Contrasting flowers at a ruffled neckline. The puffed sleeves, the softly gathered bodice are fashion's last word. A rustling rayon taffeta slip shimmers through the filmy sweeping skirt. Dance your way to glory in this romantic gown! It's perfect for graduation, too! **$3.98**
Length, about 59 inches.
Sizes: 12-14-16-18-20.
To Fit Bust: 30-32-34-36-38 in.
State size and color. Shipping weight, 1 pound 6 ounces.
31 L 2049—Petal Pink 501, Sky Blue 202, White or Orchid 416.

Whispers in the Dark

YOU—pretty as a picture in a formal of misty Celanese Rayon Ninon agleam with rayon satin stripes! Proud puffed sleeves, softly shirred bodice slashed in a V, a gay flower. High Princess waistline nipped by tieback belt. In street length, too! **$3.98**
Sizes: 12-14-16-18-20.
To Fit Bust: 30-32-34-36-38 in.
State size and color.
Shipping weight, 1 lb. 4 oz.
Formal Length—about 59 in.
31 L 2052—Patou Rose 504, Romance Aqua 918 or White.
Street Length—about 45 in.
31 L 2053—Navy Blue or White.

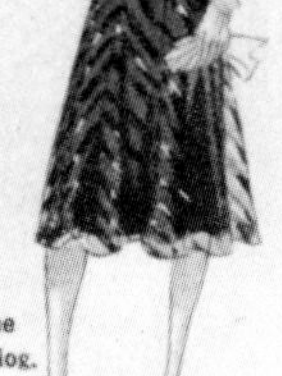

Dresses on these two pages are sent direct from New York to you. Pay postage only from our nearest Mail Order House. Numbers after colors refer to Sears Color-Graph facing first index page in back of book.

Measure Carefully. See Page F in Back of Catalog.

...TO PUT COLOR IN YOUR LIFE

Splurge right now on blouses like these that turn the simplest skirt into a "party" or casual affair. It's the American way of many changes at small cost.

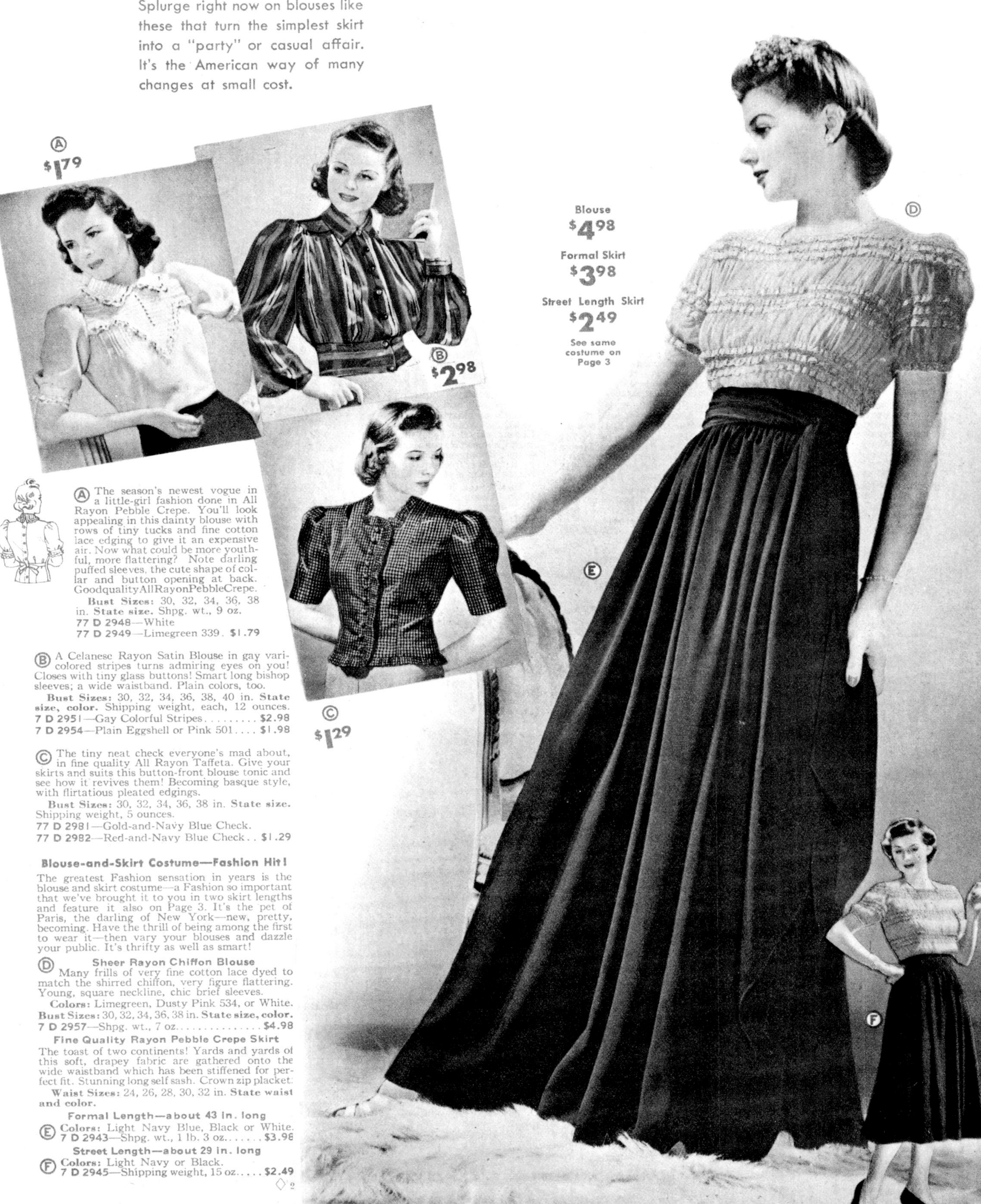

Ⓐ The season's newest vogue in a little-girl fashion done in All Rayon Pebble Crepe. You'll look appealing in this dainty blouse with rows of tiny tucks and fine cotton lace edging to give it an expensive air. Now what could be more youthful, more flattering? Note darling puffed sleeves, the cute shape of collar and button opening at back. Good quality All Rayon Pebble Crepe.

Bust Sizes: 30, 32, 34, 36, 38 in. **State size.** Shpg. wt., 9 oz.
77 D 2948—White
77 D 2949—Limegreen 339. **$1.79**

Ⓑ A Celanese Rayon Satin Blouse in gay vari-colored stripes turns admiring eyes on you! Closes with tiny glass buttons! Smart long bishop sleeves; a wide waistband. Plain colors, too.

Bust Sizes: 30, 32, 34, 36, 38, 40 in. **State size, color.** Shipping weight, each, 12 ounces.
7 D 2951—Gay Colorful Stripes......... **$2.98**
7 D 2954—Plain Eggshell or Pink 501.... **$1.98**

Ⓒ The tiny neat check everyone's mad about, in fine quality All Rayon Taffeta. Give your skirts and suits this button-front blouse tonic and see how it revives them! Becoming basque style, with flirtatious pleated edgings.

Bust Sizes: 30, 32, 34, 36, 38 in. **State size.** Shipping weight, 5 ounces.
77 D 2981—Gold-and-Navy Blue Check.
77 D 2982—Red-and-Navy Blue Check.. **$1.29**

Blouse-and-Skirt Costume—Fashion Hit!

The greatest Fashion sensation in years is the blouse and skirt costume—a Fashion so important that we've brought it to you in two skirt lengths and feature it also on Page 3. It's the pet of Paris, the darling of New York—new, pretty, becoming. Have the thrill of being among the first to wear it—then vary your blouses and dazzle your public. It's thrifty as well as smart!

Ⓓ **Sheer Rayon Chiffon Blouse**

Many frills of very fine cotton lace dyed to match the shirred chiffon, very figure flattering. Young, square neckline, chic brief sleeves.

Colors: Limegreen, Dusty Pink 534, or White.
Bust Sizes: 30, 32, 34, 36, 38 in. **State size, color.**
7 D 2957—Shpg. wt., 7 oz............... **$4.98**

Fine Quality Rayon Pebble Crepe Skirt

The toast of two continents! Yards and yards of this soft, drapey fabric are gathered onto the wide waistband which has been stiffened for perfect fit. Stunning long self sash. Crown zip placket.

Waist Sizes: 24, 26, 28, 30, 32 in. **State waist and color.**

Formal Length—about 43 in. long

Ⓔ **Colors:** Light Navy Blue, Black or White.
7 D 2943—Shpg. wt., 1 lb. 3 oz....... **$3.98**

Street Length—about 29 in. long

Ⓕ **Colors:** Light Navy or Black.
7 D 2945—Shipping weight, 15 oz..... **$2.49**

◇ 2

Mix-Ups!

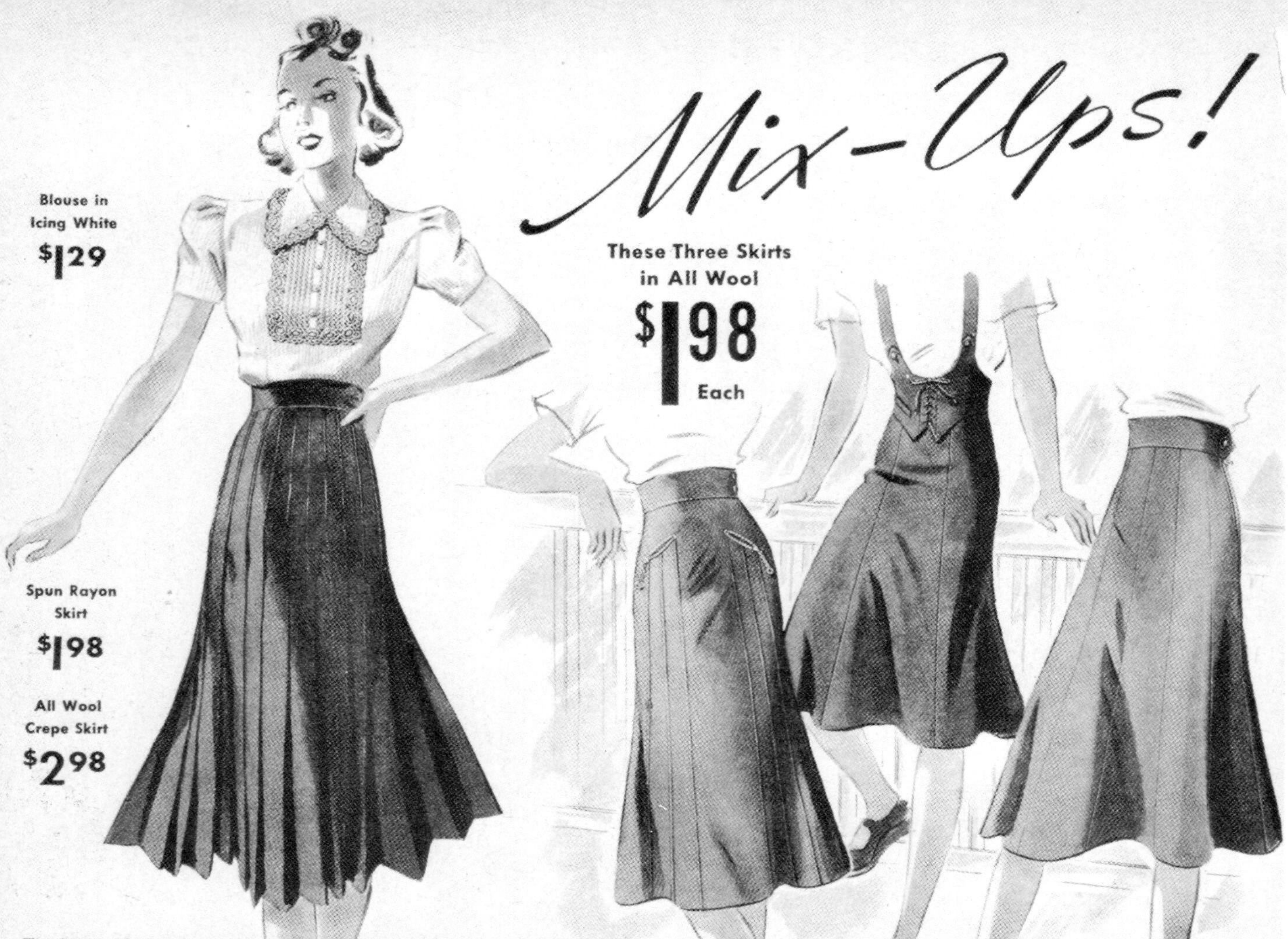

Blouse in Icing White
$1.29

Spun Rayon Skirt
$1.98

All Wool Crepe Skirt
$2.98

These Three Skirts in All Wool
$1.98 Each

The Skirt—Pleated all around! **Anne Williams** selects it because it is so new, so graceful in motion, so slim-hanging, straight-lined. Precisely tailored-stitched pleats. Crown zip placket.

Even Sizes: 24 to 34-in. waist. **State size and color.** Shipping weight, 1 lb.

Spun Rayon Herringbone Weave
A fine quality fabric; so soft and supple.
77 L 2531—Lt. Gray or Navy . . **$1.98**

Fine Quality All Wool Crepe
77 L 2530—Lt. Navy, Black, Strawberry Rose 515 . . . . **$2.98**

The Blouse—with new fashion features and one of the prettiest we've ever seen. Becoming collar, square vestee front, dainty lace edgings and fagoting inserts. Little glass ball buttons. Fine quality Rayon Pique; washfast.

Even Sizes: 30 to 40-in. bust. **State size.** Shpg. wt., 8 oz.

77 L 2547—White . **$1.29**

SIZE SCALE. These are body measurements. Sears make all necessary allowances for size to give perfect fit.

Waist:	24	25	26	27	28	29	30	31	32	34	36	38	40 in.
Hip:	32	34	35	36	37	38	39	40	41	43	45	47	49 in.
Lengths:	29	29	30	30	30	30	31	31	31	32	32	32	32 in.

$1.98 Wool Flannel

Fine quality All Wool Flannel or good quality Sanforized-Shrunk Cotton Twill skirt with Crown zip-up pockets . . . a bright idea! Young and smart and fun to wear! Slenderizing tucks, front and back. Crown zip placket. **Even Sizes:** 24 to 34-in. waist. **State size, color.** Size Scale, left. Shpg. wt., 14 oz.

All Wool Flannel
77 L 2532—Light Navy or Sparkling Burgundy 916 . **$1.98**

Sanforized Cotton Twill
Fabric shrinkage not more than 1%
77 L 2533—Navy Blue, or White **$1.00**

$1.98 Wool Flannel

Juniors love suspender skirts—this new version offers choice of two fabrics. Note the clever laced corselette effect, with tiny pocket, the smart flare of the six-gored skirt. Suspenders cross in back, button in front.

Junior sizes: 11 to 19 years to fit waist 24 to 32 inches. See Size Scale, left. **State size, color.** Shpg. wt., 1 lb.

Fine All Wool Flannel
77 L 2534—Royal Blue 917, Romance Aqua 918 . . . . . **$1.98**

Good Quality Half Wool Flannel, Balance Rayon and Cotton.
77L2535—NavyorWine. **$1.29**

$1.98 Wool Flannel

Ten-gored, dramatically flared, tailored to a T in two chic fabrics. Skirts with this much style usually cost so much more! Marvelous at creating a wasp waisted, long limbed effect. Goes with any type of blouse, dressy or tailored. Crown zip placket.

Even Sizes: 24 to 34-in. waist. See Size Scale, left. **State size, color.** Shpg. wt., 14 oz.

Fine All Wool Flannel
77 L 2536—Navy or Rust-Brown 611 . . . . **$1.98**

Good Rayon Sharkskin
77 L 2537—White or Pink Each **$1.59**

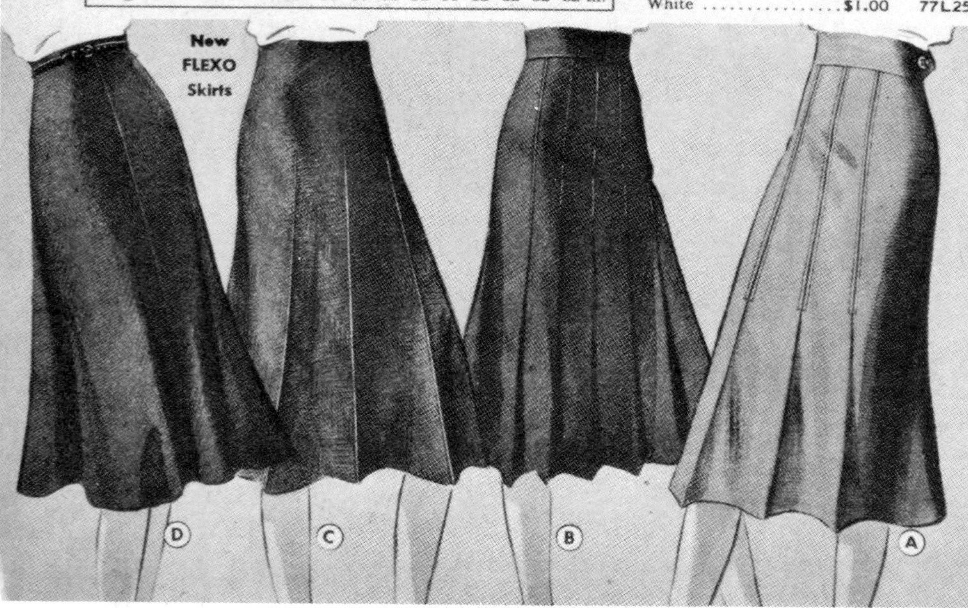

Ⓐ Three good quality fabrics for regular and larger figures. **Even Sizes:** 26 to 40-in. waist. **State size, color.** Shpg. wt., 1 lb. **$1.00 And up**

All Wool Crepe
77 L 2544—Lt. Navy or Woodrose 533 . . . . . **$1.98**

Half-Wool Flannel. Balance Rayon and Cotton.
77 L 2545—Navy, Wine, Brown **$1.29**

Imported Belgian Linen
Oyster White.
77 L 2546 . . . . **$1.00**

Ⓑ A real value! In 3 fabrics. Pleated front and back. **Even Sizes:** 24 to 34-in. waist. **State size, color.** Shpg. wt., 1 lb. **$1.59 And up**

Fine All Wool Flannel
77 L 2541—Lt. Navy or Med. Gray **$1.98**

Fine All Wool Crepe
77 L 2542—Duck Blue 921, Saddle Brown 923 . . . **$1.98**

Good Rayon Sharkskin
77 L 2543—Choice of White, Sunburst Yellow 922, Aqua **$1.59**

FAMOUS FLEXO SKIRTS

Flexo skirts fit any figure! Bias cut, hidden elastic waistband; Crown zip placket. Shipping weight, 1 pound.

Ⓒ Tweed, 55% rayon, 45% wool. Tucked, front, back. Larger sizes, too. **Colors:** Fr. Blue, Lt. Gray, or Tan. **State size, color.**
77 L 2539—**Reg. Sizes:** Small to fit waist (25-27); Med. (28-30); Large (31-33) inches. Each **$2.59**
77 L 2540—**Stout:** (34-36); **Extra Stout** (37-39) inches. Each **$2.98**

Ⓓ Our very finest All Wool Flannel Skirt—flared all around. Narrow leather-like belt. Fits smoothly; no gaping.

Sizes: Small to fit waist (25-27); Med. (28-30); Large (31-33) inches. **State size, color.** See Size Scale, left.
77 L 2538—Black or Navy. Each **$2.98**

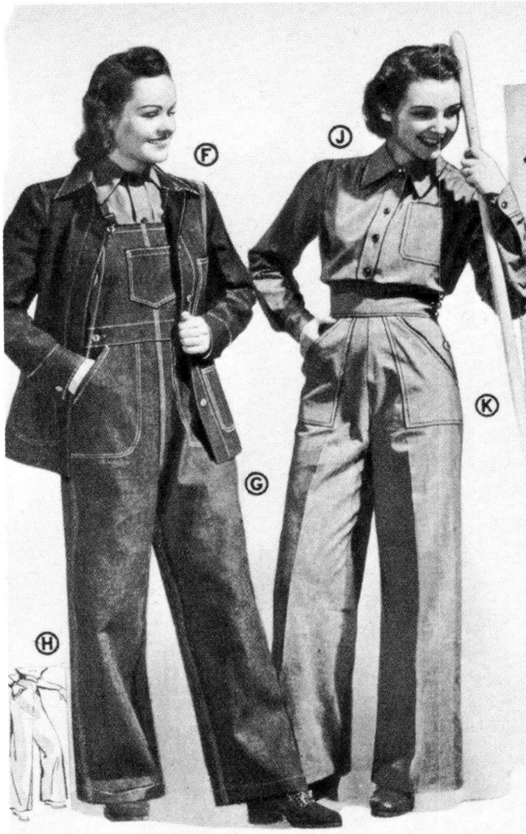

SANFORIZED-SHRUNK WORK-PLAY CLOTHES

(Maximum Fabric Shrinkage 1%)

Garments of **Indigo Blue Overall Denim** made to fit the feminine figure but with details of men's overalls—double stitching, metal buttons, buckles, pockets. Bar-tacked. **State size.**

Ⓕ **Jacket. Bust Sizes:** 32, 34, 36, 38, 40, 42, 44 in. Shipping wt., ea., 1 lb. 1 oz.
27 D 9727—98c: 2 for $1.89

Overalls or Slacks. Waist Sizes: 26, 28, 30, 32, 34, 36, 38 in. Shpg. wt., ea., 1 lb. 4 oz.

Ⓖ **27 D 9726—Overalls**
Each...**98c;**...2 for **$1.89**

Ⓗ **27 D 9729—Slacks**
Each.................**89c**

Shirts and slacks in **Indestructo** chambray, same material as our 4-Star Feature work clothes shown at right. Wears and washes beautifully. Specially cut for women. Double stitched seams, generous pockets. Exceptional values. Blue only.

Ⓙ **27 D 9728 — Shirt, . . 79c**
Bust Sizes: 32, 34, 36, 38, 40 42, 44 in. **State size.** Shipping weight, 11 ounces.

Ⓚ **27 D 9730 — Slacks, 98c**
Waist Sizes: 26, 28, 30, 32, 34, 36, 38 in. **State size.** Shipping weight, 14 ounces.

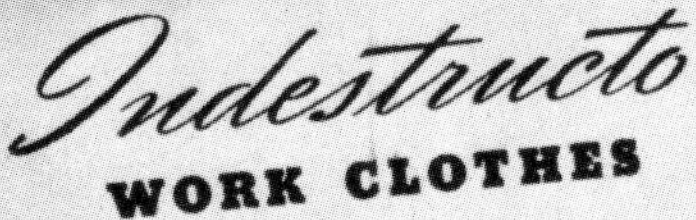

Indestructo

WORK CLOTHES

FOUR-STAR FEATURES

- Sears Wonder Fabric
- Sanforized-Shrunk (Maximum Fabric Shrinkage 1%)
- Tested For Durability
- Outwears Them All!

Indestructo is Sears own wonder cloth. A closely woven end-to-end Cotton Chambray, the sturdiest, longest-wearing Chambray of its weight to come out of our laboratory! Yet soft—tailors nicely. Sanforized-Shrunk for lasting fit. See Page 480 for complete story of the wonder fabric!

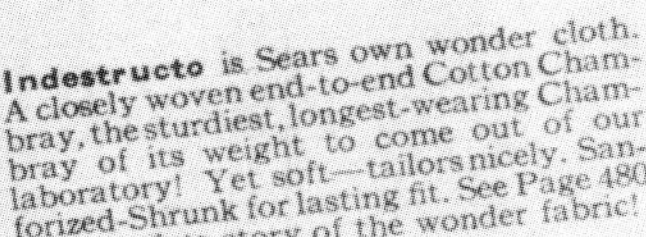

Ⓐ **Getting Down to Business!** **89c**

When you've got an honest-to-goodness job on hand, this is the quick on-and-off work dress to tackle it in. Three enormous pockets in the apron front, roomy cut, ties at waist. Toss it in the tub without a thought—it's made of Indestructo, wonder fabric described above.

Colors: Blue, or Green.
Size: Ex. Small, Small, Medium, Large.
Bust: 30-32 34-36 38-40 42-44
State size and color.
27 D 9725—Shipping wt., 14 oz.....89c

Ⓑ **Complete Coverage**

Sturdy work dress for factory or home giving absolute protection, freedom, comfort! Cut full with action back, new yoke. Convertible collar, open front, 4 pockets, double stitched seams. New cotton wash fabric, Indestructo—see above.

Colors: Blue or Green. **State size, color.** Shpg. wt., each, 1 lb. 1 oz.
27 D 9720—Women's Size Range: 32 34, 36, 38, 40, 42, 44 only. See Size Scale, Page 80. Each.......... **$1.00**
27 D 9721—Stout Size Range: 45, 47, 49, 51, 53 only. See Size Scale, Page 79. Each.......... **$1.19**

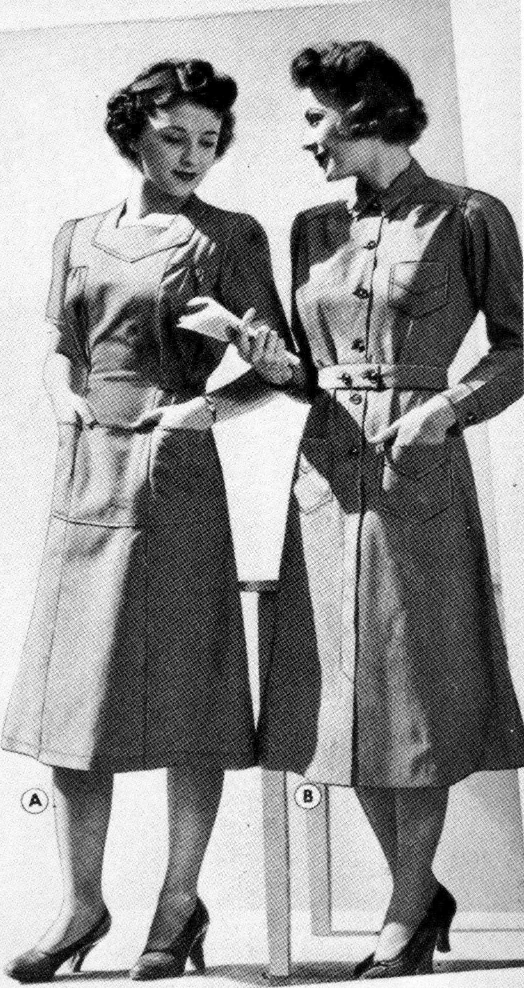

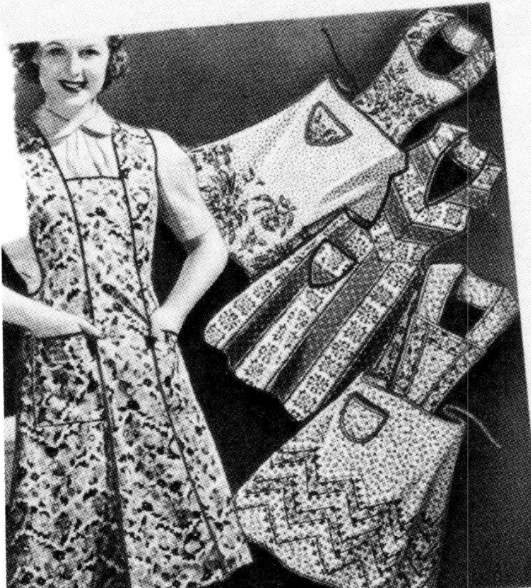

2 Aprons for 79c

Better washfast Percale. One floral, one check print. **State size.** Shpg. wt., set, 2 lbs. 14 oz.

Sizes: Small (34-36); Medium (38-40); Large (42-44).
27 D 9717—2 for.....79c

Extra-Large Sizes: (46-48); Stout (50-52).
27 D 9718—2 for 95c

3 Aprons for 59c

Gay, pretty aprons at a 'way low price! Colorful bindings, handy pockets. Better washfast Percales in border prints, florals, stripes.

One Size Fits Average Figure. Shpg. wt., set of three, 10 oz.
27 D 1940—Assorted prints. Set of three..**59c**

SUPER VALUE!

Good Quality Percales

57c Each 2 for $1.09

Ⓒ Remarkable value for such good washfast Percale in a flattering button-down-the-front coat dress! White pique and ric-rac on V-neckline. Handy pockets.
Misses' Size Range: 12, 14, 16, 18, 20, 22. **State size;** Size Scale, Page 80. Shpg. wt., ea., 10 oz.
27 D 9724—Assorted Prints
Each......**57c;**......2 for **$1.09**

Ⓓ Amazingly low priced for a lovely floral print dress of washfast Percale. Lace-edged collar. **State size.** Shipping weight, ea., 9 oz.
Women's Size Range: 34, 36, 38, 40, 42, 44 only. Size Scale, Pg. 79.
Stout Size Range: 45, 47, 49, 51, 53 only. See Size Scale, Page 79.
27 D 8598—Navy Ground
27 D 8599—Lavender Ground
Each......**57c;**......2 for **$1.09**

Ⓔ Clever one-piece bolero-effect dress! Smart two tone piping—a becoming square neckline that's softly shirred. Good quality washfast Percale in a floral print.
Misses' Size Range: 12, 14, 16, 18, 20 only. Size Scale, Page 80. **State size.** Shpg. wt., ea., 8 oz.
27 D 8595—Copen Blue
27 D 8596—Rose-wine
Each.......**57c;**.......2 for **$1.09**

SEARS ◇ PAGE 383

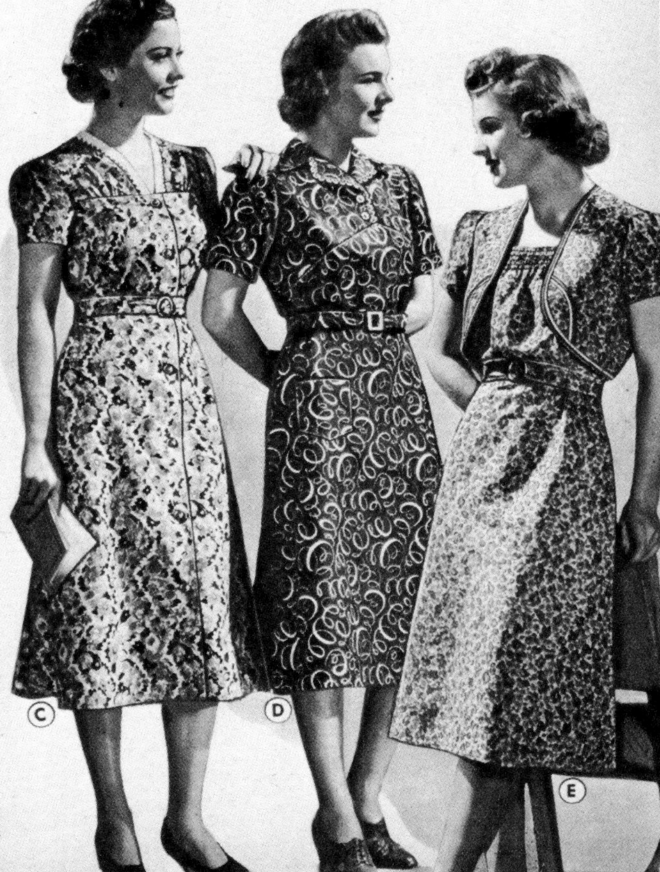

good Colors get together

TOGETHER . . . that one word is your color cue for Fall and Winter fashions. Each of the new shades is fresh and arresting in itself . . . but real excitement begins when they meet. Combine three shades in a single dress, like the tri-colored triumph at the left . . . or pick some resonant shade and echo it again and again in your costume, as shown in the color tableaux below. Outstanding accents of the Season are these . . Sears *Bittersweet*, *Wintergreen* and *American Beauty*. Use them as we do here . . or dare to be different and work out your own color plan. Accessories are described on accessory pages.

Bittersweet . . . . . sister shades to your beloved rust. Lighter, brighter, and redder. Excellent against black, brown, navy and all greens.

Wintergreen . . . . headed for fame; it's becoming to blondes, brunettes, silver heads and reds! Sharp accent for brown, rust, blacks.

American Beauty . . well named! It's a beauty. Newest of the blue-red shades. Bright companion to all blues and blacks.

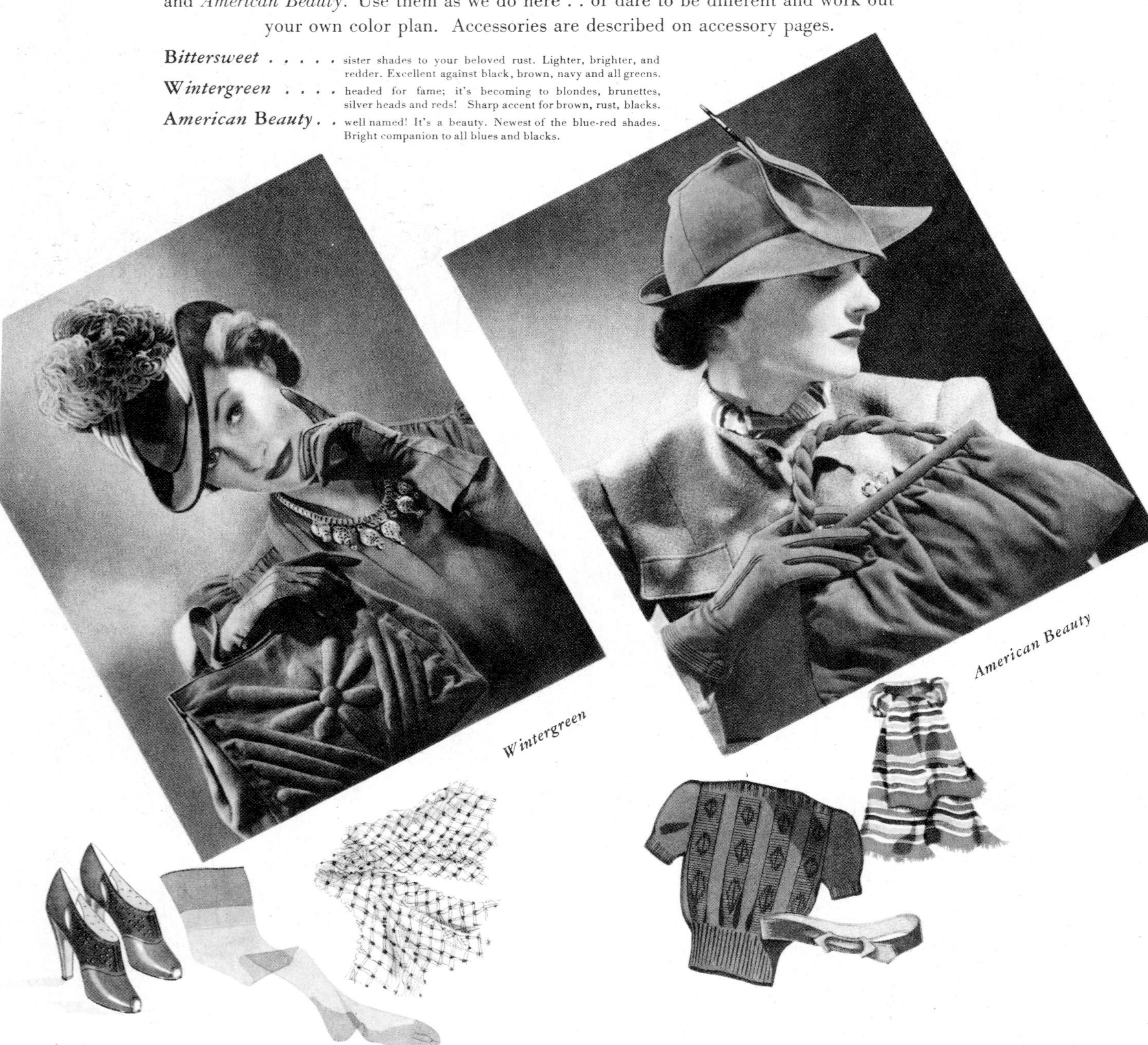

Wintergreen

American Beauty

Ⓐ
Ⓑ
Ⓒ
COLOR . . . Dramatically Draped in a New and Exciting Oriental Turban
COLOR . . . in a Merry Plaid Bow Perched on a Gay Little Hat Perfect With Any Hair-Do!

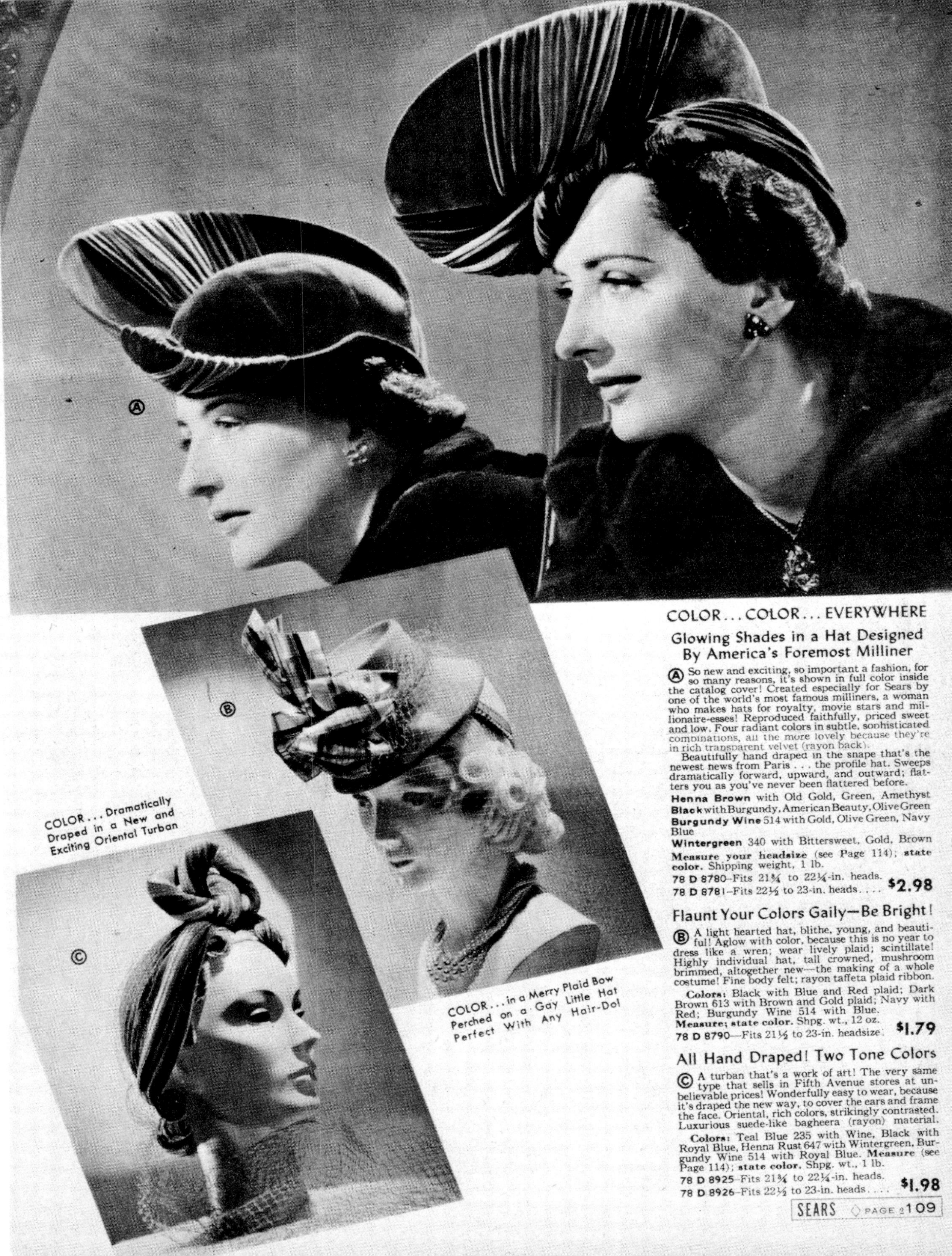

COLOR . . . COLOR . . . EVERYWHERE

Glowing Shades in a Hat Designed By America's Foremost Milliner

Ⓐ So new and exciting, so important a fashion, for so many reasons, it's shown in full color inside the catalog cover! Created especially for Sears by one of the world's most famous milliners, a woman who makes hats for royalty, movie stars and millionaire-esses! Reproduced faithfully, priced sweet and low. Four radiant colors in subtle, sophisticated combinations, all the more lovely because they're in rich transparent velvet (rayon back).

Beautifully hand draped in the shape that's the newest news from Paris . . . the profile hat. Sweeps dramatically forward, upward, and outward; flatters you as you've never been flattered before.

Henna Brown with Old Gold, Green, Amethyst
Black with Burgundy, American Beauty, Olive Green
Burgundy Wine 514 with Gold, Olive Green, Navy Blue
Wintergreen 340 with Bittersweet, Gold, Brown

Measure your headsize (see Page 114); **state color.** Shipping weight, 1 lb.

78 D 8780–Fits 21¾ to 22¼-in. heads.
78 D 8781–Fits 22½ to 23-in. heads **$2.98**

Flaunt Your Colors Gaily—Be Bright!

Ⓑ A light hearted hat, blithe, young, and beautiful! Aglow with color, because this is no year to dress like a wren; wear lively plaid; scintillate! Highly individual hat, tall crowned, mushroom brimmed, altogether new—the making of a whole costume! Fine body felt; rayon taffeta plaid ribbon.

Colors: Black with Blue and Red plaid; Dark Brown 613 with Brown and Gold plaid; Navy with Red; Burgundy Wine 514 with Blue.
Measure; state color. Shpg. wt., 12 oz.
78 D 8790—Fits 21½ to 23-in. headsize. **$1.79**

All Hand Draped! Two Tone Colors

Ⓒ A turban that's a work of art! The very same type that sells in Fifth Avenue stores at unbelievable prices! Wonderfully easy to wear, because it's draped the new way, to cover the ears and frame the face. Oriental, rich colors, strikingly contrasted. Luxurious suede-like bagheera (rayon) material.

Colors: Teal Blue 235 with Wine, Black with Royal Blue, Henna Rust 647 with Wintergreen, Burgundy Wine 514 with Royal Blue. **Measure** (see Page 114); **state color.** Shpg. wt., 1 lb.

78 D 8925–Fits 21¾ to 22¼-in. heads.
78 D 8926–Fits 22½ to 23-in. heads **$1.98**

SEARS ◇ PAGE 2109

Velvet

BRINGS OUT THE SPARKLE IN YOUR EYES

Ⓐ Transparent rayon velvet for flattery . . . makes your skin look radiant! Shirred bumper brim hat; dainty muff to match. **$1.98 SET**

Colors: Black, Brown 613, Burgundy Wine 514, Royal Blue 218. Hat fits 21½ to 23 inches. **Measure your headsize** (see Page 114); **state color.**

78 D 9110–**2-piece set.** Shipping weight, 1 lb. 3 oz. **$1.98**
78 D 9111–**Hat only.** Shpg. wt., 14 oz. . $1.19

Ⓑ 1940 is one year you won't want to be without a turban! Get yours early! Hand draped **$1.00 EA.**

Colors: Black, Brown 613, Burgundy Wine 514, Navy. **Measure** (see Pg. 114); **state color.** Shpg. wt., ea., 12 oz.

Transparent Rayon Velvet
78 D 8845—Fits 21¾ to 22¼ in. $1.00
78 D 8846—Fits 22½ to 23 in. $1.00

Rayon Bagheera Cloth (Napped Jersey Weave)
78 D 8847—Fits 21¾ to 22¼ in. $1.00
78 D 8848—Fits 22½ to 23 in. $1.00

Ⓒ The new shirred transparent rayon velvet in a hat that looks like $5, at the least! Young, gay, altogether new! Grosgrain "little-girl" streamers. **$1.89**

Colors: Brown 613, Burgundy Wine 514, Black, Navy. **Measure your headsize** (see Page 114). **State color.** Shpg. wt., 1 lb.

78 D 9015—Fits 21½ to 23 in. headsize.

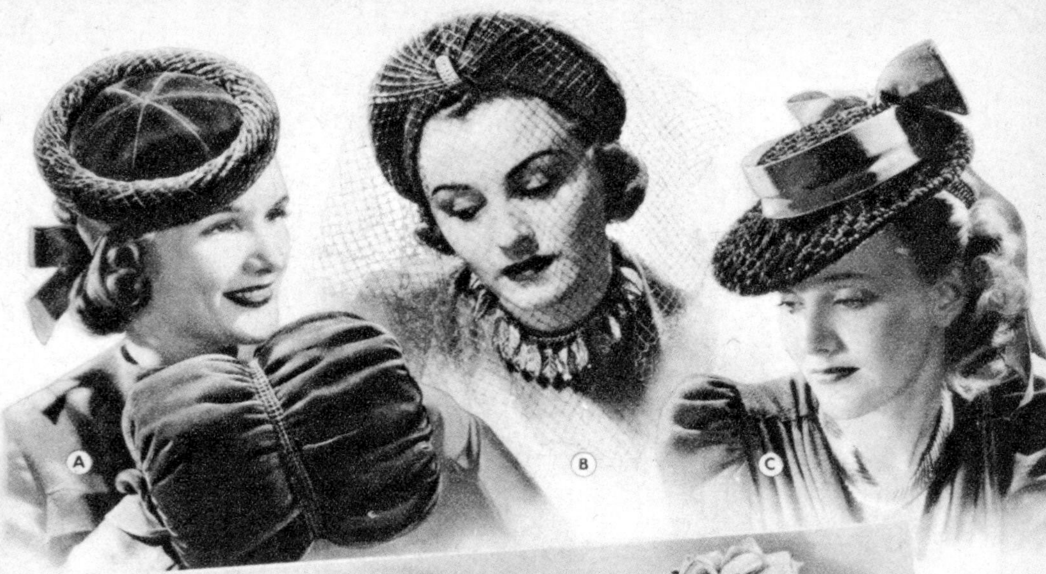

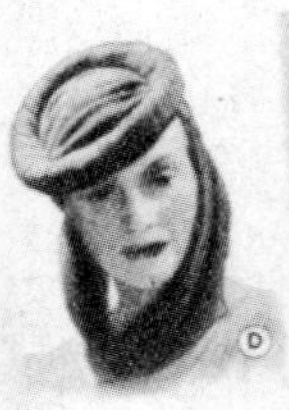

Yes! YOU CAN WEAR THESE!

Different, but Definitely Flattering!

Ⓓ High drama . . . for the lady who believes hats should be exciting! Drape the wimple the way it suits you best; the effects you can create are marvelous! Richest of colors, vivid, vibrant, in a new suede-effect rayon cloth. Goes with any hair-do. **89c**

Colors: Black, American Beauty 515, Teal Blue 235, Gold 720, Bittersweet (see Page 4). **Measure** (see Page 114); **state color.** Shipping weight, 14 oz.

78 D 9175—Fits 21¾ to 23 in headsize.

Ⓔ The snood hat, romantic Paris fashion! New, easy to wear! Has a practical purpose, too; the snood holds curls in place, anchors the hat to your head. Grosgrain ribbons in lilting multi-colors; rolled bumper brim; remarkably becoming! Good body felt. **$1.39**

Colors: Black, Navy, Henna Rust 647, Burgundy Wine 514. **Measure your headsize** (see Page 114); **state color.** Shipping weight, 12 oz.

78 D 8835—Fits 21¾ to 23-in. headsize.

Hats May Be Bought On Easy Terms. See Page 11.

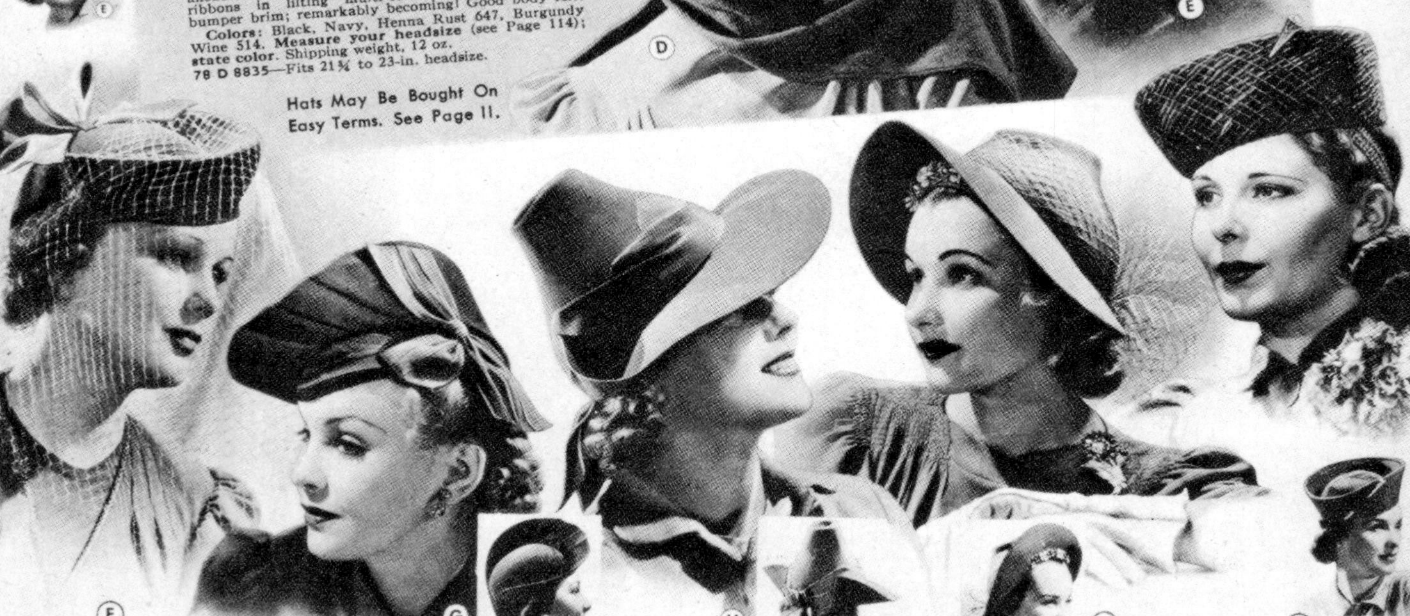

Ⓕ Decidedly dressy, definitely new! The forward tilt, the deep back, the narrow look are advance fashion! And complimentary to most faces! Good felt body; you'll like it. **$1.19**

Colors: Black, Navy, Burgundy Wine 514 with deep Blue veil and bow, Brown 613 with Rust veil and bow. **Measure your headsize** (see Page 114); **state color.** Shipping weight, 12 oz.

78 D 9040–Fits 21¾ to 22¼ in.
78 D 9041–Fits 22½ to 23 in.

Ⓖ Forward, and upward! Stunning version of the profile hat with the high-sweeping line that's so striking, yet so easy to wear. Cleverly placed contrasting bow accents the line of the hat. Good body felt. Looks very expensive. **$1.79**

Colors: Black, Henna Rust 647, Navy, Burgundy Wine 514. **Measure** (see Page 114); **state color.** Shipping weight, 14 ounces.

78 D 8910—Fits 21¾ to 22¼ in.
78 D 8911—Fits 22½ to 23 in.

Ⓗ High-rising crown, new! Dipping "different" brim, designed to be as smart from one side as the other! Comfortable to wear; becoming to all ages. American Classic! Good body felt. **$1.00**

Colors: Henna Rust 647, Laurel Green 313, Navy, Burgundy Wine 514, Black. **Measure** (see Pg. 114); **state color.** Shipping weight, 1 pound.

78 D 9160–Fits 21½ to 22 in.
78 D 9161–Fits 22¼ to 22¾ in.

Ⓙ A beguiling bonnet, if there ever was one! Young and disarming, with enchanting flowers perched above the brow. Turn the brim back—it's off-the-face. Bouffant veil bow. Good felt. **$1.19**

Colors: Black, Teal Blue 235, Burgundy Wine 514, Bittersweet (see Page 4). Matching veil. **Measure** (see Page 114); **state color.** Shpg. wt., 14 oz.

78 D 8965–Fits 21¾ to 22¼ in.
78 D 8966–Fits 22½ to 23 in.

Ⓚ High, and wide! Does so much to make faces look young! **$1.00 EA.**

Choice of 2 fabrics. **Colors:** Black, Burgundy Wine 514, Royal Blue 218, Henna Rust 647. Fits 21¾ to 23 in. **Measure** (see Page 114); **state color.** Shpg. wt., ea., 12 oz

78 D 9115—Rayon velvet
78 D 9180—Rayon bagheera

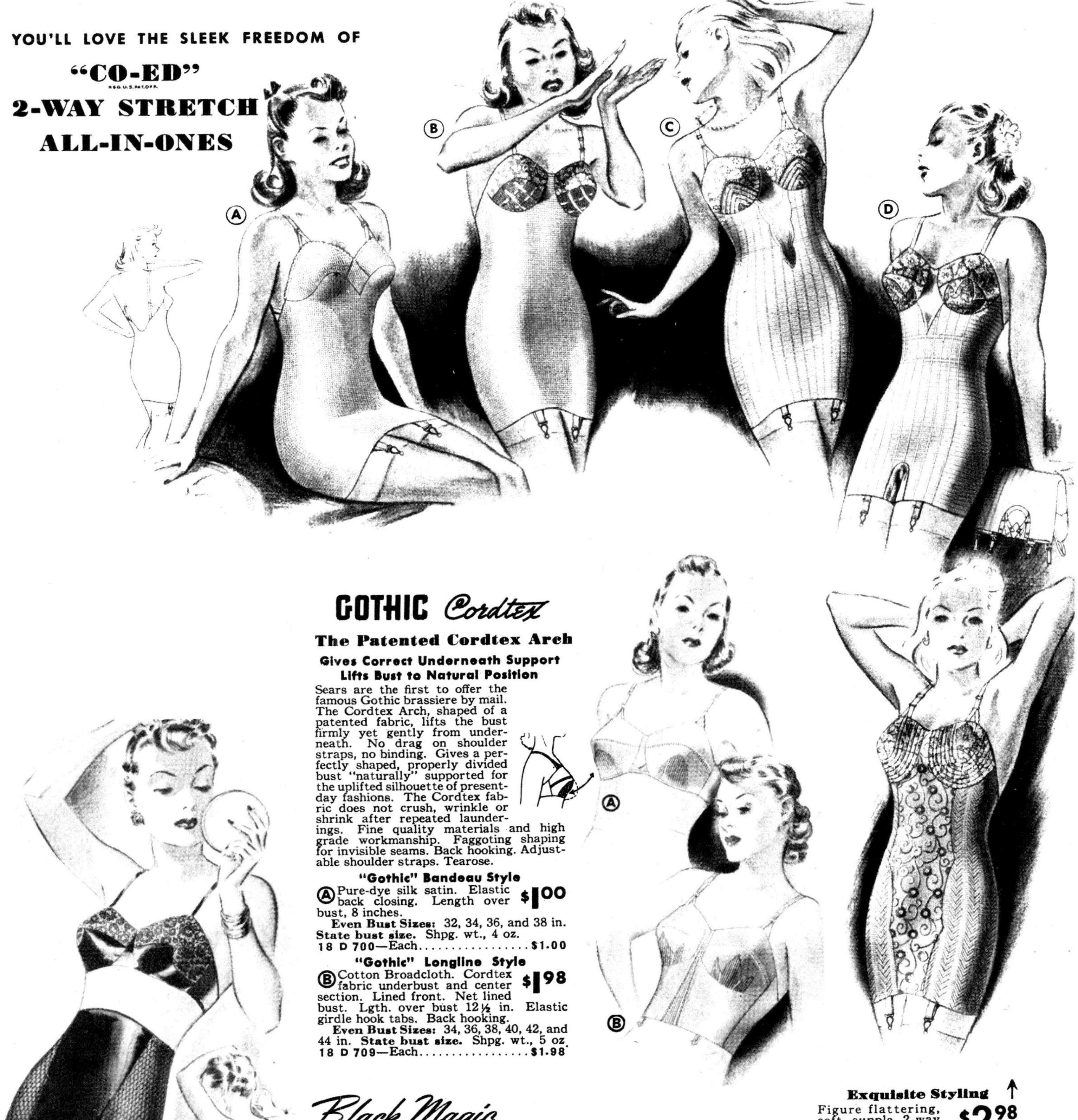

YOU'LL LOVE THE SLEEK FREEDOM OF

"CO-ED"

REG. U.S. PAT. OFF.

2-WAY STRETCH ALL-IN-ONES

GOTHIC Cordtex

The Patented Cordtex Arch

Gives Correct Underneath Support Lifts Bust to Natural Position

Sears are the first to offer the famous Gothic brassiere by mail. The Cordtex Arch, shaped of a patented fabric, lifts the bust firmly yet gently from underneath. No drag on shoulder straps, no binding. Gives a perfectly shaped, properly divided bust "naturally" supported for the uplifted silhouette of present-day fashions. The Cordtex fabric does not crush, wrinkle or shrink after repeated launderings. Fine quality materials and high grade workmanship. Faggoting shaping for invisible seams. Back hooking. Adjustable shoulder straps. Tearose.

"Gothic" Bandeau Style

Ⓐ Pure-dye silk satin. Elastic back closing. Length over bust, 8 inches. **$1.00**

Even Bust Sizes: 32, 34, 36, and 38 in. **State bust size.** Shpg. wt., 4 oz.

18 D 700—Each................$1.00

"Gothic" Longline Style

Ⓑ Cotton Broadcloth. Cordtex fabric underbust and center section. Lined front. Net lined bust. Lgth. over bust 12½ in. Elastic girdle hook tabs. Back hooking. **$1.98**

Even Bust Sizes: 34, 36, 38, 40, 42, and 44 in. **State bust size.** Shpg. wt., 5 oz.

18 D 709—Each................$1.98

Black Magic

FOR THE NEW 1940 FASHIONS

Glamorous Sleek Fitting Evening Bra or Girdle

You'll love this perfect fitting bra—the tearose for daytime, black for evenings! Shimmering silk faced, rayon back satin and fine net lined lace. Low evening back with double elastics; hook attaches to girdle. Lgth. over bust, 8 in. $1.00 value. **Bra 69c**

Even Bust Sizes: 32 to 38 in. **State size.** Shpg. wt., 4 oz.

18 D 665—Black. Each...69c

18 D 655—Tearose. Each..69c

Flattering! Lovely step-in! Front and back of up-and-down-stretch lustrous rayon and cotton satin Darleen super-elastic. 2-way stretch open weave Power Net elastic sides. Not a bone in it's body. You'll want one of each color. Lgth. 14½ in. **Girdle $1.98**

For Medium to Tall Figures—Fits Hips 7 to 10 Inches Larger Than Waist

Waist Sizes: 24, 26, 28, 30, 32, 34 in. **State waist and hip measure.** Shpg. wt., 12 oz.

18 D 552—Black. Each..$1.98

18 D 553—Tearose. Each 1.98

Exquisite Styling ↑

Figure flattering, soft, supple, 2-way stretch Lastex. Has hidden removable, light boning in its gorgeous, brocaded rayon and cotton satin Darleen super-elastic front panel. Beautifully stream lines the figure. It's style and fine quality that usually sells for $5.00 anywhere else. Lovely ribbon trim uplift style lace bust, net lined. Adjustable forked satin shoulder straps. Flat garters. Length over bust to garter, 24 in. Tearose color. **$2.98**

For All Figures

Bust Sizes: 32, 34, 36, 38 in. **State bust and hip measure;** read How to Measure on Page 145. Shipping weight, each, 14 ounces.

18 D 119...............$2.98

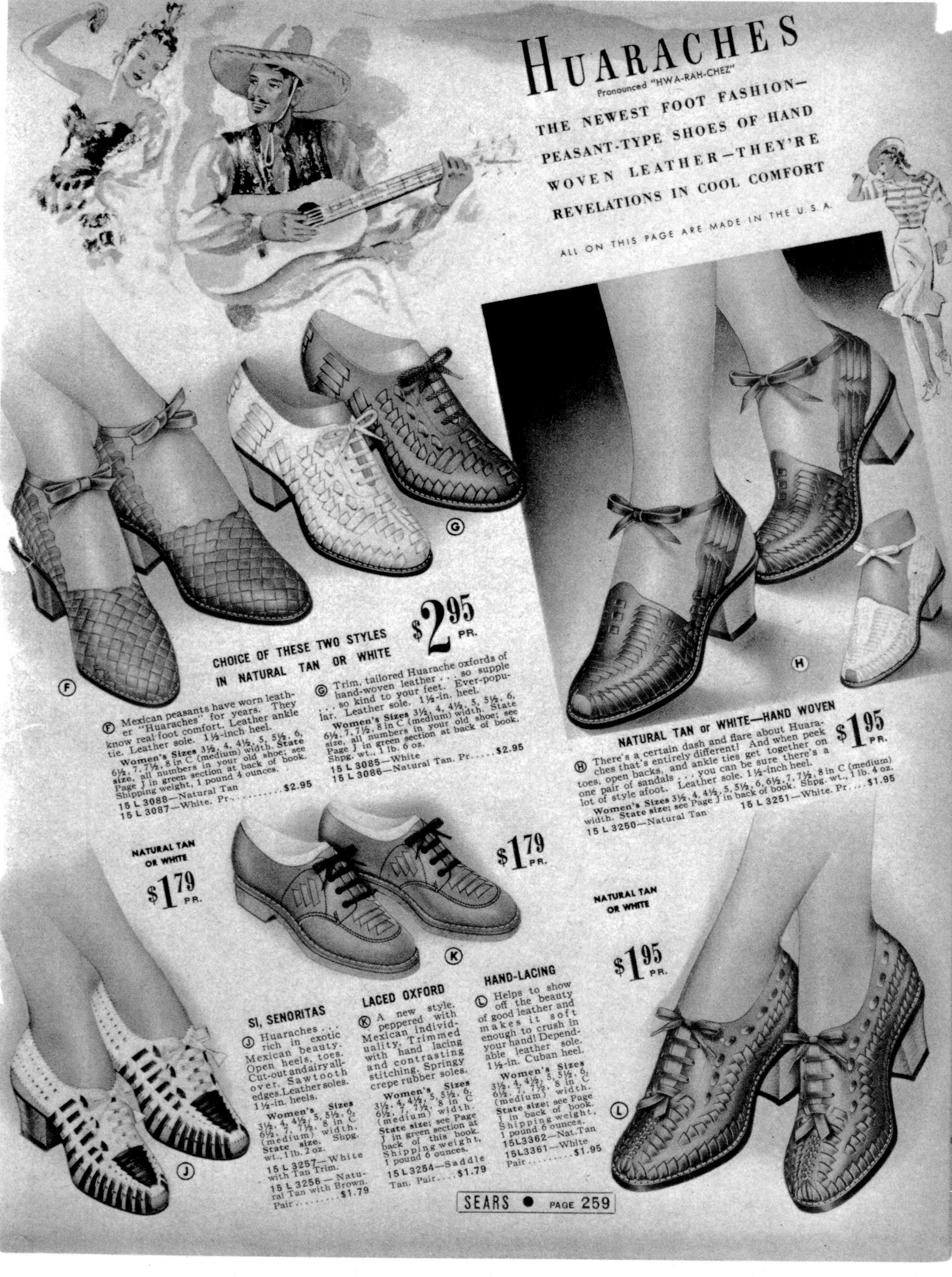
HUARACHES
Pronounced "HWA-RAH-CHEZ"
THE NEWEST FOOT FASHION—
PEASANT-TYPE SHOES OF HAND
WOVEN LEATHER—THEY'RE
REVELATIONS IN COOL COMFORT
ALL ON THIS PAGE ARE MADE IN THE U.S.A.
G
CHOICE OF THESE TWO STYLES IN NATURAL TAN OR WHITE
$2.95 PR.
F
F Mexican peasants have worn leather "Huaraches" for years. They know real foot comfort. Leather ankle tie. Leather sole. 1½-inch heel.
Women's Sizes 3½, 4, 4½, 5, 5½, 6, 6½, 7, 7½, 8 in C (medium) width. State size, all numbers in your old shoe; see Page J in green section at back of book. Shipping weight, 1 pound 4 ounces.
15 L 3088—Natural Tan
15 L 3087—White. Pr. $2.95
G Trim, tailored Huarache oxfords of hand-woven leather . . . so supple . . . so kind to your feet. Ever-popular. Leather sole. 1½-in. heel.
Women's Sizes 3½, 4, 4½, 5, 5½, 6, 6½, 7, 7½, 8 in C (medium) width. State size, all numbers in your old shoe; see Page J in green section at back of book. Shpg. wt., 1 lb. 6 oz.
15 L 3085—White
15 L 3086—Natural Tan. Pr. $2.95
H
NATURAL TAN or WHITE—HAND WOVEN
$1.95 PR.
H There's a certain dash and flare about Huaraches that's entirely different! And when peek toes, open backs, and ankle ties get together on one pair of sandals . . . you can be sure there's a lot of style afoot. Leather sole. 1½-inch heel.
Women's Sizes 3½, 4, 4½, 5, 5½, 6, 6½, 7, 7½, 8 in C (medium) width. State size; see Page J in back of book. Shpg. wt., 1 lb. 4 oz.
15 L 3250—Natural Tan
15 L 3251—White. Pr. . . . $1.95
NATURAL TAN OR WHITE
$1.79 PR.
$1.79 PR.
K
NATURAL TAN OR WHITE
$1.95 PR.
SI, SENORITAS
J Huaraches . . . rich in exotic Mexican beauty. Open heels, toes. Cut-out and airy all-over. Sawtooth edges. Leather soles. 1½-in. heels.
Women's Sizes 3½, 4, 4½, 5, 5½, 6, 6½, 7, 7½, 8 in C (medium) width. State size. Shpg. wt., 1 lb. 2 oz.
15 L 3257—White with Tan Trim.
15 L 3256—Natural Tan with Brown. Pair $1.79
LACED OXFORD
K A new style, peppered with Mexican individuality. Trimmed with hand lacing and contrasting stitching. Springy crepe rubber soles.
Women's Sizes 3½, 4, 4½, 5, 5½, 6, 6½, 7, 7½, 8 in C (medium) width. State size; see Page J in green section at back of this book. Shipping weight, 1 pound 6 ounces.
15 L 3254—Saddle Tan. Pair. . . . $1.79
HAND-LACING
L Helps to show off the beauty of good leather and makes it soft enough to crush in your hand! Dependable leather sole. 1½-in. Cuban heel.
Women's Sizes 3½, 4, 4½, 5, 5½, 6, 6½, 7, 7½, 8 in C (medium) width. State size; see Page J in back of book. Shipping weight, 1 pound 6 ounces.
15L3362—Nat. Tan
15L3361—White
Pair $1.95
J
L
SEARS • PAGE 259

Voted Most Popular
NAILHEADS VOTED MOST SENSATIONAL
A AND C WIDTHS
F
$2.88 PR.
G
$2.98 PR.
J
$2.88 PR.
Gored Slip-on
(F) You'll adore this soft calfskin shoe. Leather sole. Goodyear Welt construction. 1½-in. heel; rubber lift.
Women's Sizes 5, 5½, 6, 6½, 7, 7½, 8, 9 in A (narrow) width. Sizes 3½, 4, 4½, 5, 5½, 6, 6½, 7, 7½, 8, 9 in C (medium) width. State size and width. Shpg. wt., 1 lb. 8 oz.
15 D 2682—Brown.
15 D 2683—Black. Pair $2.88
Cossack Boot
(G) Smacking of the "Old World" in the smartest young American way—a boot of fine leather. Goodyear Welt. Contrasting cuff. Leather sole, 1½-in. heel.
Women's Sizes 3½, 4, 4½, 5, 5½, 6, 6½, 7, 7½, 8 in C (medium) width. State size. Shpg. wt., 1 lb. 10 oz.
15 D 2124—White, Brown Cuff.
15 D 2125—Beige, Brown Cuff.
Pair $2.98
CREPE SOLES VOTED MOST LIKELY TO SUCCEED
H
$2.49 PR.
A AND C WIDTHS
Classic Saddle
(H) Beloved on campus. White leather, brown saddle. Goodyear Welt. Red rope and natural crepe rubber sole and heel.
Women's Sizes 5, 5½, 6, 6½, 7, 7½, 8, 9 in A (narrow) width. Sizes 3½, 4, 4½, 5, 5½, 6, 6½, 7, 7½, 8, 9 in C (medium) width. State size and width, see Page J in back of book. Shpg. wt., 1 lb. 12 oz.
15 D 2103—White. Pair ... $2.49
Debonair Dutchees
(J) Your feet will sparkle with tiny lights from the nail-heads on the soles of these oxfords. Burnt toast (light tan color) leather uppers; Goodyear Welt. Crepe rubber soles and heels.
Women's Sizes 3½, 4, 4½, 5, 5½, 6, 6½, 7, 7½, 8, 9 in C (medium) width. State size, see Page J in back of book. Shpg. wt., 1 lb. 14 oz.
15 D 2117—Pair $2.88
DUTCHEES VOTED THE SWEETEST
$1.98 PR.
$1.88 PR.
$1.98 PR.
$1.98 PR.

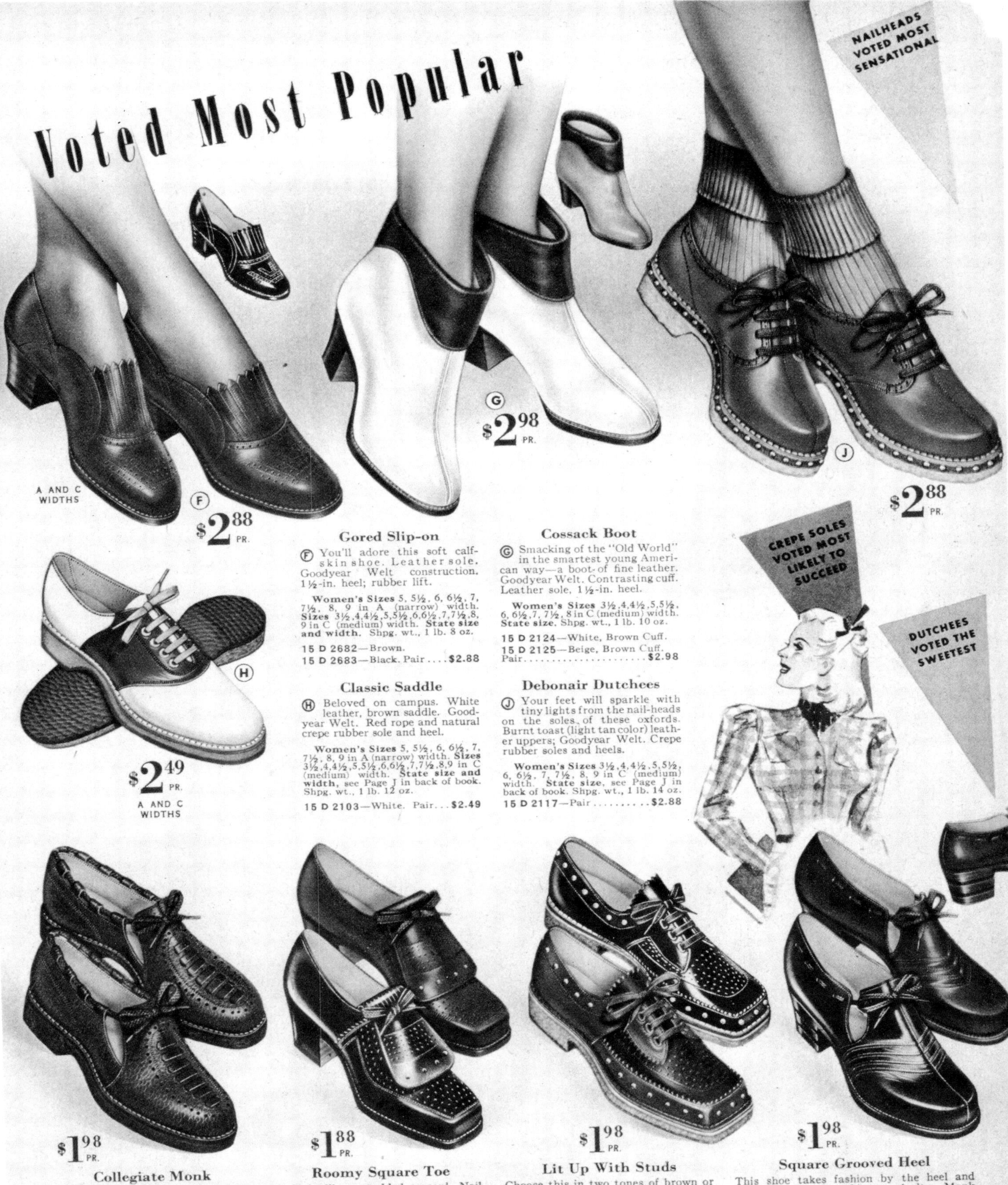

Collegiate Monk

Bound all around with "camisole" lacing through the top, this high throated tie ranks first in the fashion class. Brown crushed leather with interlacing on vamp. Springy crepe rubber sole and heel for cushioned steps.

Women's Sizes 3½, 4, 4½, 5, 5½, 6, 6½, 7, 7½, 8 in C (medium) width. **State size,** see Page J in back of book. Shipping weight, 1 pound 12 ounces.

15 D 2678—Brown. Pair **$1.98**

Roomy Square Toe

It looks like a studded season! Nailheads accent the shawl tongue of this popular shoe. Foot-conforming wall last . . . plenty comfortable. Quality leather upper, leather sole. 1½-inch heel with rubber lift.

Women's Sizes 3½, 4, 4½, 5, 5½, 6, 6½, 7, 7½, 8 in C (medium) width. **State size.** Shipping weight, 1 pound 8 ounces.

15 D 2139—Brown.
15 D 2140—Black. Pair **$1.88**

Lit Up With Studs

Choose this in two tones of brown or in all black leather for campus chic. It borrows the scow last from brother and adds studs for coeducational charm. Crepe rubber sole, heel.

Women's Sizes 3½, 4, 4½, 5, 5½, 6, 6½, 7, 7½, 8 in C (medium) width. **State size,** see Page J in back of book. Shipping weight, 1 pound 12 ounces.

15 D 2142—Black.
15 D 2141—Two-Tone Brown. Pr. **$1.98**

Square Grooved Heel

This shoe takes fashion by the heel and there's no question of its popularity. Monk tie of smooth leather, "Dutch girl" walled last. Leather sole. 1½-inch heel.

Women's Sizes 3½, 4, 4½, 5, 5½, 6, 6½, 7, 7½, 8 in C (medium) width. **State size,** see Page J in back of book. Shipping weight, 1 lb. 12 oz.

15 D 2149—Brown **15 D 2150**—Black
Pair **$1.98**

ENJOY ROSY CHEEKS . . KEEP YOUNG AND PEPPY

Snow Boots FOR WINTER FUN!

SEARS EASY PAYMENT PLAN LETS YOU AFFORD THE BETTER THINGS SEE PAGE II

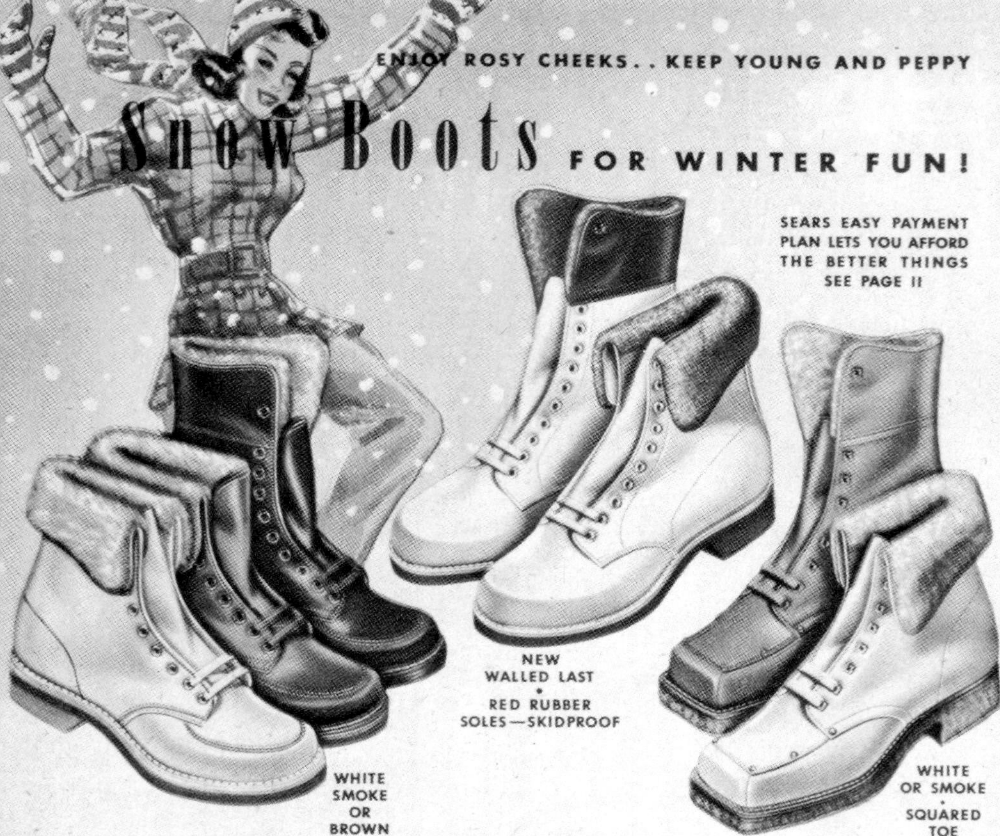

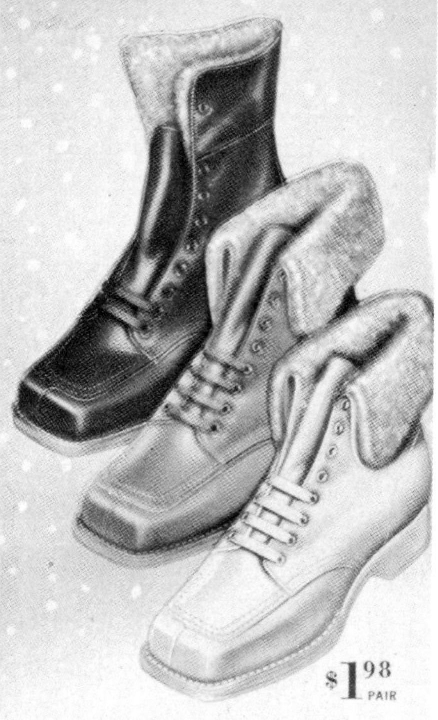

SHEEPSKIN CUFFS ON SOFT PLIABLE ELK GRAIN LEATHER "SNOW TOPS"

When the Snow Flies!

Be sure of warm feet in cozy snow boots. They are made over the roomy, moccasin, walled last with full, protective tongues. Uppers of fine grade elk-grained leather; sheepskin cuffs. Sport rubber soles and heels; leather insoles and counters. $1.79 PAIR

Women's Sizes 2½, 3, 3½, 4, 4½, 5, 5½, 6, 6½, 7, 7½, 8 in D (medium wide) width. **State size**, see Page J in back of book. Shipping weight, 2 lbs. 4 oz

15 D 2045—White
15 D 2046—Smoke
15 D 2047—Brown. Pair $1.79

Brighten Frosty Days

The Dutch walled last is perfect for sports shoes. Here are snow boots in this extra comfortable style. Uppers are fine elk-grained leather with cuffs smartly contrasting in red leather when worn up. Cozy shearling cuff is nice and warm around your ankles. Skid-proof red rubber soles and heels. $1.98 PAIR

Women's Sizes 2½, 3, 3½, 4, 4½, 5, 5½, 6, 6½, 7, 7½, 8 in D (medium wide) width. **State size**, see Page J in back of book. Shipping weight, 2 pounds 2 ounces.

15 D 2035—White. Pair $1.98

Be Young This Winter!

Our finest snow boots. Grand for hiking, tobogganing and all winter sports wear—square toe, wall lasted. Of best grade elk-grained leather. Vamps are youthfully studded with nailheads. The up-or-down cuffs are soft, warm, sheep's wool. Soles and heels are thick, spongy crepe rubber. $2.98 PAIR

Women's Sizes 2½, 3, 3½, 4, 4½, 5, 5½, 6, 6½, 7, 7½, 8 in C (medium) width. **State size**, see Page J in back of book. Shipping weight, 2 lbs. 5 oz.

15 D 2007—White
15 D 2039—Smoke. Pair $2.98

Square toe styles have taken the fashion world by storm. Sears bring you this popular idea in wall lasted, moccasin type snow boots that will be all the rage this season. Roomy toed and wonderfully comfortable. The uppers are good quality elk-grained leather. Full tongues help keep out cold and dampness. Cuffs of fluffy sheep's wool are cuddly around your ankles. The soles and heels are firm, durable rubber. Outstanding value at Sears low price. Even if you've never been outdoors-minded you'll want to get these and learn to enjoy the crisp, healthful, winter weather.

Women's Sizes 2½, 3, 3½, 4, 4½, 5, 5½, 6, 6½, 7, 7½, 8 in D (medium wide) width. **State size**, see Page J in back of book. Shipping weight, 2 pounds 2 ounces.

15 D 2205—White
15 D 2206—Smoke
15 D 2207—Brown
Pair $1.98

THE NEW SQUARE TOE

Snow Boots

. . ARE THE THING FOR WINTER SPORTS —FOR SCHOOL, TOO!

THE LABEL OF QUALITY

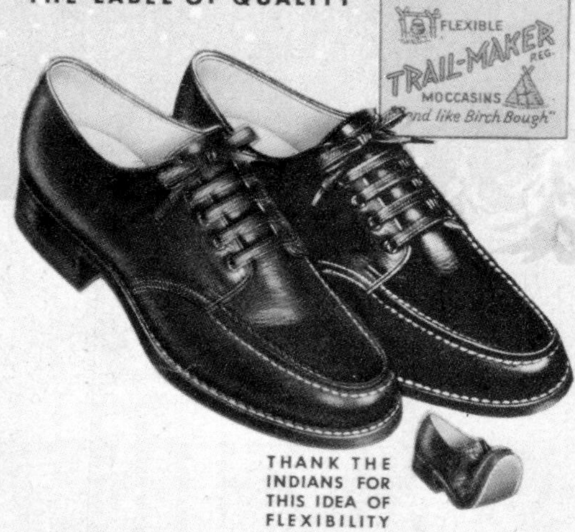

① GROOVED SKI HEELS
② THICK TAP SOLES
③ RIVETED SHANK

THANK THE INDIANS FOR THIS IDEA OF FLEXIBILITY

Snug Ankle Strap Boot

It's a honey! The grandest shoe you can find for wintry days. White elk-grained leather upper. Inlay and ankle strap are smooth brown leather. Soft shearling "up-or-down" cuff. Double leather Goodyear welt sewed sole. 1-inch grooved ski heel and all the other features illustrated at left. $2.88 PAIR

Women's Sizes 2½, 3, 3½, 4, 4½, 5, 5½, 6, 6½, 7, 7½, 8 in C (medium) width. **State size.** Shipping weight, 2 lbs. 2 oz.

15 D 2543—White with Brown Trim
Pair $2.88

When The Snow's Deep

Eight eyelet boots to give you complete protection in deep snow. Fleecy sheep's wool cuffs. The uppers combine smoke and brown colors in fine quality smooth leather. Full tongue gives ample protection. Sturdy leather sole. Comfortable new squared toe. 1-inch groove ski-type heel. $2.49 PAIR

Women's Sizes 2½, 3, 3½, 4, 4½, 5, 5½, 6, 6½, 7, 7½, 8 in C (medium) width. **State size**, see Page J in back of book. Shipping weight, 1 pound 12 ounces.

15 D 2542—Brown and Smoke. Pr. $2.49

Just Made For Outdoors!

Genuine hand sewn moccasin specially designed for active wear. The upper is full elk-grained leather, smooth and wonderfully strong. The moccasin type toe is soft and roomy. The sole of excellent quality leather . . . bends like a birch bough. 1-inch heel; rubber lift. $2.88 PAIR

Women's Sizes 3½, 4, 4½, 5, 5½, 6, 6½, 7, 7½, 8, 9 in C (medium) width. **State size**, see Page J in back of book. Shipping weight, 1 pound 14 ounces.

15 D 2156—Black
15 D 2155—Brown. Pair $2.88

TWO-WAY TOPPER
ALWAYS IN SEASON
COMBINATION TOPCOAT/OVERCOAT
The All Wool Lining Zips In and Out!
From a Handsome Easy-Weight Topcoat to a Snug Warm Overcoat in Less Than 15 Seconds!
$17.75 Cash
ONLY $2.50 DOWN
See Page 11
Sears 4 STAR FEATURE

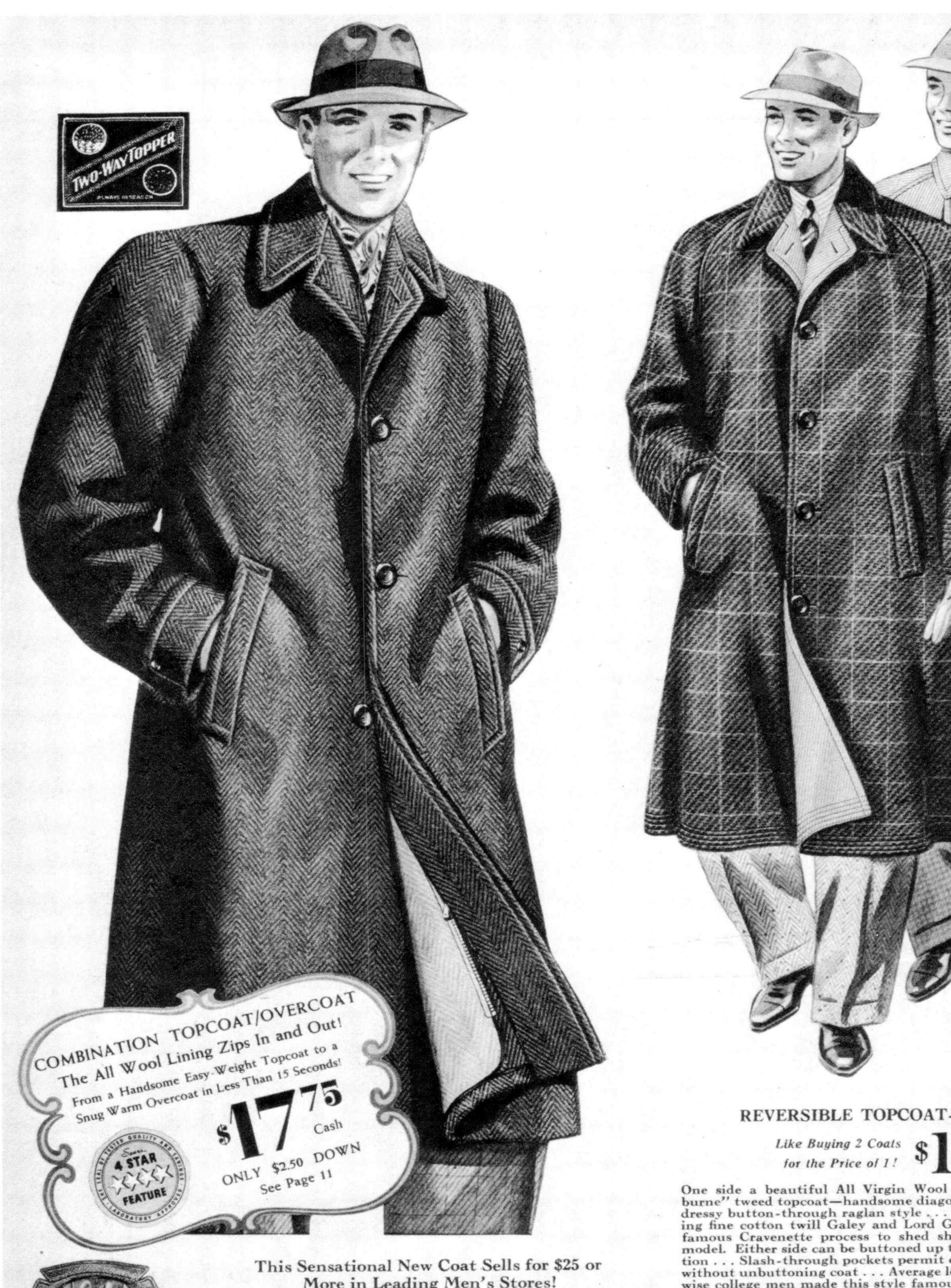

REVERSIBLE TOPCOAT-RAINCOAT

Like Buying 2 Coats for the Price of 1! **$11.00 CASH**

One side a beautiful All Virgin Wool showerproofed "Rockburne" tweed topcoat—handsome diagonal-overplaid pattern—dressy button-through raglan style . . . Other side a harmonizing fine cotton twill Galey and Lord Gabardine—treated with famous Cravenette process to shed showers—smart fly front model. Either side can be buttoned up to neck for extra protection . . . Slash-through pockets permit entrance to suit pockets without unbuttoning coat . . . Average length, 48 inches. Stylewise college men made this style famous!

Meet any kind of weather in a marvelous new reversible that's worth $17.50 easily! A spectacular fashion hit direct from big Eastern campuses where the college men know how to dress right for any occasion without straining their budgets. Warmth, comfort and rich shading in the luxurious showerproofed All Wool Tweed topcoat, lots of natty-looking protection in the Cravenetted cotton gabardine raincoat—and you have either one by a simple reverse that takes only seconds! Splendid tailoring, a wealth of style, many months of deep satisfaction—one of the best buys you'll ever make anywhere!

Sizes: 33 to 42-inch chest. **State chest measurement taken over vest; also age, height and weight.** See Easy Measuring Instructions on Page G in back of book. Shipping weight, 3 lbs. 14 oz.

65 D 8316—Medium Gray Reversible $11.00
65 D 8317—Medium Green Reversible 11.00
65 D 8318—Medium Brown Reversible 11.00

This Sensational New Coat Sells for $25 or More in Leading Men's Stores!

Luxurious All Wool "Rumson" Cheviot—in new Herringbone pattern and striking shades . . . Removable All Wool lining in attractive camel tan shade . . . Talon slide fastener works smoothly to make the coat a topcoat or overcoat in a jiffy! . . . Average length, 47 inches. A 4-Star Feature.

Most practical development in clothing history! **Two coats in one!** Lining in, a warm overcoat. Lining out, a comfortable topcoat with all the fine features of our regular *Fashion Tailored* topcoat with yoke and sleeve lining of lustrous Earl-Glo rayon. New "Dorchester" model; smart set-in sleeves, military collar.

Sizes: 33 to 42-inch chest. **State chest measure taken over vest; also age, height and weight.** See Easy Measuring Instructions on Page G in back of book. Shpg. wt., 5 lbs. 14 oz.

65 D 8374—Medium Gray Two-Way Topper $17.75
65 D 8376—Dark Green Two-Way Topper 17.75
65 D 8378—Med. Dk. Brown Two-Way Topper 17.75

These Men's Topcoats are Shipped from Chicago, Philadelphia, or Minneapolis. You Order and Pay Postage from Your Nearest Mail Order House.

IN THE 1939 SPORTLIGHT...

NEW..PRACTICAL..SMART

Summer Togs

Everything at Sears Sold on Easy Terms...See Page 5

Cool Sports Coat of "Sportflash" Cloth

$3.49 Famous cotton fabric in popular checks of bright new summer shades . . . Sanforized-Shrunk for permanent fit. (1% Maximum fabric shrinkage.) . . . Unlined . . . Sportsback. Smart with odd slacks.

Colorful woven-in pattern. 2-button notch lapel model; 3 patch pockets.

Sizes: 34 to 44-in. chest. **State chest and sleeve length measures as shown on Page F in back of book.** Shipping weight, 1 lb. 8 oz.

45 L 7377—Brown **$3.49**
45 L 7378—Green **3.49**

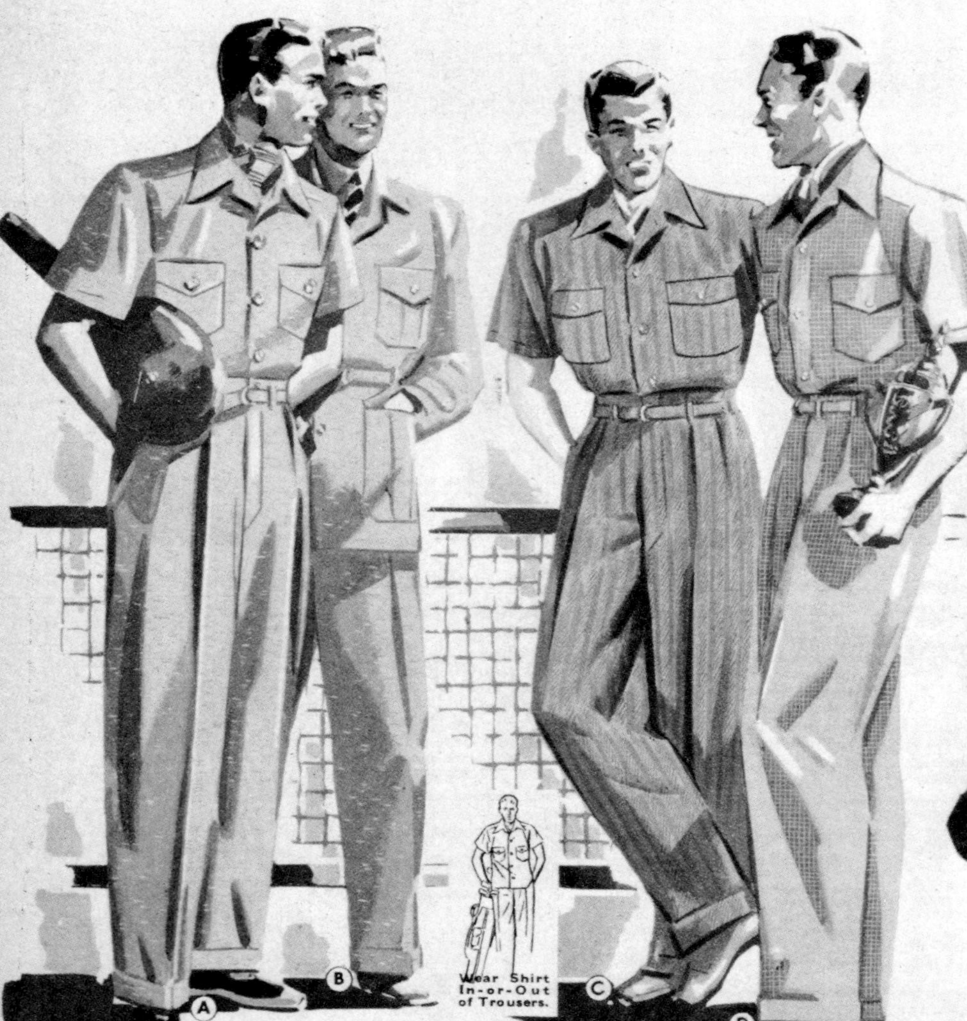

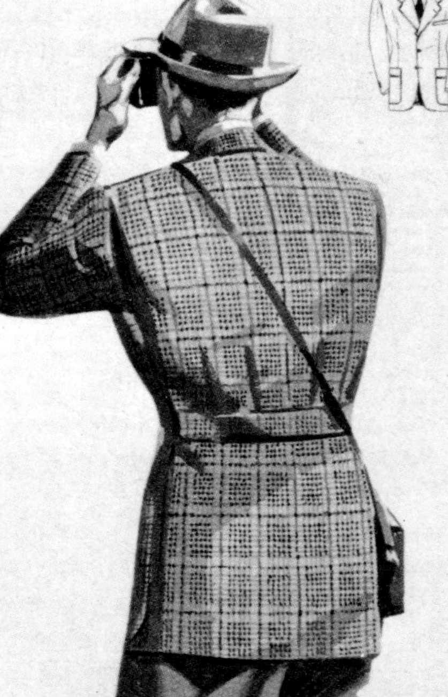

Now—Matchea Outfits! New Style and Comfort!

Ⓐ "The Ensenada"

$1.88 • Sports sensation from fun loving coast of lower California. Nationally advertised last summer at $2.95 to $3.50.

2-Pc. Outfit

A cool, airy weave of natural tan shade porous cotton, Sanforized-Shrunk for lasting fit. Maximum fabric shrinkage 1%. Easily laundered at home. Shirt with wooden buttons, two pockets. Slacks have setdown belt loops, self belt with rings, pleats.

Shirt sizes: 36 to 46-in. chest. **Pants sizes:** waist, 28 to 42 in.; all inseams 29 to 34-in. **State chest, waist, and inseam sizes.** Shipping weight, 2 pounds 8 ounces.

41 L 4780—Shirt and Pants **$1.88**

Ⓑ **Bush Coat** . . . Sports back, adjustable cuffs, all-around belt with ring buckles, 4 pockets, wooden buttons. Av. lgth., 30 in.

Sizes: 36 to 46-in. chest. **State size.**

41 L 451—Bush Coat. Shpg. wt., 2 lbs. **$1.39**

Ⓒ "The Riviera"

$3.95 Lustrous Herringbone Deerfield suiting—featherweight, colorfast, finely spun of superb quality cotton. Self belt has eyelets and buckle.

Ⓓ "The Pasadena"

$2.98 Attractive Basket Weave (self check) cotton suiting. A light, breezy summer fabric—easy to launder . . . Self belt with rings.

Matched outfits are sweeping the country, and Sears give you the smartest to be found at savings of at least $1.50 to $2! Jaunty, short-sleeved Polo coat-style shirt, worn in or out. Trousers are swagger slack style; self belt, double pleats, 20-inch cuffs. Pockets and waistband lining of durable twill. Sanforized-Shrunk (not over 1% fabric shrinkage no matter how often they're washed). Handsomely designed, made to keep you *cool.* **Available only in matched sets of shirt and trousers.**

Sizes for "Riviera" and "Pasadena"

34 to 44-in. chest. 28 to 40-in. waist. 29 to 34-in. inseam. **Be sure to state chest, waist and inseam measures; also age, height and weight.** Shipping weight, 2 lbs. 6 oz.

45 L 7380—Tan
45 L 7382—Light Blue
45 L 7384—Gray **$3.95**

45 L 7390—Light Tan
45 L 7392—Light Gray **$2.98**

Newest All Wool Sports Coat

$7.95 Luxurious All Wool Cassimere in striking Hounds Tooth check with overplaid . . . Latest 3-button notch lapel model with flapped patch pockets, "Free Swing" back.

Beautifully tailored and lined with Earl-Glo rayon. Wear it with sport slacks for an ensemble outfit.

Sizes: 34 to 44-in. chest. **State chest and sleeve measurements as shown on Page F in back of book.**

45 L 7375—Spring Green. Shpg. wt., 2 lbs. **$7.95**
45 L 7376—Medium Brown **7.95**

YOU'RE DRESSED FOR SPORT
IN A
TWIN SET
Zip Front Coat
and
Slipover

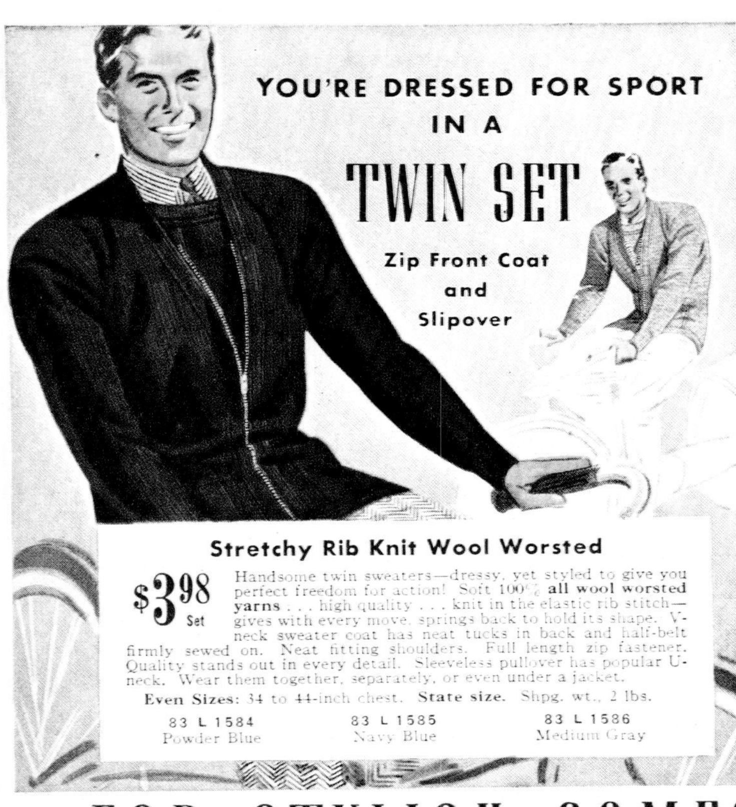

Stretchy Rib Knit Wool Worsted

$3.98 Set Handsome twin sweaters—dressy, yet styled to give you perfect freedom for action! Soft 100% **all wool worsted yarns** . . . high quality . . . knit in the elastic rib stitch—gives with every move, springs back to hold its shape. V-neck sweater coat has neat tucks in back and half-belt firmly sewed on. Neat fitting shoulders. Full length zip fastener. Quality stands out in every detail. Sleeveless pullover has popular U-neck. Wear them together, separately, or even under a jacket.

Even Sizes: 34 to 44-inch chest. **State size.** Shpg. wt., 2 lbs.

83 L 1584 Powder Blue — 83 L 1585 Navy Blue — 83 L 1586 Medium Gray

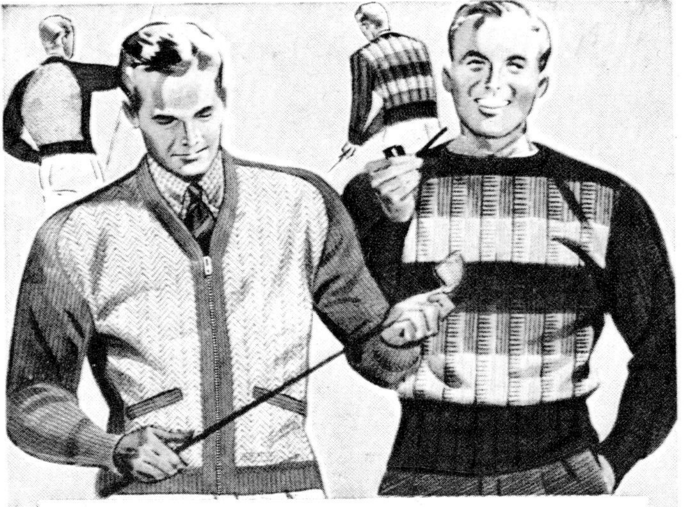

New Utility Sweater

$1.98 Each Gray heather herringbone cloth front and back. Contrasting knit sleeves and trim. Contains 50% wool, balance cotton. Crown zip front.

Even Sizes: 36 to 44-inch chest. **State size.** Shpg. wt., 1 lb. 8 oz.

83 L 1563 Lt. Gray with Dk. Gray Trim — 83 L 1564 Lt. Gray with Navy Trim

All Wool Worsted

$1.98 Each Knit in the link-and-link stitch of 2-ply all wool worsted yarns. Medium weight crew neck pullover. Contrasting stripes. Wear it anywhere—it will always be "right!"

Even Sizes: 34 to 44-in. chest. **State size.** Shpg. wt., 1 lb. 2 oz.

83 L 1514 Royal, Powder Blue and Silver. — 83 L 1515 Brown, Rust and Eggshell

FOR STYLISH COMFORT ON LAND OR SEA

Buy Everything at Sears on EASY TERMS . . See Page 5

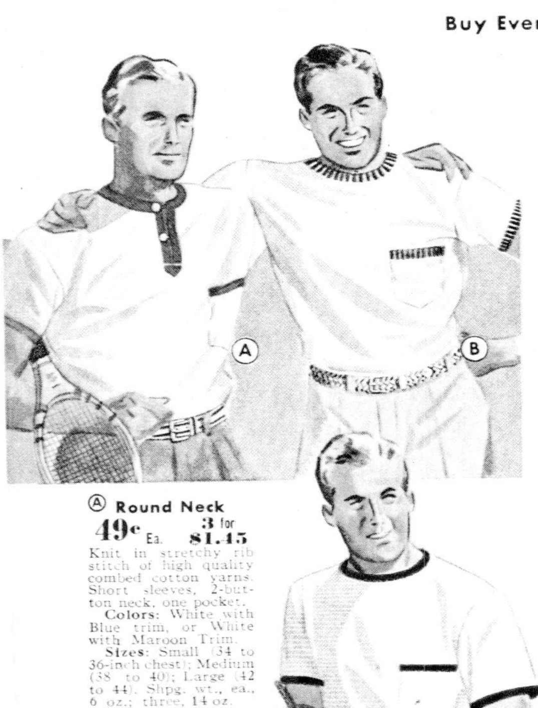

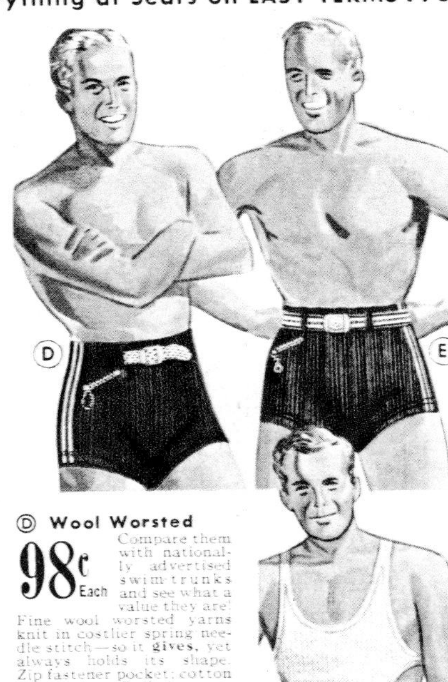

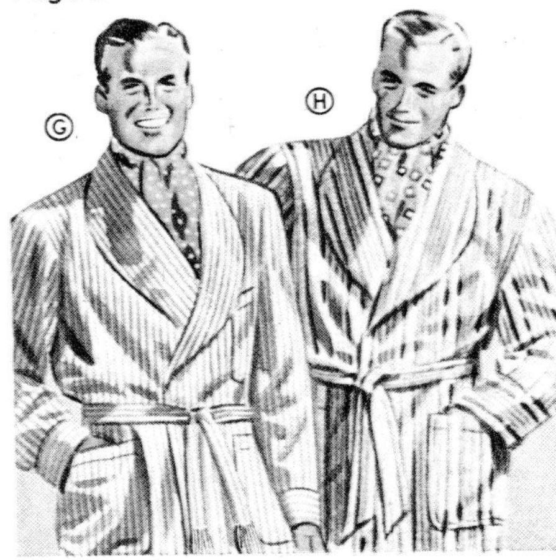

Ⓐ **Round Neck**

49c Ea. 3 for $1.45

Knit in stretchy rib stitch of high quality combed cotton yarns. Short sleeves, 2-button neck, one pocket.

Colors: White with Blue trim, or White with Maroon Trim.

Sizes: Small (34 to 36-inch chest); Medium (38 to 40); Large (42 to 44). Shpg. wt., ea., 6 oz.; three, 14 oz.

83 L 2040

State size and color.

Ⓑ **Crew Neck**

29c Ea. 3 for 85c

Ideal hot weather "T" shirt! Smooth balbriggan fabric knit of fine combed cotton yarns. Lightweight. Crew neck . . . short sleeves. Contrasting trim.

Colors: White with Blue; or White with Maroon.

Sizes: Small (34 to 36-inch chest) Medium (38 to 40); Large (42 to 44). Shpg. wt., ea., 6 oz.; three, 14 oz.

83 L 2041

State size and color.

Ⓒ **Cool Mesh Knit**

39c Ea. 3 for $1.15

Fine combed cotton yarns in this elastic mesh knit "T" shirt. Medium weight. Contrasting trim.

Colors: White with Blue trim, or White with Maroon Trim.

Sizes: Small (34 to 36-inch chest); Medium (38 to 40); Large (42 to 44). Shpg. wt., ea., 7 oz.; three, 1 lb. 1 oz.

83 L 2043

State size and color.

Ⓓ **Wool Worsted**

98c Each Compare them with nationally advertised swim trunks and see what a value they are! Fine wool worsted yarns knit in costlier spring needle stitch—so it **gives**, yet always holds its shape. Zip fastener pocket; cotton web belt. Built-in supporter.

Colors: Navy Blue, Royal Blue or Maroon.

Even Sizes: 28 to 42-inch waist. Shipping weight, 7 ounces.

83 L 9800

State size and color.

Ⓔ **Knit-in Lastex**

$1.59 Each You'll cut a real figure in these handsome rib knit swim trunks. Fine all wool worsted yarns knit with stretchy lastex—always shapely. Loops hold cotton web belt in place. Handy pocket with slide fastener. Built-in supporter. Slip into a pair and enjoy new swimming comfort.

Colors: Navy Blue, Maroon or Royal.

Even Sizes: 30 to 40-in. waist. Shpg. wt., 8 oz.

83 L 9801

State size and color.

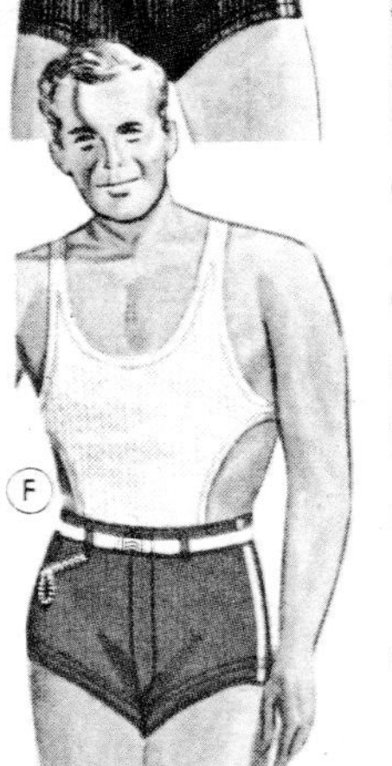

Ⓕ **2-Piece Suit**

$2.29 Each Fancy knit shirt zips on to spring needle rib knit trunks. Built-in supporter. All wool worsted yarn. **Colors:** Navy trunk, White top, Royal trunk, White top.

Even Sizes: 34 to 44-in. chest. Shpg. wt., 10 oz.

83 L 9802

State size and color.

Ⓖ **Cotton Seersucker Robe**

Washable . . . Needs No Ironing

$1.89 Each You'll wonder how you ever got along without this big comfortable wrap-around robe. Tailored of cool, **crinkly cotton seersucker** . . . the perfect hot-weather fabric. Good-looking striped patterns that are always in style. Easy to keep fresh and neat because it's **washable.** Three convenient pockets, shawl collar. Fringed sash. Perfect for home, beach wear or traveling.

Even sizes: 34 to 48-inch chest. **State size.** Shipping weight, 1 pound 6 ounces.

33 L 1985—Blue Stripe on White
33 L 1986—Tan Stripe on White

Ⓗ **Thick Terry Cloth Robe**

Washes Like a Turkish Towel

$2.98 Each No need to pamper this sturdy robe. Made of full bodied cotton terry cloth in the popular wrap-around style. The rough terry fabric makes it unusually absorbent. That's why it's just the thing to slip into after a shower or a swim. Perfect summer lounging robe, too. Attractive contrasting stripes on white grounds, or plain white. Washes like a Turkish towel—needs no ironing. Double shawl collar, matching sash. Two pockets.

Even Sizes: 34 to 48-inch chest. **State size.** Shipping weight, 1 pound 12 ounces.

33 L 1901—White, Maroon and Gray Stripes
33 L 1902—White, Yellow and Blue Stripes
33 L 1903—Plain White

Sears BIGGEST BUY IN HORSEHIDE

First Time in Our History—a Genuine Horsehide Cossack with Many Extra Value Features at a Price This Low!

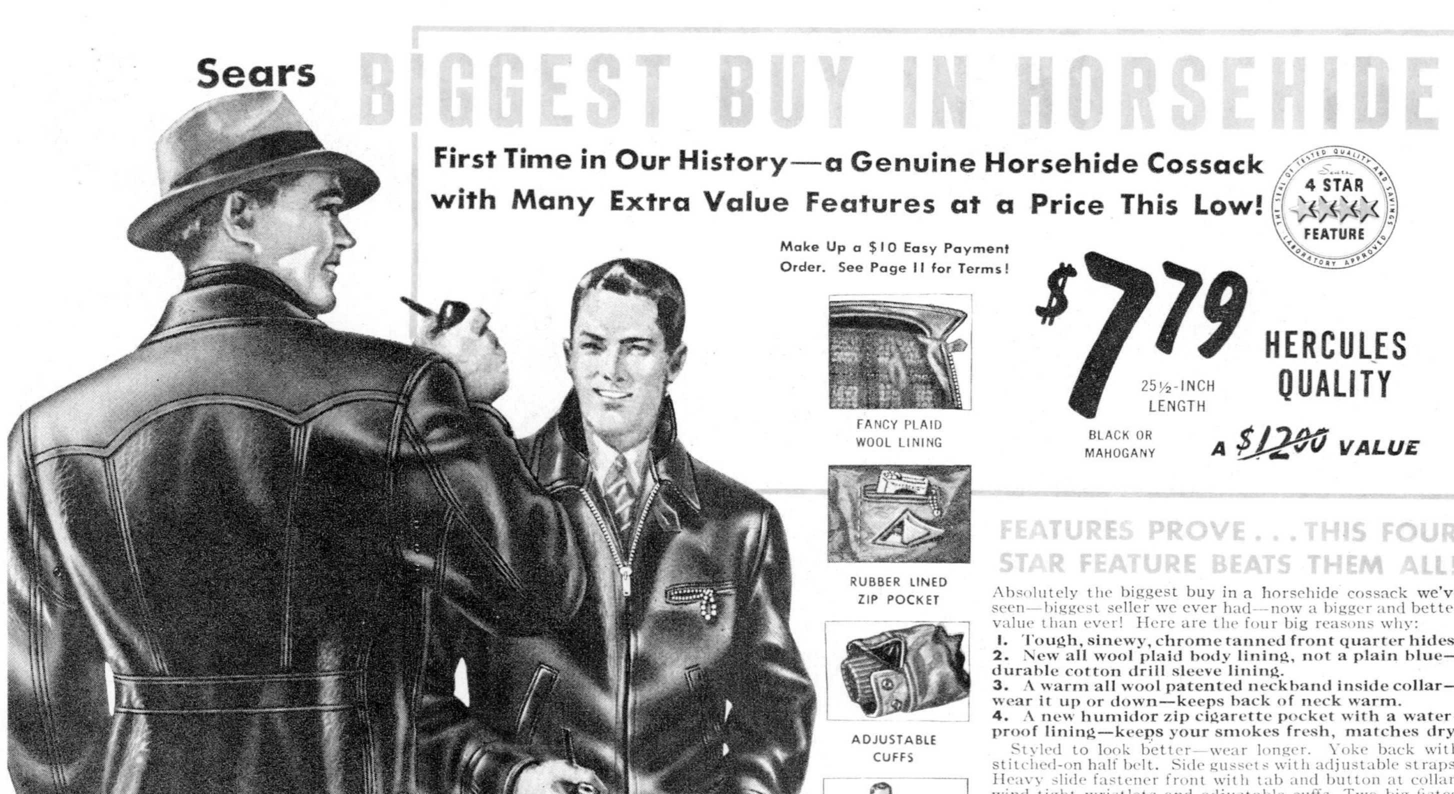

FEATURES PROVE . . . THIS FOUR STAR FEATURE BEATS THEM ALL!

Absolutely the biggest buy in a horsehide cossack we've seen—biggest seller we ever had—now a bigger and better value than ever! Here are the four big reasons why:

1. Tough, sinewy, chrome tanned front quarter hides!
2. New all wool plaid body lining, not a plain blue—durable cotton drill sleeve lining.
3. A warm all wool patented neckband inside collar—wear it up or down—keeps back of neck warm.
4. A new humidor zip cigarette pocket with a waterproof lining—keeps your smokes fresh, matches dry.

Styled to look better—wear longer. Yoke back with stitched-on half belt. Side gussets with adjustable straps. Heavy slide fastener front with tab and button at collar, wind-tight wristlets and adjustable cuffs. Two big-fisted slash pockets—cotton flannel lined. Ventilating eyelets.

Regular Sizes: Even chest sizes 34 to 48 in. 25½ inches long. **State chest measurement.** Shipping weight, 4 lbs. 12 oz.
41 D 6600—**Black** . . . $7.79
41 D 6604—**Mahogany Brown** 7.79

Extra-Long Sizes. Chest sizes as at left but 2 in. longer body, 1½ in. longer sleeves. Shipping weight, 5 lbs. 1 oz.
41 D 6603—**Black** . . . $8.79
41 D 6605—**Mahogany Brown** . . . 8.79

NONE TOUGHER THAN SEARS SELECTED FRONT QUARTER HORSEHIDES . . WINDPROOF! CRACKPROOF! SCUFFPROOF!

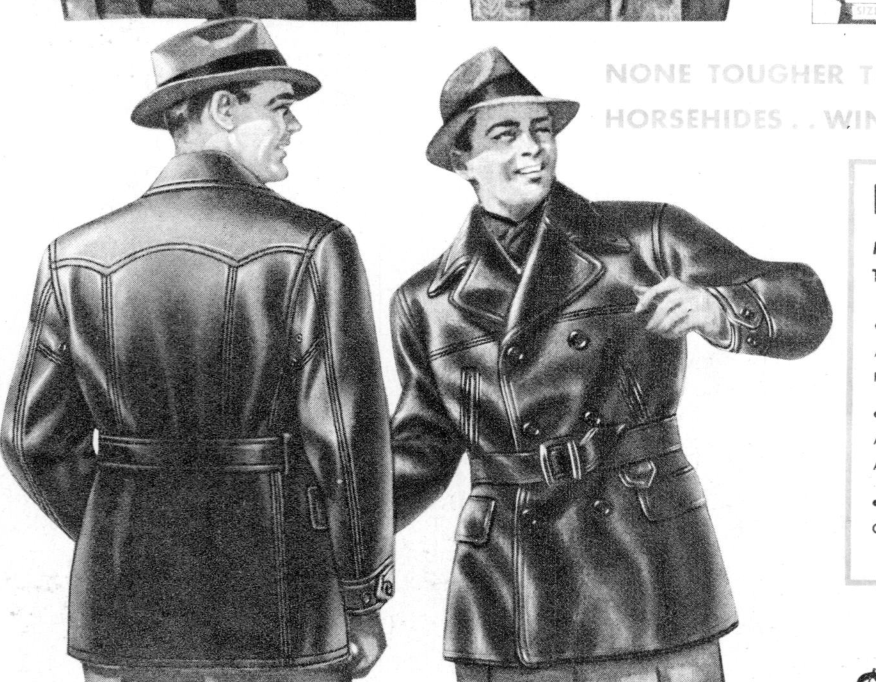

FULL 32-INCH WARMLY-LINED HORSEHIDE COATS

$9.95 Black — **chrome tanned front quarter hides in good-looking 32-inch double breasted styles with panel back and durable corduroy lining** — $10.95 Brown

Hercules quality—in a roomy comfortable construction that's as strong as the horsehide itself! Double breasted style gives double protection across the chest. Fancy yoke back and all-around belt. Lined with durable corduroy (blue in the black coat; brown in the mahogany).

Husky, warm moleskin cloth lining in sleeves . . . unbreakable buttons sewed on with imported linen thread—special Sears features! Double leather collar with corduroy faced neckband. Two big cotton flannel lined muff pockets. Two roomy lower flap pockets. Ventilation eyelets under arms.

Sizes: Even chest sizes 34 to 48 in. **State chest measurement.** See How to Measure on Page 469. Shipping weight, 6 lbs. 4 oz.

41 D 617—**Black Horsehide Coat** $9.95
41 D 618—**Mahogany Brown Horsehide Coat** . . . 10.95

ROOMY BLOUSE STYLE

Made Two to Four In. Longer Than Ordinary Leather Jackets

- WINDTIGHT COLLAR, CUFFS AND WAISTBAND OF ONE-HALF WOOL (BALANCE COTTON)
- EXTRA PROTECTION AT HIPS, WAIST AND NECK!
- NEW SLIDE FASTENER CIGARETTE POCKET!

$6.98 Full 27 In. Long

FRONT QUARTER HORSEHIDE—MELTON LINED

thick, warm 65% wool (balance cotton) navy blue lining in body . . tough, durable blackdrill in sleeves

Plenty of reasons why you'll be proud to own this good-looking husky horsehide blouse. The comfort of a longer, 27-inch style—with warm durable trim to keep it snug at waist, wrists, neck.

Cotton flannel lined slash pockets . . . a new handy zip cigarette pocket. Easy-action heavy slide fastener front with tab and button at neck. Air holes under arms. A mighty good jacket for hardest work!

Sizes: Even chest sizes 34 to 48 inches. **State chest measurement.** See How to Measure on Page 469. Shpg. wt., 4 lbs. 7 oz.

41 D 602—**Black Horsehide Blouse** $6.98

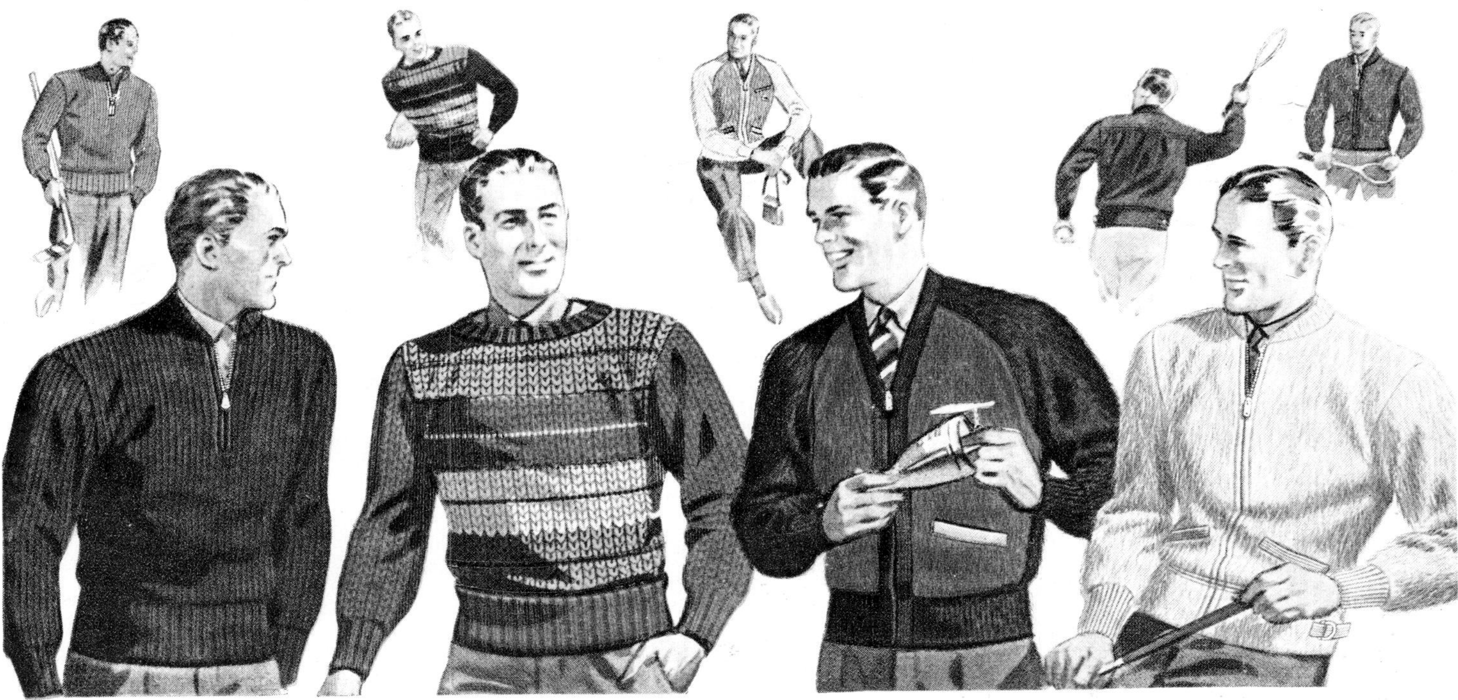

MEDIUM WEIGHT WOOL

close tight knit . . priced for big saving . . zip neck

Fine textured baby shaker stitch. Military collar with Crown slide fastener. Snug cuffs and bottom.

$1.59 Each

Even Sizes: 34 to 46-inch chest. **State size.** Shpg. wt., each, 14 oz.
83D1500—Navy 83D1501—Black

46% Wool . . . Balance Cotton

Same style and sizes as above. Shipping weight, 1 pound 2 ounces.
83 D 1555–Tan Mixture
83 D 1633–Navy Blue
83 D 1634—Gray

98¢ Each

NEW WOOL CARDIGAN

heavyweight . . livened with bold contrasting stripes

Here's the type of sweater that takes top honors on the sports scenes where the style pace is set. Handsome, rugged . . . and low-priced, too. New barrel neck fits high and emphasizes broad shoulders. Wool in the cardigan stitch assures long wear.

$1.49 Each

Ground Colors: Royal or Maroon.

Even Sizes: 34 to 44-inch chest. See "How to Measure" on Page 460. Shipping weight, each, 14 ounces.
83 D 2012—**State size and color.**

NAPPED WOOL MOHAIR

backed with cotton . . zip front . . leather pocket top

You can see it's a winner! 28% mohair wool lends a rich sheen to backing of sturdy cotton and rayon. Tightly knit and brushed to a luxuriously soft surface. Raglan shoulders . . . contrasting sleeves, back and bottom. Zip chest pocket. Two slash pockets. Crown slide fastener. Shpg. wt., 1 lb. 8 oz.

$2.98 Each

Colors: Royal with Navy Blue, or Dark Gray with Silver.

Even Sizes: 36 to 44-inch chest.
83 D 2007—**State size, color.**

VELVET-SOFT DEEP NAP

mohair wool and cotton . . zip front and shirred back

Sports or dress . . . this sweater is at home anywhere! Solid colors take a new richness from the silk-like nap. Shirred action back and slash pockets. Adjustable tabs at waist. Knit of 50% mohair wool, balance cotton. Full Crown slide fastener. Military collar.

$2.98 Each

Even Sizes: 36 to 44-inch chest. **State size.** See "How to Measure" on Page 460. Shipping wt., 1 lb. 8 oz.

83D1677 Royal Blue | 83D1678 Maroon | 83D1679 Gray

"Supreme Brand"

TWIN SWEATERS

$2.98 A Set

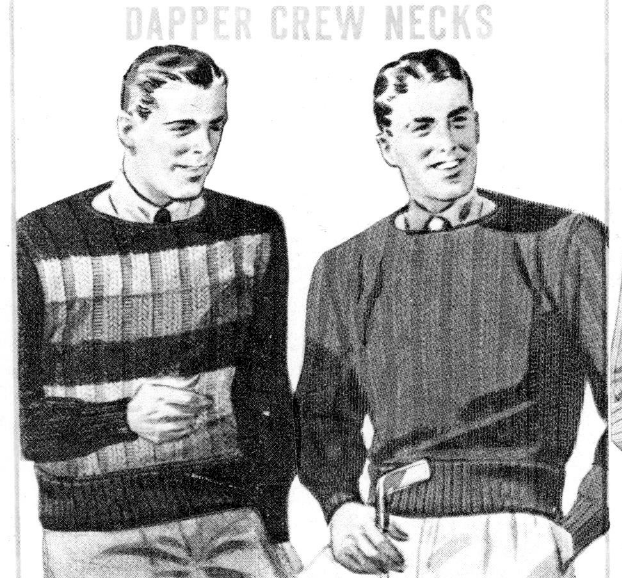

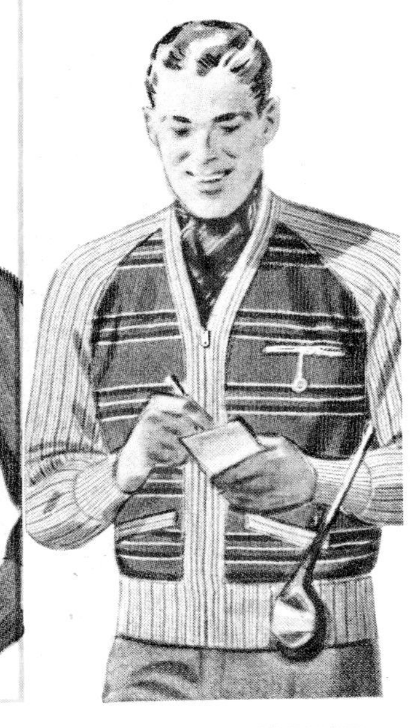

IT'S WOOL, EVEN AT THIS PRICE!

sturdy yarns closely knit . . full zip front . . smart contrasting color trim

If you want one of the most distinguished sweater combinations of the year, here's your buy! Both coat and sleeveless pullover are knit of WOOL yarns . . . both marked by a distinct drop stitch effect. Coat has the easy-fitting raglan sleeves. Contrasting sleeves and trim. V-neck style with full length Crown slide fastener. Slash pockets add an extra smart touch. Wear them separately or together.

Colors: Navy and Royal Blue, or Royal Blue and Gray.

Even Sizes: 34 to 44-inch chest. See "How to Measure" on Page 460. Shipping weight, set, 1 pound 12 ounces.
83 D 2010—**State size and color.** A Set.......... **$2.98**

PANEL KNIT ALL WOOL WORSTED

2-ply yarns in the link-and-link stitch contrasting stripes or solid colors

Two of the season's most handsome pullovers . . . choice of plain colors or bright contrasting stripes. Medium weight crew neck styles, knit of 2-ply All Wool Worsted . . . tight-twisted yarns, famous for long wear. Snug cuffs and bottom.

$1.98 Each

Even Sizes: 34 to 44-inch chest. See "How to Measure" on Page 460. **State Size.** Shipping weight, each, 1 pound 2 ounces.

Contrasting Colors
83 D 1514—Royal Combination
83 D 1515—Brown Combination

Plain Colors
83 D 1617—Royal Blue
83 D 1618—Navy Blue
83 D 1619—Dark Green

STYLE PACE-MAKER

wool worsted . . new striped front . . rib knit

High color at its best! Full Crown slide fastener . . . zip chest pocket. Raglan sleeves.

$2.98 Each

Colors: Royal and Gray or Navy and Royal. Shpg. wt., 1 lb. 4 oz.

Even Sizes: 36 to 44-inch chest.
83 D 2011—**State size, color.**

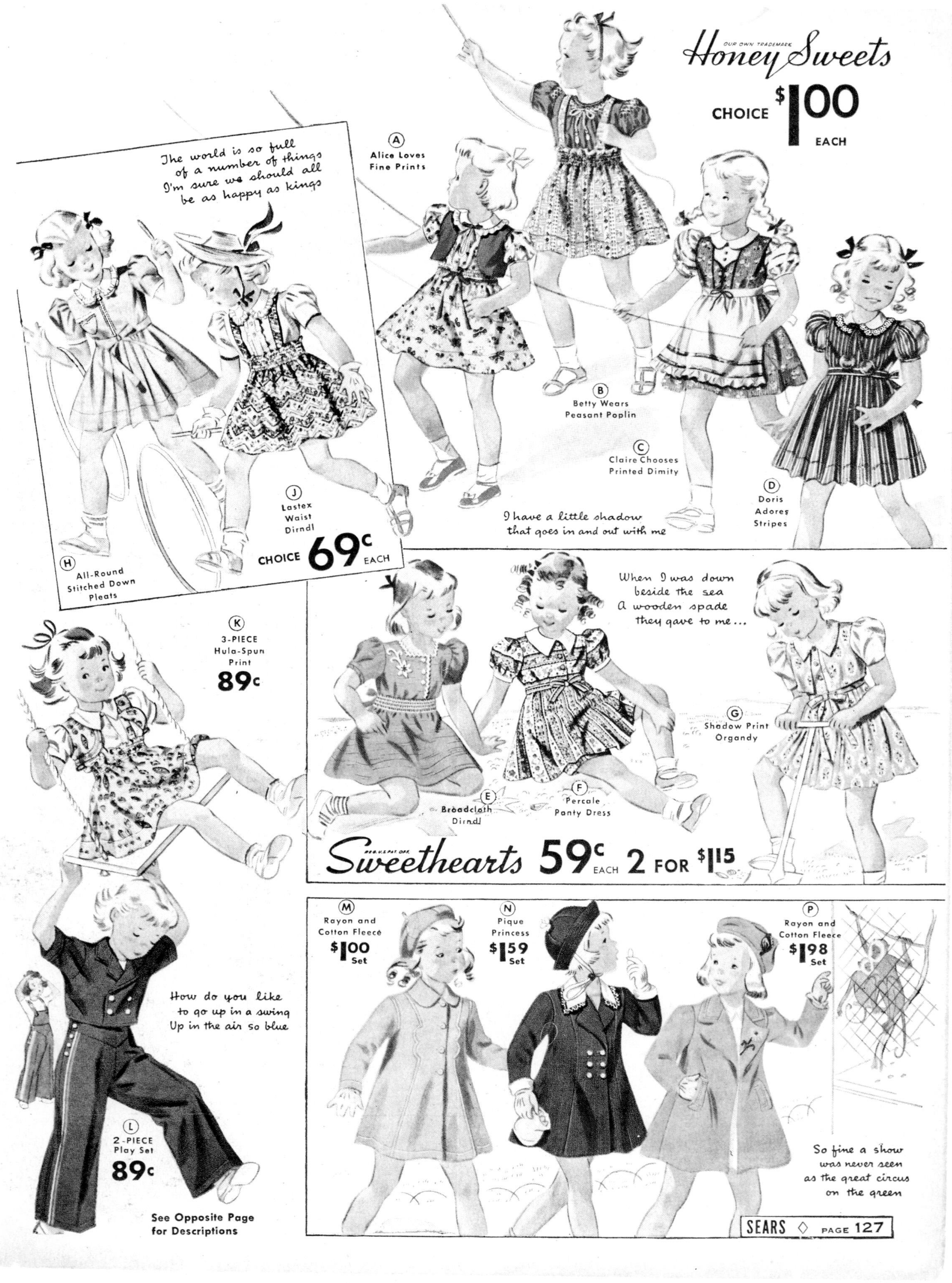

OUR OWN TRADEMARK
Honey Sweets
CHOICE $1.00 EACH
The world is so full
of a number of things
I'm sure we should all
be as happy as kings
(A) Alice Loves Fine Prints
(B) Betty Wears Peasant Poplin
(C) Claire Chooses Printed Dimity
(D) Doris Adores Stripes
I have a little shadow
that goes in and out with me
(J) Lastex Waist Dirndl
CHOICE 69c EACH
(H) All-Round Stitched Down Pleats
(K) 3-PIECE Hula-Spun Print
89c
When I was down
beside the sea
A wooden spade
they gave to me...
(G) Shadow Print Organdy
(E) Broadcloth Dirndl
(F) Percale Panty Dress
Sweethearts 59c EACH 2 FOR $1.15
(M) Rayon and Cotton Fleece $1.00 Set
(N) Pique Princess $1.59 Set
(P) Rayon and Cotton Fleece $1.98 Set
How do you like
to go up in a swing
Up in the air so blue
(L) 2-PIECE Play Set
89c
See Opposite Page
for Descriptions
So fine a show
was never seen
as the great circus
on the green
SEARS ◇ PAGE 127

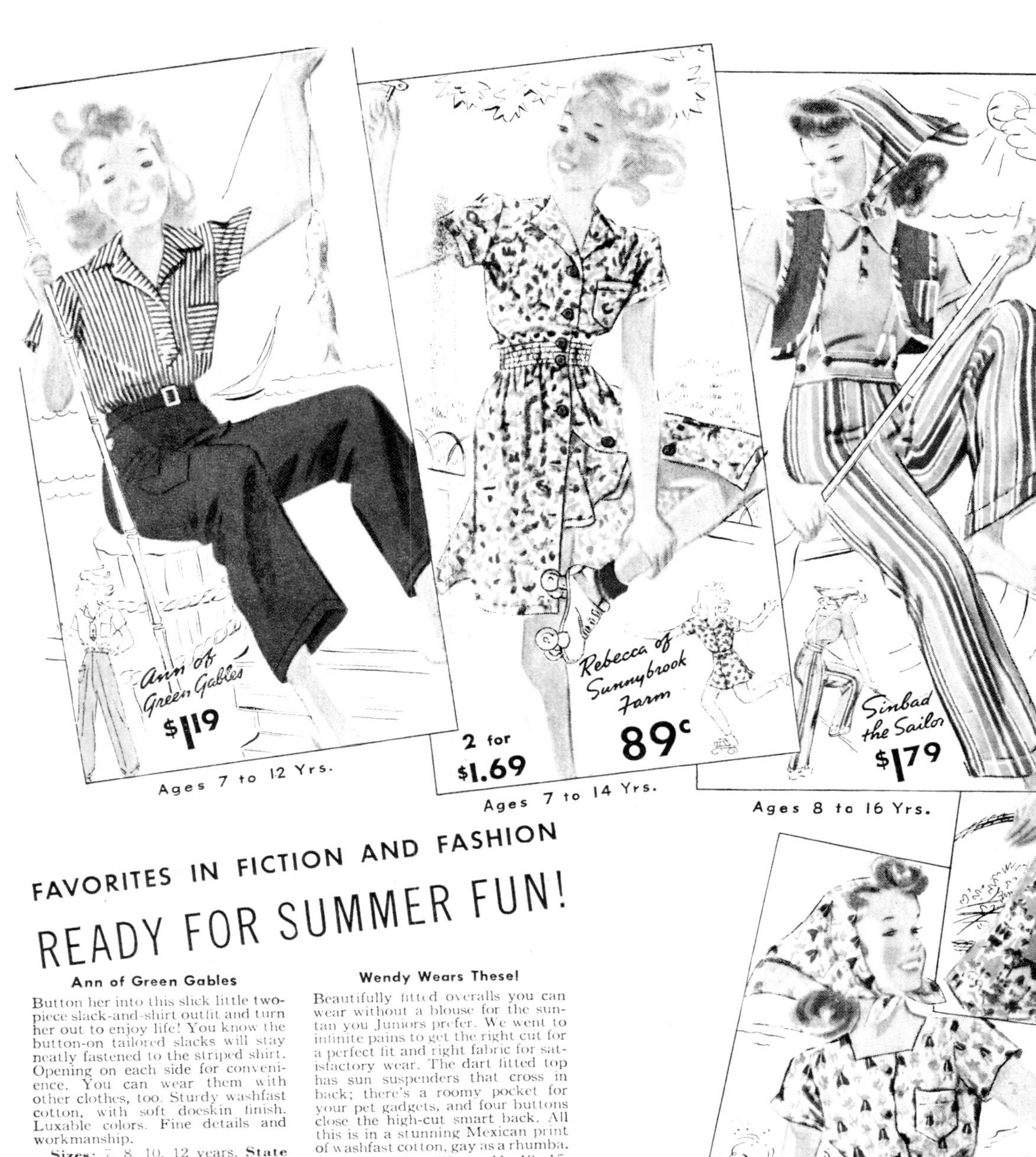

Sizes 11 to 19

Becky Thatcher

$1.19

Sizes 11 to 19

Heidi $1.98

FAVORITES IN FICTION AND FASHION

READY FOR SUMMER FUN!

Ann of Green Gables

Button her into this slick little two-piece slack-and-shirt outfit and turn her out to enjoy life! You know the button-on tailored slacks will stay neatly fastened to the striped shirt. Opening on each side for convenience. You can wear them with other clothes, too. Sturdy washfast cotton, with soft doeskin finish. Luxable colors. Fine details and workmanship.

Sizes: 7, 8, 10, 12 years. **State age-size.** Shipping wt., 1 lb. 2 oz.

27 L 4105—Navy Blue 214.
27 L 4106—Terra Cotta Rust 605.
Two-Piece Outfit **$1.19**

Rebecca of Sunnybrook

Hurrah for outdoors and a playsuit like this! It's a well cut shirt and shorts in one piece; separate skirt with Lastex shirred waistline, buttoning down the front so you can get it off in a hurry for active sports. Expensive details—the shorts have a new convenient side opening, and the Lastex "gives" in active play. A bright Mexican print; good cotton Percale. Luxable colors. Big value!

Sizes: 7, 8, 10, 12, 14 years. **State age-size.** Shipping weight, each 12 ounces.

27 L 4107—Wine print.
27 L 4108—Navy Blue print.
Playsuit. . . .**89c**; . . . .2 for **$1.69**

Sinbad the Sailor

FOUR good-looking garments combined in one exciting ensemble—separate them to use so many different ways. You get striped slacks with boyish elastic suspenders, wide waistband, hip pocket; plain tailored shirt with convertible collar; gay little sleeveless bolero and a peasant scarf to tie up your hair or go about your neck. All of good quality cotton hopsacking; smart, rugged, washfast fabric, a plain natural color with brilliant stripes in Luxable colors.

Sizes: 8, 10, 12, 14, 16 years. **State age-size.** Shipping weight, 1 pound 10 ounces.

27 L 4109—Colorful Stripe. **$1.79**

Wendy Wears These!

Beautifully fitted overalls you can wear without a blouse for the suntan you Juniors prefer. We went to infinite pains to get the right cut for a perfect fit and right fabric for satisfactory wear. The dart fitted top has sun suspenders that cross in back; there's a roomy pocket for your pet gadgets, and four buttons close the high-cut smart back. All this is in a stunning Mexican print of washfast cotton, gay as a rhumba.

Junior Miss Sizes: 11, 13, 15, 17, 19 years. **State size.** Shipping weight, 12 ounces.

77 L 2700—Wine Print **95c**

Becky Thatcher

Smart Juniors have great fun in a 3-piece playsuit like this—and wise mothers buy several at such a thrifty price. The shorts-and-shirt are in one piece, with becoming square neckline; the button down skirt has a Lastex shirred waistline; the triangle scarf goes over your head in the Hollywood fashion. Take off the skirt for active play. All good quality cotton washfast pique, bright as a sunny day, with quaint figures in vivid Luxable colors.

Junior Miss Sizes: 11, 13, 15, 17, 19. **State size.** Shpg. wt., 14 oz.

77 L 2703—Novelty Print . . **$1.19**

Heidi Inspired It

Be the best dressed Junior in your crowd in this three-piece, polka dot, rayon sharkskin outfit that you can mix with other costumes . . . for an all-summer-long wardrobe. The suspender skirt with its high waistline is held close by Lastex shirring. Flare skirt has lots of dash. The cute little separate bolero reverses the color scheme of the separate blouse. Good quality crisp rayon sharkskin.

Junior Misses' Sizes: 11, 13, 15, 17, 19. **State size.** Shipping weight, 1 pound 7 ounces.

77 L 2706—Navy with White dots.
77 L 2707—Aqua with White dots. **$1.98**

Numbers after color names refer to COLOR-GRAPH facing first index page.